MEDICAL LIBRARY
VARIETY CHILDREN'S HOSPITAL

SURGICAL
PEDIATRICS

SURGICAL PEDIATRICS

Edited by

Stephen L. Gans, M.D.

Chief, Pediatric Surgery Service
Cedars of Lebanon Hospital, Los Angeles

Attending Surgeon
Division of Pediatric Surgery
Childrens Hospital of Los Angeles

Associate Clinical Professor of Surgery
UCLA School of Medicine, Los Angeles

Grune & Stratton   NEW YORK and LONDON

Library of Congress Cataloging in Publication Data
Gans, Stephen L.
  Surgical pediatrics.
  Includes bibliographies.
    1. Children—Surgery. 2. Physician and patient.
I. Title. [DNLM: 1. Surgery—In infancy & childhood. WO 925 G199s 1973]
RD137.G35   617'.98   72-8721
ISBN 0-8089-0778-6

© 1973 by Grune & Stratton, Inc.
All rights reserved. No part of this publication may be reproduced or transmitted in
any form or by any means, electronic or mechanical, including photocopy, recording,
or any information storage and retrieval system, without permission in writing from
the publisher.

        Grune & Stratton, Inc.
        111 Fifth Avenue
        New York, New York 10003

Library of Congress Catalog Card Number 72–8721
International Standard Book Number 0-8089-0778-6
Printed in the United States of America

To my wife, Elizabeth,
and my three sons,
Will, Gary, and Jon

Preface

"Give me blood and the proper amount of fluids and electrolytes; add plenty of oxygen to the anesthesia, and I will show you that I can tolerate a terrific amount of surgery. You will be surprised at the speed of my recovery, and I shall always be grateful to you." These words put into the mouth of an infant "with no language but a cry" by Willis Potts * have stated the objectives which have prompted the preparation of this book. From a broader viewpoint, we would add, "Please get me safely to a well-equipped and properly staffed hospital environment, thoroughly evaluate my condition and prepare me for operation carefully, monitor and manage me through all hazardous situations, guard me from infections, and throughout this experience protect my sensitive mind and alleviate the dreadful anxiety of my family."

If the reader is only concerned with the technical aspects of surgical procedures, he will get little use from this book. Excellent volumes are available for that purpose. This is a book about supportive care for

* Potts, Willis. *The Surgeon and the Child.* Philadelphia: W.B. Saunders, p. vi, 1959.

the infant or child who needs surgery, presented in recognition of the fact that a brilliantly conceived and perfectly executed operation may result in disastrous failure without skillful and commensurate efforts in medical management. The crossroads of pediatric and surgical care are at the bedside of the seriously ill child with a surgical problem. This text should be particularly useful for the house officer or pediatrician who participates in the care of surgical patients, and for the general surgeon or other surgical specialist whose background in general pediatric care is not broad enough to make him completely familiar with these practices. Moreover, even though the pediatric surgeon may have experts at hand to take over various aspects of medical management, the final responsibility is still in his hands, and possession of this kind of knowledge for direction and moderation is most necessary.

The impressive rate of progress in this field has made it virtually impossible for one man to master the whole subject, much less to put it all together in one volume in sufficient time so that the material is still relatively current. Therefore, this book is the result of a cooperative effort involving experts with wide experience in each subject, each adding his personal style of expression. Some duplication has occurred, and we think it desirable in selected instances. For example, there are many different methods of calculating the proper amounts of fluids and electrolytes for intravenous therapy, and all are gross approximations. Three acceptable methods are proposed in this book. Other duplications are for purposes of emphasis and represent the overlapping of various disciplines or specialties with occasional differences in points of view.

Inasmuch as the contributors have been urged to express ideas and methods formed by their own experiences, as well as those gained from other sources, the use of references varies from author to author. Some have no references; in a few chapters detailed bibliographies are appended; in most, however, a few selected references for additional readings are listed.

We wish to acknowledge with great appreciation the efforts of all the contributors. We are also most grateful for the cooperation, encouragement and assistance of our publisher. A final word of thanks goes to our secretaries, Mildred Kosloff and Janelle Coluzzi, for their patient and painstaking efforts.

Stephen L. Gans, M.D.

Contributors

Arnold G. Coran, M.D.
Chief of Pediatric Surgery, Los Angeles County–USC Medical Center; Assistant Professor of Surgery, USC School of Medicine, Los Angeles, California

John B. Das, M.D.
Research Associate in Surgery, Children's Hospital Medical Center; Principal Associate in Surgery, Harvard Medical School, Boston, Massachusetts

Angelo J. Eraklis, M.D.
Associate in Surgery, Children's Hospital Medical Center; Assistant Professor of Surgery, Children's Hospital Medical Center, Harvard Medical School, Boston, Massachusetts

Richard S. Farr, M.D.
Head of the Department of Clinical Immunology, Allergy and Chest Diseases, National Jewish Hospital, Professor of Medicine, University of Colorado Medical School, Denver, Colorado

Robert M. Filler, M.D.

Chief of Clinical Surgery, Children's Hospital Medical Center; Associate Professor of Surgery, Children's Hospital Medical Center, Harvard Medical School, Boston, Massachusetts

Eric W. Fonkalsrud, M.D.

Professor and Chief of Pediatric Surgery, UCLA School of Medicine, Los Angeles, California

Gerald S. Gilchrist, M.B., B.Ch., D.C.H.

Consultant in Pediatrics and Hematology, Mayo Clinic; Associate Professor of Pediatrics, Mayo Medical School, Rochester, Minnesota

Benjamin M. Kagan, M.D.

Director, Division of Pediatrics, Cedars-Sinai Medical Center; Professor of Pediatrics, UCLA School of Medicine, Los Angeles, California

C. Everett Koop, M.D., Sc.D.

Surgeon-in-Chief, The Children's Hospital of Philadelphia; Professor of Pediatric Surgery, The University of Pennsylvania, Philadelphia, Pennsylvania

Donald A. Lackey, M.D.

Director of Neonatology, Cedars of Lebanon Hospital Division, Cedars-Sinai Medical Center; Assistant Clinical Professor of Pediatrics, UCLA School of Medicine, Los Angeles, California

Leonard M. Linde, M.D.

Professor of Pediatrics, UCLA School of Medicine, Los Angeles, California

Percy Minden, M.D.

Staff Physician, Department of Clinical Immunology, Allergy and Chest Diseases, National Jewish Hospital; Associate Professor of Pediatrics, University of Colorado Medical School, Denver, Colorado

Thomas S. Morse, M.D.

Associate Professor of Surgery (Pediatric), Department of Surgery, Ohio State University College of Medicine; Attending Staff, Children's Hospital and University Hospital, Columbus, Ohio

Lawrence K. Pickett, M.D.

William H. Carmalt Professor, Clinical Surgery and Pediatrics, Yale University School of Medicine, New Haven, Connecticut

Marc I. Rowe, M.D.

Professor of Surgery and Pediatrics, Chief, Division of Pediatric Surgery, University of Miami School of Medicine, Miami, Florida

Harry J. Sacks, M.D.
> Director of Clinical Pathology, Cedars-Sinai Medical Center; Clinical Professor of Pathology, USC School of Medicine, Los Angeles, California

Joseph W. St. Geme, Jr., M.D.
> Professor and Head, Department of Pediatrics, Harbor General Hospital Campus, UCLA School of Medicine, Los Angeles, California

Robert M. Smith, M.D.
> Director of Anesthesia, Children's Hospital Medical Center, Boston, Massachusetts

Sheldon L. Spector, M.D.
> Staff Physician, Department of Clinical Immunology, Allergy, and Chest Diseases, National Jewish Hospital; Assistant Professor of Medicine, University of Colorado Medical School, Denver, Colorado

Howard S. Traisman, M.D., F.A.A.P.
> Associate Professor of Pediatrics, Northwestern University Medical School; Attending Endocrinologist and Head of Diabetes Clinic, Children's Memorial Hospital, Chicago, Illinois

Miriam G. Wilson, M.D.
> Chief, Genetics Division, Department of Pediatrics, Los Angeles County–USC Medical Center; Professor of Pediatrics, USC School of Medicine, Los Angeles, California

Morton M. Woolley, M.D.
> Head, Division of Pediatric Surgery, Department of Surgery, Childrens Hospital of Los Angeles; Associate Clinical Professor of Surgery, USC School of Medicine, Los Angeles, California

Contents

Section I

External Influences

1

The Surgeon, Physician, Child, and Family: Interpersonal Relationships

C. Everett Koop, M.D., Sc.D.

When dealing with a child, the pediatrician or surgeon never has one patient. At least one other member of the family must always be taken into consideration; frequently both parents are involved and, on occasion, even grandparents and other relatives. What can be said to the child in reference to preparation for hospitalization may not be the things that the parents want to hear, except as they are being taught how to prepare their child for hospitalization. The child's questions, if he will ask them, are about lengths of hospital stay, needles, pain; parents are concerned with risk, prognosis, and expense. There is a difference between being prepared for hospitalization and being prepared for a surgical procedure. For the child, hospitalization means spending time in a new environment, separated from home and parents and facing what is sometimes the fearful unknown. Preparation for a surgical procedure, on the other hand, involves all of the things that go into preparing for hospitalization, but in addition, both the child (if he is old enough) and the family must be prepared for some of the unique things about a surgical procedure such as the incision, intravenous fluids, and the stitches.

Preparation of the child and family for what lies ahead can be one of the most rewarding aspects of pediatric practice. It is most gratifying to be able to take a frightened child and his concerned parents and, by simple explanation, instill confidence, eliminate fear, and guide them through what otherwise might be a very trying time. A tremendous dividend is paid when the family is properly prepared for an operative procedure: the elimination of the suspicion of doctors, hospitals, and medicine in general. I firmly believe that with the proper family preparation, malpractice litigation could be virtually eliminated.

BEFORE THE FAMILY MEETS THE SURGEON

Except in unusual situations, surgeons have their patients referred to them. Therefore, the first inkling of the possibility of the need for surgery is presented to the family by a nonsurgeon, usually the family physician or pediatrician. Such referrals may be for either emergency surgery or elective surgery. The patient's problem may be something completely understood by the referring physician, or it may be something he is not certain about and for which he feels the need for surgical consultation. These are certainly times when the family looks to the familiar physician for guidance. Sometimes the family has had surgical experience with another member of the family and has its pet surgeon in whom it already has confidence. The referring physician must decide whether that surgeon has the competence necessary for the situation at hand. The surgeon who took Aunt Hattie's gallbladder out so that she didn't turn a hair might not necessarily be the surgeon who should repair an esophageal atresia, explore an infant to ascertain the cause of jaundice, or to remove a Wilms' tumor of prodigious size. The referring physician's confidence in the surgeon is the beginning of a successful relationship between the surgeon and the family of the pediatric patient.

We all probably tend to oversimplify things as we attempt to assuage the anxiety of the families with which we deal. One of the certain ways to get the surgical relationship off on the wrong foot is for the referring physician to commit the surgeon to a course of action which the surgeon himself may not think is wise. This occurs most often in an emergency situation when anxiety is at a higher pitch than it is for the elective procedure, as, for example, when a child suffers with abdominal pain. Abdominal pain in a child alerts any thinking individual to the possibility of appendicitis, and yet those who deal with children regularly know of the frequency of other causes for abdominal pain, as well as the comparative rarity of appendicitis. When the referring physician makes a flatfooted diagnosis of appendicitis and commits the surgeon, who has not yet seen the patient, to immediate operation, and promises a smooth convalescence and successful conclusion, there is no room in which the surgeon can maneuver; there is no easy way out of a mistaken diagnosis. If the physician commits the surgeon to appendectomy and the surgeon, in all honesty, cannot agree with the diagnosis, the parents' confidence in their own physician is undermined, even though they might be relieved at not having to face an operation. How much better for the referring physician to inform the family that he is suspicious that the abdominal pain might have surgical implications and that he would like a surgical consultation. The physician and surgeon can then work as a team and the patient can be properly studied before diagnosis is firmly established.

In elective procedures, also, it is well to let the surgeon have a little leeway in such matters as the timing of operation, the length of hospitalization, and what is to be expected during convalescence. It is very difficult for the surgeon to live up to the promises made by the referring physician who underestimated the seriousness of the operation and the difficulty of recovery. Nonsurgeons seem particularly prone to promising outstanding cosmetic results, again for the understandable reason of allaying the family's anxiety. If minimizing a procedure and its sequelae is bad, exaggerating the gravity of a situation (as in the case of a doctor misinforming the family that the mortality rate for any operation for Hirschsprung's disease is 50 percent) either extreme must be avoided.

MEETING THE SURGEON

Any parent who reads the *Ladies' Home Journal* or the *Reader's Digest* knows enough about medicine that the surgeon can no longer act the part of the magician. The family is entitled to explanations and expects them. The more they know of the things they should know, the more likely they are to feel part of the surgical team and to take in stride, without anxiety, some of the natural postoperative occurrences.

Presenting explanations to parents about the approaching operation on their child is like walking a tightrope. Enough has to be said, on the one hand, to gain their confidence and to increase their understanding; on the other hand, the surgeon must avoid sharing his own anxieties with the family. Introducing parents to every possible complication should be avoided, unless complication seems very likely and foreknowledge on the part of the family would be to everyone's benefit.

In emergency surgery, special efforts must be made to establish confidence and to emphasize the consequences of delay. A suitable waiting area must be provided for the patient's parents and specific arrangements should be made by the surgeon to meet the family postoperatively to discuss the outcome of the surgical procedure. This appointment should be kept promptly. It provides the doctor with an opportunity to prepare the parents for some of the things that they might see when they first visit their child postoperatively: intravenous fluids, blood transfusion, oxygen tent, and monitoring equipment. These modalities of therapy and surveillance are considered by the laity, even today, to be associated only with the most serious of illnesses. Explanations at this time to the family need be only minimal, and definitive discussion of some situations can be postponed awaiting the outcome of a histologic report from the laboratory or a later evaluation of the patient in the recovery room or intensive care unit. It is at this time that the family frequently wants to know how it can be informed of up-to-the-minute news on the child. This, of course, is a matter of individual preference on the part of the surgeon, but one satisfactory and manageable technique is to tell the family that if there is any unexpected development or change from the normal postoperative course, the surgeon will be in touch with them, and that, otherwise, they ought to consider no report as being indicative of a postoperative course in conformity with what is to be expected.

When the family reports to the surgeon for consultation concerning the possibility of elective surgery, the situation is quite different from that of emergency surgery. There is usually a lapse of time between the referral and consultation, and during this interval the family no doubt checks out the surgeon with others who have known him and may even discuss with other parents just what is to be expected. As a result, such consultation is, with most people, a much more relaxed affair, and the surgeon can make his explanations with some confidence that they will be heard and understood. Although it is possible to tell parents too much, surgeons are much more frequently guilty of telling them too little.

Where is the child during this interview with his parents? There is no pat answer to this question, but, in general, I prefer to have the patient on hand while I talk to his family, for a number of reasons. First of all, he won't feel that we are moving against him behind his back. Since I need as much confidence from this youngster as I can get in the days to come, this is an important beginning. Secondly, the simple explanation I give the child's parents can frequently be understood by the patient himself, permitting him to ask questions spontaneously and also permitting me to ask the patient if there is anything he would like to know about what I have said.

The minimum amount of information to which a family is entitled is an explanation of why, how, and when. In the process of saying these things I try to make it a point to relieve any possible guilt feelings on the part of the parents by stating that the situation at hand was beyond anyone's control.

When I see a youngster with an undescended testicle, for example, I may very well show the family the asymmetry of the scrotum and demonstrate the fact that I can or cannot feel the testicle under the abdominal skin suprapubically. I suggest that they dress their youngster and then sit down quietly with me while I tell them some of what I know about undescended testicles, some of which they may already be familiar with, but which I would like to review for the sake of completeness. What I have to say is a monologue and goes something like this: "Everything on your youngster's left side is perfectly normal, but on the right, as you know, his scrotum is empty, his testicle can be felt up in his lower abdomen, it cannot be brought down, and I can feel a hernia. Now, don't be upset that this is anything special in your boy. Over 90 percent of children who have an undescended testicle have a hernia in association with it. We could wait from now to the end of time and your boy's undescended testicle would never come down spontaneously. There is no medical management that would bring his testicle into the scrotum. Now, you should know that if you do nothing about this undescended testicle at all, your youngster would grow up to be a normal sexual male and a normal reproductive male, because he needs only one testicle and he already has one which has descended and is normal.

"However, if your boy were my boy, there are at least four reasons why I would not be happy to have him go through life with an undescended testicle, if it were possible to correct the situation. The first of these reasons is, to my way of thinking, the most important one, and that is the psychological reason. Your boy will reach the age when he will be undressing at school or at camp or at a swimming club in front of other young boys who will all have two testicles. I am not concerned about the kidding he will have about this, but I am concerned about the misinformation that he will pick up and never bring home to his family.

"Secondly, I have already mentioned that he has a hernia and this will soon be knocking on your door for attention. His hernia would be fixed at the same time his testicle is brought down.

"The third reason is not a very important reason, but I mention it to you because so frequently parents have heard something about this and I want to be sure that you have no misconceptions. Although it is true that undescended testicles do have a higher incidence of tumor formation, if that were the only reason to bring down this testicle I am not sure I would think it necessary.

"My fourth reason is a very practical one. The testicle your boy has on his good left side will take care of all of his sexual and reproductive needs, but it's nice to have a spare one in case something happens to it.

"The operation is not one which carries a high risk and whether your boy is treated as an outpatient or is in the hospital overnight, when he is discharged he will have no external sutures, no dressings, and his activity need not be restricted."

Young children might be frightened at some of the things that are said and even cry occasionally. This provides the occasion for the surgeon to interrupt his discussion with the family and to put things in terms that the child will understand. For example, "Nobody really likes to come to the hospital, but you will be here for only a very short period of time. Let me tell you the things about it that you won't like.

You will have to have a blood count, which means you will be stuck in the finger with a needle, but that doesn't hurt any more than when your mother pricks her finger while she is sewing on a button. Then, before you have your operation you will be given a shot just like your doctor gives you a shot when you go to his office for a checkup. After you get that shot, your mouth will feel dry and you will get sleepy. Put your head down and go to sleep and when you wake up your operation will all be over and your mother and father will be there."

Older children sometimes want to know why an undescended testicle has to be brought down. It can be explained that the day will come when he will want to be like all of his friends and that this is a better time to do such an operation than at the time when he would really appreciate it more. Occasionally, a child will ask, "Do you have to cut me open?" In reply, the surgeon can say, "Yes, but I also will sew you up and both the cutting and the sewing will be done while you are sound asleep and feel no pain. After the operation, the place where you had your incision may feel a little tight when you move around, but most boys your age are out playing the day after their operation."

Families need guidance on deciding the date of admission. The natural tendency is for people to postpone experiences they would rather not face, such as a hospitalization. When told that one of the most difficult things about having a child operated upon is the anxiety produced while waiting for it to be accomplished, parents generally realize that an early admission is preferable to postponement. Naturally, for certain elective procedures, it is important to discuss how the child benefits from having the surgery performed at a particular time. Surgeons working in a referral center, whose patients come from considerable distances, sometimes make it a practice of planning a consultation with the child and his family and admitting the patient to the hospital immediately thereafter. If this arrangement is to be successful, it is essential that the referring physician make a significant contribution to the preparation of the child and the family for hospitalization. It is also necessary that the surgeon's secretary, who makes the necessary arrangements, be knowledgeable on matters of preparation of the family so that she can smooth out the rough spots both before and after consultation. For elective surgery, an arrangement like this is applicable only to such conditions as hernias, undescended testicles, or subcutaneous lesions. It should be stressed to the family that consultation and admission so scheduled is for the family's convenience. If the surgeon's secretary senses in the family any hesitancy to accept the idea of immediate admission, the sensible thing to do is back off and give the family an interval between decision for operation and hospital admission.

For elective admissions, it is also important that the surgeon not state his case for early admission without being flexible enough to make adjustments to family, social, or economic problems. Again, parents need guidance in making their decision when alternative possibilities exist. For example, a pregnant woman whose child requires elective surgery may be anxious to have her pregnancy come to its natural conclusion before becoming involved with a new problem. Actually, most women can better cope with an operation on their child while they are pregnant than they can when they have an additional baby to care for.

When an elective admission has been set up and then must be postponed because of an intercurrent respiratory infection, gastroenteritis, or other illness, the parents frequently need reassurance that delaying the operation will not be detrimental to its outcome.

PREPARING THE CHILD AND HIS FAMILY FOR HOSPITALIZATION

If the physician realizes that the family's anxiety about a hospital admission is due largely to fear of the unknown, his major effort should be to make the unknown known. Parents should be prepared for all of the red tape that hospital admission entails. It would be well for physicians and surgeons who admit patients to hospitals to review admission procedures periodically, since administrative procedures frequently change, and what the physician promises may not be what the family experiences. Some hospitals use a preadmission form which the family returns to the hospital by mail some time before admission. This introduces the family to the kind of questions hospitals ask and also provides the opportunity to answer them at a time when the tensions of the admissions procedure do not contribute to the family's anxiety.

Since children do not have the same concept of time as adults, it is well for the family not to start preparing the child for separation from them and his home too far in advance of the actual occurrence. There is no hard and fast rule to follow, but keep in mind that intelligent parents know their child far better than does an advising physician. Usually, one or two days is sufficient advance notice and many parents are able to make the stay in the hospital an enjoyable experience for the child by playing doctor or nurse with him beforehand.

Parents must be truthful, to the best of their knowledge, about hospital procedures. If they present hospitalization as an adventuresome experience, without transmitting their own anxiety, and within the bounds of honesty, the whole affair might be quite pleasant for the child. Naturally, parents need guidance in these matters and the physician can describe to the family the specific studies that he will be ordering. He might also indicate which things will be unpleasant for the child, such as blood counts or intravenous sticks. It is also important to stress the positive things that the child will enjoy, if he is old enough, such as the hospital's play program, a leisure-time activity supervisor, and television.

Parents who have not experienced hospital procedure before,

should be told that the history and physical examination, as well as a number of the studies will be done by members of the house staff, and this is the time to transmit to the family the physician's confidence in those who work at his direction. In all of his discussions with the parents, the surgeon must be sensitive to their personalities and choose the best technique of presenting material he thinks it is important for them to know. A flip manner of presentation may be just the right approach for some parents, but for others, who view a hospital stay as an extremely serious and potentially dangerous affair, such a presentation would be abrasive, if not an insult.

Many hospitals provide written instructions for families about to bring a child into the hospital, and some of these are extremely good. Other such instructions are commercially available, and present in story form some of the things that the child might reasonably expect in the hospital.

Many mothers wish to live in with their children. Except for the times when a child is in the recovery room or the intensive care unit, there are many advantages to having a mother not separated from her child, but there are disadvantages as well. If a mother is determined to stay with her child, she should be warned that the children whose mothers do not stay are usually those who come to the operating room properly premedicated, drowsy, or asleep. Mothers who remain with their children after preoperative medication is given, who talk with them, hold them, and accompany them to the elevator to the operating room are performing a disservice rather than an act of love. If this is properly explained to the mother, and she leaves the child after he has had his preoperative medication, sedation is accomplished and the child should have no unpleasant recollection of his trip to the operating room or induction of anesthesia.

Many parents have more questions about anesthesia than they do about the contemplated surgery itself. Just as the surgeon resents the promises made by the referring physician that he himself cannot fill, the surgeon must not yield to the temptation to make promises for the anesthesiologist that *he* cannot fulfill. It is far better to state that the goal of the medical team is to have the youngster go through his operating room experience without unpleasant memory and to transmit confidence in the anesthesiologist, rather than to go into details of technique and anesthetic agent.

FINANCES

Someone in the surgeon's office, either the surgeon himself or his representative, should discuss with the family the financial obligations it will take on in reference to hospitalization and surgery. This presupposes knowledge of such things as third party insurance carriers and state programs. Although the surgeon will not be billing for more than his surgical procedure, he or his representative is the ideal person to outline what the family's total financial obligation might be, what will be covered by insurance, and what will not. Many parents are naive about such things and many of them will be encountering the hospital situation for the first time. They should be told that the hospital bill is separate from the surgical fee and, if there is a separate fee for anesthesia, this should also be made clear. The same is true of preliminary outpatient studies that might not be covered by insurance.

If it becomes obvious that the family is not in a position to undertake the financial burden that the contemplated hospitalization will bring, the surgeon or his representative must offer to assist in arranging help from a crippled children's program or some other source, such as the hospital's clinic. Under these circumstances, it is extremely important that the parents not believe that their child will be relegated to the position of a second-class citizen; every effort should be made to make it clear that the care will be excellent in any circumstance. From the answers to questionnaires filled in by parents after hospitalization, it is clear that the overall impression of the hospitalization is frequently marred by something totally apart from the psychological impact on their child or the effect of the surgical procedure. More often than not, it is an unexpected financial obligation. Many times it is the unexpected aspect of the obligation, rather than the obligation itself, which is so irritating.

FOLLOW-UP

Surgeons readily accept their obligation for follow-up on their postoperative patients. When long-term repeated follow-ups are necessary, there should be an understanding between referring physician and surgeon concerning this responsibility. After short-term hospitalization for elective operative procedures, and particularly after operative procedures done on an outpatient basis, the family often has a sense of unreality about the whole affair. Even though the surgeon may feel confident that a follow-up examination is not necessary, the parents will derive tremendous psychological benefit from such a follow-up visit and from the assurance from their surgeon, whom they never got to know very well, that all is as it should be.

THE RELATIONSHIP BETWEEN THE REFERRING PHYSICIAN AND THE SURGEON

When a patient is referred by a physician to a surgeon who eventually refers the patient back to that physician, certain things need clarification for all concerned if the whole experience is to be as smooth as possible. The family should know who is responsible for what. If the surgeon is a pediatric surgeon and wants to take the entire care of the patient himself during the hospitalization and postoperative course, the family should be aware of this. If the situation is one in which the referring physician continues to share the responsibility for hospital care of the patient and essentially takes care of preoperative and post-operative orders exclusive of the surgical procedure itself, the family should also know this. If the pediatrician and surgeon are not working side by side in the same hospital, it is necessary that the surgeon notify the pediatrician either by telephone or letter what he has diagnosed and what he plans to do about it. Ideally, the referring physician should be notified of the date of contemplated surgery and should be informed postoperatively of what has been accomplished and what degree of success has been achieved. The reasons for this are very practical. In spite of the fact that the referring physician and the surgeon may each know full well where his own responsibility starts and ends, the family does not and very frequently refers surgical problems back to the physician. If the physician isn't properly informed of plans and ac-complishments, he is either unable to answer questions or he answers them incorrectly. In the former case, the family members feel that their child has been let down (and the whole medical profession suffers from their criticism). In the latter case, the family is misled and may be-come equally disillusioned with the medical profession.

If the surgeon is doing the follow-up after a surgical procedure, he should make it clear to the referring physician and to the family exactly what he considers to be his responsibility. When he believes his responsibility has come to an end, both family and referring phy-sician should be notified so that the patient and his problems do not fall between two authorities without proper care.

2

Transportation of Sick and Injured Children

Thomas S. Morse, M.D.

Transportation has been a neglected subject in the treatment of critically ill and injured patients. In many parts of the country, it is finally beginning to receive the attention it deserves. Within the past decade, standards for emergency ambulance services have been determined,[1] a curriculum for training emergency medical technicians has been developed,[2,3] and the medical requirements for ambulance design and equipment have been published.[4,5,6] The special requirements of infants and children have been detailed,[7] and, in a few areas, ambulances specifically designed for the transport of infants have been put in operation.[8]

Efforts are being made to adapt to civilian needs the techniques developed by the military during the Korean and Vietnam wars to provide medical aid for and evacuation of wounded soldiers. The Departments of Defense and Transportation are exploring, in a joint project, the use of military helicopters, equipment, doctors, and personnel for civilian use in urban and rural areas.[9] The lessons learned in airplane evacuation of military patients returning from overseas have been made available for civilian benefit.[10,11] The principles of safe removal of the injured from wrecked vehicles have been spelled out.[12]

Encouraging as these developments may be, much more remains to be done. In many parts of the country, a huge gap exists between what is known about management of the critically injured and what is delivered to them in the way of professional treatment.[13] More than half of all vehicles used for transportation of sick children fail in some important way to meet the minimum published standards.[14] Only a minority of the attendants have had any formal training at all, the majority being unskilled volunteers. The mortality due to accidents has been shown to be far higher in rural areas than in urban areas.[15] While the effects of shorter distances, shorter transportation times, and more sophisticated personnel and facilities at the end of the ambulance ride are important, there can be no doubt that part of the increased urban salvage is due to better ambulance equipment manned by people with better training.[16]

For many critically ill or injured children, transportation continues to be poorly conceived, hastily arranged, and often conducted in a communication vacuum. All too often, faulty transportation compounds the problems of the child whose life it is supposed to save.

What goes wrong? The two most frequent complications are respiratory failure and hypovolemic shock. Other preventable catastrophes are aspiration of vomitus, compression of the spinal cord from inadequate immobilization of neck or back injuries, compounding of simple fractures, overdistention of the bladder, bacterial contamination, and dangerous loss of body heat. No physician willingly inflicts these disasters on his patients. Their repeated occurrence suggests a tendency on the part of physicians to underestimate the hazards of transportation and, therefore, to fail to take responsibility for providing adequate safeguards.

Children are transported to a hospital either by rescue squads from the scene of an accident or by ambulance from another hospital. One might expect the mortality to be higher when a rescue squad transports a child, since usually no physician has seen the child before transportation is completed. Actually the mortality is lower when a rescue squad brings the child directly to a hospital than when a physician arranges transfer from one hospital to another. Perhaps the most important reason for this is that many rescue squad members receive effective training in the management of emergency transportation. They expect emergencies, they plan for them, and, most important, they assume responsibility for the patient from the moment of first contact until the trip is completed. The physician, arranging transportation from one hospital to another, usually deals with the problem only sporadically, usually has had no formal training in transportation, frequently underestimates the potential hazards involved, and often washes his hands of responsibility for the patient when the ambulance ride begins. The result is that during this critical period *no doctor assumes responsibility for the welfare of the patient.*

The remainder of this chapter deals specifically with the role of the physician in planning, initiating, and supervising the interhospital transport of critically ill or injured infants and children. While different clinical situations demand special considerations, certain fundamentals pertain to every transport situation.

FUNDAMENTALS

Determination of Transportability

No matter how desirable it may be to move a patient, it is futile to do so if he cannot be expected to survive the trip. Children who are in respiratory distress or shock must be considered not transportable until these conditions have been corrected. Children who are bleeding externally are not transportable until bleeding is controlled and blood loss has been replaced. Experience has frequently shown the rewards of a brief period of initial stabilization, during which these essential objectives are achieved before transport is begun.

Communication

It is inexcusable to pack a child off in an ambulance before the sender has spoken on the phone with the physician who will assume charge of the child on arrival. Time after time, as receiving physicians, we have been in a position to make valuable suggestions regarding immediate care and preparation for safe transport. Time after time we have been denied this opportunity because we first heard that a child was coming after he had been sent on his way. Failure of doctor-to-doctor communication prior to the start of the trip is probably the single most important factor leading to preventable death during transport.

Written Record

In addition to telephone communication, the receiving physician should be given a written record summarizing the hospital course and the preparations for transfer. Laboratory data, x-rays, and signed parental consent-to-treatment forms should accompany the child. In many instances, blood samples from the infant and mother should be included.

Ambulance Equipment

The standards for ambulance design and equipment are published. In a few fortunate localities the physician can be sure these standards are scrupulously met. In most areas, however, he will do well to check personally the availability of the equipment and supplies his patient may need during the trip.

Patient's Attendant

The driver cannot be expected to do anything but drive the ambulance. A second person must accompany the patient and attend to his needs. If this person is a skilled, trained attendant who has been properly briefed as to the child's condition, the patient is fortunate indeed. In many instances the physician should give serious consideration to the idea so eloquently expressed by Segal,[7] "If a physician's services are needed for intensive care before and after the journey, it would seem unlikely that they can safely be dispensed with during the trip." In Segal's experience, as in our own, the fewest deaths occur in ambulances when a *doctor* accompanies the child from hospital to hospital.

In any event, the attendant must be prepared and equipped to prevent and, failing prevention, to recognize and deal with any or all of the following emergencies.

Respiratory Failure
  Vomiting and aspiration
  Other forms of airway obstruction
  Flail chest and sucking wounds
  Pneumothorax and hemothorax
  Central respiratory depression

Circulatory Failure
  Shock due to bleeding
  Shock due to dehydration
  Cardiac tamponade

Complications of Fractures
  Spinal cord compression
  Compounding of simple fractures
  Overdistention of bladder

Gastric Distention

Convulsions

Bacterial Contamination

Hyperthermia and Chilling

RESPIRATORY FAILURE

Respiratory failure is the most frequent serious problem encountered in transporting children. It is especially hazardous in the patient who is obtunded by head injury, shock due to hemorrhage or dehydration, brain tumor, meningitis, poisoning, electrolyte imbalances, or chronic debilitating illnesses. It also occurs in those with inflammation or anomalies of the airway, those with foreign bodies in the esophagus or bronchi, those with hemothorax, pneumothorax, rib fractures, or sucking wounds of the neck or thorax, those with massive abdominal distention, and those who are liable to vomit and aspirate. The latter category, those who are liable to vomit and aspirate, includes nearly every child sick enough or sufficiently severely injured to warrant a ride in an ambulance.

A child with respiratory failure is not transportable until every effort has been made to relieve the problem before the trip begins. Gastric distention, which occurs more frequently in injured children than in adults, should be suspected and prevented or relieved with an indwelling nasogastric tube. Of all tubes, catheters, and cannuli which can be inserted into children, the nasogastric tube may well be the most important. After the stomach has been emptied, provisions should be made to aspirate the tube periodically because the stomach may not remain empty if obstruction or paralytic ileus is present, or if, as so frequently happens, the anxious child swallows more air than he usually would.

The child should not be positioned or restrained in such a way that he cannot turn his head if vomiting occurs, and proper suction equipment must be available to clear away vomitus promptly. Semiconscious or unconscious children should be transported in a lateral recumbent position to prevent aspiration. If obtunded enough to accept an oral airway, the child should have one of the proper size.

If the need for an indwelling endotracheal tube or a tracheostomy is in question, often a brief delay will clarify the question and prevent a disaster en route.

If a pneumothorax or hemothorax is suspected, its presence can promptly and safely be confirmed by needle aspiration of the chest, followed by insertion of an indwelling chest tube which can be aspirated periodically with a syringe and stopcock in the absence of more sophisticated equipment. Recent studies suggest that neonates with pneumothorax secondary to the airblock syndrome may be the exception,[17] but older children should always be treated by evacuation of the air or blood before and during transfer.

Flail chest results from multiple rib fractures which allow a significant portion of the rib cage to move inward with inspiration and outward with expiration, thus reducing the tidal volume. Modern hospital management includes the use of positive pressure ventilation with a respirator and endotracheal tube or cuffed tracheostomy tube. In doubtful cases, consultation with a specialist at the receiving hospital may prove lifesaving. Splinting the chest with sandbags or tape will not return the ventilation to normal but may markedly improve it.

If respiration fails en route, it must be supported artificially until the cause can be corrected. An Ambu bag and mask or connection to an endotracheal tube permits the administration of environmental air or oxygen. If a mask is used, the stomach must be aspirated frequently, as large amounts of gas are invariably forced down the esophagus.

Penetrating wounds of the chest should be covered with a vaseline gauze or similar dressing so that air will not be sucked into the chest on inspiration. A method of covering the wound with a rubber surgeon's glove which has been tightly fixed to the periphery of the wound is occasionally helpful. A small portion of one fingertip can be cut from the glove to act as a one-way valve permitting the escape of air with expiration. On inspiration the glove collapses and does not allow air to be drawn in.

Properly humidified oxygen is frequently desirable, although it must be clearly understood that there is no medical or surgical condition for which oxygen is a cure. As long as oxygen is required, a continuing search for other ways to relieve the child should be conducted. Prolonged exposure to high concentrations of oxygen is toxic to infants and children of all ages, but from a practical point of view, it is essentially impossible to harm a patient in an ambulance with oxygen properly administered over a short ride. If in doubt, it is usually wise to administer it liberally. Empty oxygen tanks look just like full ones; it takes only a minute to check before the trip begins.

Restless and irrational behavior in children is usually not the result of pain or fear; it is more often due to either inadequate ventilation or inadequate circulation. Proper treatment calls for attention to the airway and the blood volume rather than administration of narcotics.

CIRCULATORY FAILURE

Hemorrhagic Shock

No child in shock should be considered transportable until the hypotension has been corrected. The usual error in the treatment of shock is to give too little replacement fluid too slowly. For blood loss, the ideal replacement is properly crossmatched fresh whole blood. While this is being obtained, the following solutions in decreasing order of desirability can be used: plasma, lactated Ringer's solution, normal saline, and clinical dextran. The latter should not be administered in amounts greater than 40 ml per kg of body weight because greater volumes may interfere with coagulation. Children who are in shock from bleeding have lost at least 20 ml of blood per kg. This amount can safely be administered as fast as it can be pumped in. Usually more is required. As long as hypotension persists, more blood should be pumped in. Once normal blood pressure has been achieved, an additional 10–15 ml of blood per kg should be given because vasoconstriction permits the blood pressure to return to normal before the blood volume has been fully restored. If the physician fails to realize that hypotension disappears before the blood volume is fully restored, he may stop replacement while the patient is still precariously depleted, and the child may slip into shock again if only a few milliliters of additional blood loss occurs.

A second common error in the treatment of hemorrhagic shock is failure to stop external bleeding. No bank blood or other fluid is as useful to the child as his own blood. For every drop which can be preserved, less will have to be replaced. Pumping vessels should be clamped and ligated if they can be clearly seen and if one can be sure he will not damage adjacent structures. Blind clamping deep in a wound may do more harm than good and should not be attempted. This is especially true of wounds of the neck, axillae, and forearms. Direct pressure over the wound is almost always preferable to the use of tourniquets. In the rare instance when a tourniquet is necessary, a blood pressure cuff should be used. The cuff should be inflated to a pressure 40–60 mm Hg higher than the child's normal arterial pressure and the time of application carefully noted. Usually the cuff should not be inflated for more than one to one and one-half hours. Tourniquets made of rags and sticks may do great harm because if too tight they may produce nerve damage, and if too loose they may promote, rather than decrease, blood loss by obstructing venous return while allowing arterial bleeding to continue.

If an intravenous hypodermic needle has been used initially, it should be replaced as soon as possible with an indwelling plastic venous catheter, either of the percutaneous type or of the type inserted via a cutdown. Needles are too unreliable to trust in ambulances. Lives have been lost because needles became dislodged and could not be replaced in transit.

If the child has been resuscitated from shock, or if there is a possibility that he may develop shock in transit, the attendant must have the following items available in the ambulance: a blood pressure cuff of appropriate size, a stethoscope and a manometer, an indwelling plastic cannula which can be trusted to remain in working order during the trip, and a generous supply of appropriate replacement fluids. The amount of blood and fluids to send along with the child depends on many variables, but for massive bleeding one should think in terms of about 200 ml of blood per kg of body weight and twice this amount of lactated Ringer's solution. It is far better to arrive with a box of unopened bottles than with a child who has been allowed to bleed to death in transit.

Intravenous fluids do not run well in conventional ambulances because the bottle cannot be elevated high enough above the patient. Hence, the attendant must be prepared to deliver the fluid under pressure. A few ambulances have electric pumps for this purpose. If the blood is contained in a flexible plastic bag, a blood pressure cuff wrapped around it and inflated is effective. Otherwise, the attendant must have three-way stopcocks and a generous supply of syringes.

Acidosis develops rapidly during shock. In the absence of laboratory data, it is appropriate to administer one ml of undiluted sodium bicarbonate for every 10 ml of blood or plasma.

Valuable time can be saved at the receiving end if a sample of the child's blood in a properly labeled tube is sent with him. Neonates should be sent with a tube of cord blood and a properly labeled sample of the mother's blood. The receiving physician should be told the child's blood type over the phone so that the blood bank can be prepared.

Shock Resulting from Dehydration

Shock resulting from dehydration, such as from vomiting, diarrhea, or burns, is just as urgent an emergency as shock resulting from bleeding. Plasma is the ideal initial replacement fluid for shock due to dehydration. Plasma equivalent to one-fourth of the blood volume, i.e. plasma in the amount of 20 ml per kg, should be given as rapidly as possible. This should be followed by electrolyte solution appropriate to the condition causing the dehydration.

Cardiac Tamponade

Cardiac tamponade occurs when a penetrating wound of the heart allows blood to escape into the pericardial sac. It should be suspected whenever shock persists in the presence of a puncture wound of the chest or upper abdomen. Aspiration of the blood may be lifesaving, and should be attempted, because the salvage rate of children with penetrating cardiac wounds is very high if they can be operated upon before prolonged circulatory failure has occurred. A needle introduced under the tip of the xiphoid process and angled 45 degrees upward and 45 degrees laterally toward the left may save a life.

HEAD INJURIES

Most preventable catastrophes result not from mismanagement of the head injury itself, but from failure to support ventilation and circulation or failure to suspect associated injuries. If respiration or circulation fail en route, they must be supported as described in the previous sections. Until proven otherwise, every obtunded child with a head injury should be treated as if he has a broken neck. (See *Spinal Injuries,* below.) Except in rare instances, head injuries do *not* produce shock. Hypotension strongly suggests additional injuries, most commonly extensive blood loss through lacerations or internal injuries such as rupture of the spleen or liver. Intravenous fluids should be given very sparingly to children with isolated head injuries, but an intravenous catheter should always be placed prior to transport and blood or lactated Ringer's solution sent along so that if shock from associated injuries develops it can be managed and intractable convulsions treated intravenously.

Convulsions not only are evidence of injury or disease, but are harmful in and of themselves. They should be briefly and carefully observed, and any evidence of localization to a side of the face or body or to a single extremity noted as an aid in future treatment. Following this brief observation period, they should be stopped, if possible, with a slow intravenous injection of enough Valium or sodium amytal to control them.

The child with a serious head injury invariably should have his stomach emptied and the nasogastric tube left in place. He should travel with his head just slightly elevated to minimize intracranial venous pressure, and should be in the lateral position to prevent aspiration of vomitus. The one exception to this is the child with profuse bleeding from a compound skull fracture. In some instances, blood pouring from a scalp wound is actually coming through a skull fracture from a tear in a large intracranial venous sinus. The blood loss can be markedly reduced by elevating the head 7–10 inches above the level of the heart, being careful not to flex the neck which might be broken. Even if the child is initially hypotensive, the shock will be much easier to control if the venous blood loss is reduced by this simple maneuver. With a dressing on the head and the scalp wound undisturbed, the danger of air embolization is negligible compared to the risks entailed in allowing the child to exsanguinate by lowering his head to the level of his heart.

There are two considerations which determine how the receiving neurosurgeon will treat the child. These are the presence of localizing neurologic signs and a change in the level of consciousness. Sophisticated neurologic examination is beyond the scope of most attendants, but anyone can note weakness or paralysis of an extremity, asymmetry of the face, convulsions affecting only part of the body, and whether or not the child responds in the same way to painful stimulation of all extremities. Also, no great skill is required to record how a patient reacts to simple questions and commands so that these same questions and commands can be repeated later to check changes in consciousness. These simple observations are vitally important because localizing signs suggest a lesion amenable to emergency neurosurgical correction, and a decrease in the level of consciousness demands intensification of medical management, with the use of such measures as hyperosmolar intravenous injections and hypothermia or surgical intervention. Frequently it is not the physical findings at a given moment but the reliable history of change which enables the specialist to act quickly to save the child's life.

In summary, the essentials are oxygen, suction, an oral or endotracheal airway, an Ambu bag, a nasogastric tube, an intravenous life line and a supply of replacement fluid, and equipment to monitor pulse, temperature, blood pressure, and respiration. Contact with the receiving neurosurgeon before the trip begins is absolutely essential, and radio contact during the trip is highly desirable. Observation for evidence of localized neurologic abnormalities and changes in level of consciousness may provide lifesaving information for the receiving surgeon. Critically ill children should be accompanied by a physician if at all possible.

SPINAL INJURIES

Patients with spinal injuries should be transported flat, and should be moved with gentle hand traction and extreme care to avoid flexion of the neck or back. Just a bit of extension of neck and back is desirable.

Patients suspected of neck injuries should be gently and firmly supported, and transported at about the speed of a funeral procession. Because the child cannot turn his head, special care to avoid aspiration of vomitus is necessary. In neck and spinal injuries, overdistention of the bladder may occur in a short time. Insertion of a catheter may prevent a very serious complication.

FRACTURES

Fractures should be gently, but firmly, splinted without attempt at reduction. Compound fractures should be adequately covered with dry sterile dressings. Protruding bone fragments should not be replaced beneath the skin. The state of pulses and the presence or absence of normal sensation in the injured extremity should be noted on the record which accompanies the child.

Usually children with fractures do not suffer during transit from mismanagement of the fracture itself. It seems so natural to splint fractures that this is usually done in an adequate manner. The usual serious error in the care of these children is failure to recognize associated injuries, generally to abdominal organs or to the genitourinary tract. Often the fracture is so obvious that the unwary may be distracted from a careful search for hidden, but potentially much more lethal, injuries. Rib fractures should warn of splenic rupture, pelvic fractures of injury to the bladder or urethra. Patients with fractures should be carefully and completely examined before arrangements for transfer are made.

Another common error is failure to appreciate the amount of blood which may be lost in the soft tissues surrounding major fractures. It is not unusual for a child to lose one quarter of his blood volume into the thigh around a single fracture of the femur. Children with femoral or pelvic fractures and children with more than one fracture should not travel without an intravenous lifeline and a generous supply of blood or plasma.

BURNS

Burns require the utmost care and planning if transport is to be accomplished with minimum danger. Usually, it is safer to transport a burned child within a few hours of injury than to delay for more than 24 hours. The key to safe transport is a brief period of initial stabilization, during which time appropriate fluids are started via a secure intravenous catheter, a nasogastric tube and a Foley catheter are inserted, the airway is carefully evaluated, and the wound is dressed with simple sterile dressings. The receiving surgeon can be of tremendous help in guiding the initial stabilization and should be consulted early and in detail. In evaluating the extent of the burn, one needs to know the body weight and what fraction of the head, arms, legs, trunk, front, and back are burned.

Lactated Ringer's solution or plasma should be started via an indwelling intravenous catheter, never a needle. The amount of fluid needed depends upon the magnitude of the burn and on the length of time from injury to termination of the trip. Burns of 20 percent or less usually do not require intravenous fluids immediately, but all children with burns of more than 20 percent require them before being transported. If intravenous fluids are given, *nothing* should be given by mouth. Children with burns of 20–35 percent of the body surface require about 4 ml per kg of body weight per hour, calculated from the time of injury; those with burns over 35 percent require about 6 ml per kg per hour. Whole blood is not needed initially, but up to one half of the required fluid should be plasma, if available. If the pulse becomes rapid or the blood pressure begins to fall after deficits of this magnitude have been replaced, more fluid will be needed. The important considerations are that an intravenous lifeline be maintained, that hypotension not be permitted to develop, and that an accurate record of hourly intake and urinary output be kept.

Scalding injuries seldom result in respiratory difficulties, but airway obstruction frequently develops following flame burns, particularly those occurring indoors. The obstruction progresses for 24–36 hours before receding. Hence, the sooner the child can be fully resuscitated and safely transported, the less likely is airway obstruction to be a problem in transit. If the child is hoarse, or if the respiratory rate is at all elevated, tracheal intubation should be considered before the trip begins.

The burn wound must be covered with a sterile sheet or dressing for transport. If more than 4 hours from the time of burning will elapse before the trip is over, consideration should be given to the possible need for escharotomies. These are necessary only in deep circumferential burns of the extremities or chest. If in doubt, consult the receiving surgeon.

All children with burns of 20 percent or more can be expected to develop ileus, and insertion of a large nasogastric tube before the trip begins is absolutely mandatory.

In summary, the essentials of safe burn transport include detailed consultation between sending and receiving physicians, thorough preparation and stabilization of the child, protection of the airway, nasogastric decompression, appropriate intravenous fluids, an indwelling bladder catheter, an accurate record of hourly intake and output, sterile dressings, and a slow gentle ride with a competent attendant.

TRANSPORTATION OF INFANTS

In addition to the problems of older children, infants require more in the way of protection against bacterial contamination and changes in body temperature. Their vital signs are more difficult to monitor by conventional means, and their tolerance for error in intravenous fluid administration is limited. Because so few ambulances are equipped and staffed to give optimal care to infants in transit, increasing numbers of referral centers are developing specialized vans which are essentially mobile infant intensive care units. A physician from the receiving hospital, who is familiar with the van and its equipment and familiar with the management of the conditions for which infants require transfer, accepts responsibility for the care of the infant before the trip begins. This affords him the opportunity to participate in the initial stabilization of the baby and to be sure that the trip is not begun until this important phase is completed.

The van provides a well-lighted nursery with about 60 square feet of floor space. The ceiling is high enough so that the attendant can stand up. The nursery area is insulated and supplementary heating and air conditioning units provide an ambient temperature of about 80°F.

The infant can be cared for in an intensive care incubator which is permanently mounted in the van or in a transport incubator which can be removed and carried to the nursery. Both units afford far better visibility and temperature control than do conventional transport boxes. The infant's temperature and pulse are monitored electrically, and intravenous fluids are controlled by an electric pump. Resuscitation equipment, drugs, and intravenous fluids are available in a central work area. A two-way radio provides communication between the van and the hospital. If resuscitation or other treatment becomes necessary during the trip, the van can slow or stop so that the physician can work with steady hands.

The surgical problems most frequently requiring transport in the neonatal period are congenital intestinal obstruction, myelomeningocele, omphalocele, gastroschisis, and congenital diaphragmatic hernia.

Congenital Intestinal Obstruction

The primary special concern in babies with congenital intestinal obstruction is prevention of vomiting, aspiration, and progressive abdominal distention. Except in esophageal atresia, the stomach should be emptied via a nasogastric tube which is then aspirated frequently to remove bowel contents and swallowed air. Nasogastric decompression is best accomplished with the baby in semiupright position so that the cardioesophageal junction is higher than the remainder of the stomach. The baby should be on his side so that, if vomiting occurs, he can clear his mouth and pharynx. The tube should be carefully taped in place so that the opposite nostril is not obstructed.

Infants with esophageal atresia usually have a fistula connecting the trachea with the distal portion of the esophagus. When these babies cry, they force air down through the fistula and may overinflate the stomach. They relieve themselves by "burping." When they do this in an upright position, swallowed air rushes harmlessly up the fistula and escapes via the trachea. When they regurgitate in a recumbent position, acid peptic juice precedes the air and floods the airway. Since it is not feasible to decompress the stomach with a tube, the only protection against aspiration pneumonitis is to keep the baby as nearly upright as possible, while aspirating oral secretions from the upper blind pouch continuously or at frequent intervals as needed.

Myelomenigocele, Omphalocele, and Gastroschisis

The primary aims when these conditions exist are to protect the membranes and exposed viscera from bacterial contamination and to protect the baby from loss of body heat. The anomaly should be covered with a moist saline dressing, which in turn should be covered with a bulky dry one so that evaporation and radiant heat loss are minimized. Body temperature should be monitored and not allowed to drop below normal. In the latter two conditions, gastrointestinal tract decompression should be accomplished and maintained by nasogastric tube and suction.

Congenital Diaphragmatic Hernia

With a congenital diaphragmatic hernia the problem is that a significant part of the thorax is filled with intestines. Even in their collapsed state they occupy a dangerous amount of space, and the baby may be suffocated by well-meaning attendants who try to ventilate him by mouth-to-mouth or mask resuscitation, forcing a large amount of air or oxygen down the esophagus and inflating the intrathoracic intestine. A nasogastric tube should be inserted upon diagnosis and its function diligently monitored and adjusted. All efforts at assisting ventilation must be made via an endotracheal tube. These babies are usually acidotic and frequently hypothermic. All efforts should be made to prevent or correct these conditions before and during transport.

SUMMARY

The area of transportation holds great promise for improvement, for many preventable mistakes are being made day after day. The common errors are unwarranted haste, underestimation of the patient's needs, poor communication, and failure to assume responsibility. Improvement will be made and lives will be saved when physicians take time to be sure that their patients are transportable, and that they are protected from airway obstruction, shock, vomiting, aspiration, motion of fractures, and hypothermia during the trip. Children should never be transported until sending and receiving physicians have talked together by phone and have agreed on the transport plan. Provision of proper equipment and of an attendant with sufficient training and skill to handle any emergency which might arise en route cannot be overemphasized. Above all, the sending physician must realize that, unless specific agreements to the contrary have been made, *he* is responsible for the child until the trip is completed. If he cannot otherwise guarantee the safeguards outlined above, he can only fulfill his obligation to his patient by *climbing into the ambulance and going with him.*

REFERENCES

1. American College of Surgeons, Committee on Trauma: Standards for emergency ambulance services. *Bull Amer Coll Surg* 52:131–132, 1967.
2. Farrington, J.D., and Hampton, O.P., Jr.: Curriculum for training emergency medical technicians. *Bull Amer Coll Surg* 54:273–276, 1970.
3. U.S. Government Printing Office: Basic training program for emergency medical technician–Ambulance: course guide and course coordinator orientation program (0-372-389). Washington, D.C.: Superintendent of Documents, 1969.
4. National Academy of Sciences–National Research Council: Medical requirements for ambulance design and equipment. Washington, D.C.: Division of Medical Sciences, 1968.

5. U.S. Department of Transportation: Ambulance design criteria (Report to National Highway Safety Bureau, Federal Highway Administration, prepared by Committee on Ambulance Design Criteria of Highway Research Board, Division of Engineering). Washington, D.C.: Superintendent of Documents, U.S. Government Printing Office, 1969.

6. American College of Surgeons, Committee on Trauma: Essential equipment for ambulances. *Bull Amer Coll Surg* 55:7–13, 1970.

7. Segal, S.: Transfer of a premature or other high-risk newborn infant to a referral hospital. *Pediat Clin N Amer* 13:1195–1205, 1966.

8. Baker, G.L.: Design and operation of a van for the transport of sick infants. *Amer J Dis Child* 118:743–747, 1969.

9. Gaston, S.R.: Accidental death and disability: The neglected disease of modern society, a progress report. *J Trauma* 11:195–206, 1971.

10. White, M.S.: Medical aspects of air evacuation of casualties from Southeast Asia. *Aerospace Med* 39:1338–1341, 1968.

11. Funsch, H.F.: Improved clinical care aloft. *Milit Med* 133:647–649, 1968.

12. Farrington, J.D.: Extrication of victims—surgical principles. *J Trauma* 8:493–512, 1968.

13. Hampton, O.P., Jr: The challenge of the trauma problem to organized medicine. *J Trauma* 10:926–931, 1970.

14. Accidental death and disability: The neglected disease of modern society. Washington, D.C.: National Academy of Sciences–National Research Council, 1966.

15. Waller, J.A.: Control of accidents in rural areas. *JAMA* 201:176–181, 1967.

16. Frey, C.F., Huelke, D.F., Ph.D., and Jikas, P.W.: Resuscitation and survival in motor vehicle accidents. *J Trauma* 9:292–310, 1969.

17. Grosfeld, J.L., Clatworthy, H.W., Jr., and Frye, T.R.: Surgical therapy in neonatal air-block syndrome. *J Thorac Cardiovasc Surg* 60:392–401, 1970.

3

The Environment for Pediatric Surgery

Lawrence K. Pickett, M.D.

The milieu for the practice of medicine is changing constantly, subjected to forces of social and economic origins as well as technical proficiency and progress. In a publication printed three years ago, the hospital environment for the pediatric surgical patient was described largely from the standpoint of the hospital inpatient.[1] The intervening years have brought a rather remarkable change in the nature of the hospitalized patient, and any discussion of the subject of the environment for the pediatric surgical patient must now also take into consideration the outpatient. This chapter will do just that.

THE NATURE OF PEDIATRIC SURGERY

The change in the makeup of the patient population in pediatric surgery over the decades has been quite remarkable. Several decades ago, sepsis was perhaps the major cause of hospitalization, and certainly was involved in most problems in the pediatric surgical ward. With the development of more sophisticated antibiotics, infection control, and prophylaxis, problems of infection gave way to the correction of congenital abnormalities and the treatment of neoplasia. Trauma, including accidents and poison ingestion, obviously continued to contribute to the use of pediatric beds. There has been no recent change in the makeup of the pediatric surgical population in terms of diagnosis, but the severity and intensity of the care required has certainly changed. Technologic advances have allowed the sustaining of life and the support of vital systems in a much more efficient manner. Such advances as central venous nutrition, improved respiratory support, and cardiac management have all increased the complexity of modern surgical care. Other factors have entered into the concentration of this technological complexity. More and more agencies responsible for the cost of hospital care (insurance companies, the Shield plans, and comprehensive prepaid programs), all make allowances for delivery of more care, diagnostic tests, and x-rays to outpatients than before. This tends to remove from the hospital census those children who were once brought in for convenience to avoid the expense of diagnostic work-ups and the supportive care which could have been done on the home scene were the financial assistance present. Thus, pediatrics is migrating to the office and the clinic as an ambulatory specialty, leaving the children requiring surgery and comprehensive or intensive support as the majority of the hospitalized population. The details of the technical advances and the complexities brought on by these changes will be described in other chapters of this book. The discussion in this chapter is limited to the components necessary for the housing, care, and supervision of the children undergoing surgery.

THE ARENA

There are two major arenas for pediatric surgery: the general hospital and the pediatric hospital. The environment established in these arenas varies considerably. The competition in the general hospital setting for proper children's care is frequently unfair in terms of numbers and financial support. Administrators find it very difficult to support pediatric units because of variability in the census, necessary separations by age and sex, and the extra supporting services that are required for children's care. Many communities are finding it advantageous to consolidate the many, small, struggling pediatric services so that children who must be hospitalized can be brought together in a single large facility.

A children's hospital has the advantage of being able to gear itself entirely to the world of children and provide the proper pace of life, equipment, and consideration for the families important in the care of children. Much of what is said here is based on an ideal environment, whether in a children's hospital or a general hospital, and suggests the ideal care for the child. Local ground rules and limiting factors, such as size and financial support, will alter this ideal model, but will be left unconsidered in these discussions. The ideal environment for the care of children would be a physically identifiable unit, closely associated with other central services to avoid expensive duplication. One cannot overemphasize the advantages of having available adult consultative services with professional and paraprofessional personnel or having available the extensive diagnostic x-ray, therapeutic x-ray, and radioisotope equipment of most large hospitals. When the modalities of renal dialysis and respiratory support, to name but two, are taken into consideration, it is quite evident that centralization of equipment and expertise is essential, but that its modification for optimal use with children is also essential. The ideal unit has yet to be built. The balance between emphases must be struck in any individual situation.

NEONATAL SPECIAL CARE

In all pediatric care, it is necessary to separate patients by age and sex, but as the nature of the problems becomes more intense, the need for separation becomes less important. It should be said at the outset that the neonate offers enough unique problems to warrant special consideration. Physically, there should be a close association between the delivery room and the neonatal nursery. The neonatal intensive care unit should also be near the delivery room, particularly for high-risk deliveries where the mother is being monitored and where the expectation of neonatal problems is high. There is also a place where the mother can share in the care of the newborn baby (a rooming-in arrangement). These units should also be located near the special-care nurseries where problem children can be observed. So there are three divisions of nurseries: those for the rooming-in-mothers, those for the care of the babies where the mothers are not as involved, and the neonatal special-care units where sick infants and premature infants with both medical and surgical problems can be cared for with optimal supervision, expertise in nursing care, and availability of special equipment. The neonatal special-care unit should house as many of the special pieces of equipment as possible, so that the infants can be cared for without the necessity of removing them from the unit for diagnostic or therapeutic reasons. If the unit incorporates x-ray equipment strictly for the use of the infants and an operating suite for the same purpose, these environments can be kept suitably warm and separate from the infectious potential of the general environment. Neonatal surgery and diagnostic radiology can be carried out under optimal conditions. It is not inconceivable that the nurses who function in the intensive care of neonates could also function in the operating room nurses' role with a minimum of training. Much of what falls on the nurses' shoulders in the neonatal unit at the present time is as complex as that which faces the operating room nurses in other parts of the hospital. The two roles could be successfully brought together, solving some of the staffing problems and some of the special problems related to the care of infants in a non-infant environment.

Details concerning equipment, electronic monitoring devices, and the ideal environment in which to control infection (i.e. laminar flow rooms) must be taken into consideration before construction, renovating, or improving any neonatal unit. This subject is covered in later chapters, but it should be said here that for the neonatal special care unit, the complexities of the necessary care warrant special consideration and physical isolation. Age limitation in the neonatal unit will depend on several factors, including volume and utilization. With the exception of prematurity, the majority of critical surgical problems in the neonate are resolved by thirty days of age. The need for extended parent contact with the infant increases with age and as the intensity of the care diminishes. All surgical care of the first days of life is intense. It is quite possible that the neonatal unit might serve as the intensive-care area for infants up to ninety days with convalescence elsewhere.

The neonatal environment must not only take into account intense care for the sick infant, but also convenient accessibility of the unit to the parent. The need for visiting and progressive involvement of the mother in the infant's care before it is discharged home is essential. The visiting of parents under proper infection-control conditions is to be encouraged. The course of events altering their infant's life, perhaps resulting in permanent disability, can be better understood with intelligent on-the-scene education. The emotional needs of the parents must be attended to at the same time as the physical needs of the infant. Suitable waiting rooms, consultation rooms, and discharge and mothers' education rooms should be provided.

THE INFANT AGE GROUP

As the nature of the disorders of the inpatients becomes more acute and the care necessarily more intense, the long-adhered-to division between age and sex becomes less vital. Specialty groups among the professionals involved in pediatric surgery find that the care of the patient is much improved by clustering the patients being treated for similar illnesses together, with less regard to their age and sex. For example, all orthopedic patients would be together in one location, all urologic patients in another and the patients undergoing renal dialysis and transplantation in still another. In a similar way, cardiothoracic problems from medical cardiology to postoperative cardiac surgery can best be cared for in a localized area, and the same can be said for neurological and neurosurgical patients. If a new hospital is being built, such considerations can be incorporated into the floor plan and divisions; restoration and alteration of existing space make this more difficult.

ADOLESCENT UNIT

Just as neonatal patients have unique and specific requirements that suggest a segregation of that group, so do adolescents. They have similar physical requirements as adults, but their own emotional and social needs. Beyond this division of pediatric patients, further division of care by age is unnecessary. With older children, division by sex is easily accomplished in smaller nursing units.

INTENSIVE CARE

One of the most important factors in improving results in the treatment of the critically ill pediatric patient has been the development of an intensive care unit, bridging the gap between the needs of various specialty interests. Located there is a concentration of equipment, such as monitoring equipment, respiratory support apparatus, and thermal blankets that will permit expertise in use as well as maintenance of these complexities. Nurses and paraprofessionals needed for sophisticated intensive care can also be concentrated there to the great advantage of all. Progression from the multispecialty intensive care area to the specialty cluster area depends on the usual constraints of personnel and space.

Methods of administering the intensive care area differ in various hospitals, depending mainly on the availability of a proper administrator. Cardiorespiratory care remains the common denominator of most patients in intensive care areas. Easily available blood-gas determinations on a 24-hour basis are essential. Many intensive care units are administered by pediatric anesthesiologists. They represent an obvious source of great knowledge in cardiorespiratory physiology and experience in respiratory support therapy.

It is essential that someone be responsible for deciding who is admitted to or discharged from the unit. Also, the staff should have a constant in-service educational program. Emotional support and recognition of "intensive unit" fatigue in the personnel as a fact of life is essential. Education, rotation, and spiritual counseling are all necessary ingredients to counteract the tensions of this arena.

It is quite evident that the spread of specialization is reaching out into the paramedical personnel as well as the physicians themselves. Specialties are growing among nurses and supportive personnel, making the clustering of the patients for their ministrations in an intensive care environment quite different from the conventional children's units of old. The division of age and sex can be carried out in smaller units within a specialty interest cluster.

In large departments where volume permits, the pediatric surgical patients can be separated from the pediatric medical patients. However, it is more logical that the clustering and segregation be determined by disease, diagnosis, specialty interest and treatment requirements rather than the artificial division between medicine and surgery.

OTHER SPECIAL UNITS

The support of life, with the hope of restoration to normal function, is the role of the entire hospital, but the hospital must also care for the child who is beyond redemption and who needs custodial care as death approaches. Often it is inadvisable for terminal care to be given in the home, and in such cases, the hospital should arrange for the parents to stay with the child and in the hospital where they can render much of the necessary care. It would be ideal for this area to be separate from other areas of the hospital devoted to more conventional needs.

There should also be an area available where the mother or the parents can help care for their child in nonterminal cases as well. Such case might include hospitalization for complicated diagnostic studies, hospitalization for repeated treatments of short duration (such as transfusion), or hospitalization for care beyond the capability of the home, but not requiring the expertise, equipment, and personnel of the busy intensive ward. One should consider a separate physical environment for this group of patients. The ancillary and supporting personnel for such a unit would obviously lean less heavily on the special skills of the nurse and more heavily on the functions of paramedical support, such as the clergy, the social worker, the housekeeping department, and the volunteer. Their contributions to the environment are discussed later. This "care by parent" unit can be quite self-contained with provisions and equipment for light housekeeping if the nature of the clientele demands it. Families may use the hospital cafeteria as an "escape" from the children's ward. The increasing load of hematologic patients, children undergoing cancer chemotherapy, and patients requiring sophisticated physiotherapy makes this kind of unit quite desirable.

PERSONNEL SUPPORT FOR THE PEDIATRIC SURGERY PATIENT

Many hospitals have physician training programs with interns and residents. Medical-center-based hospitals directly associated with medical schools have medical students, clinical fellows, and a host of other members of the medical care complex in training. Supervision for these various levels of training is generally adequate. The patient obviously benefits from the great knowledge and technical skills attendant with the teaching program.

The environment for the function of these trainees and students is too often inadequate. Space for conferences and seminars should be provided separate from the patient areas so that matters of academic discussion are not heard and possibly misunderstood by the patients or families.

Another liability due to the numbers of students in various levels of training is "overexposure" of the patient. An "interesting" patient, or one with a remarkable or easily demonstrated physical finding, may be subject to repeated examinations at all hours to the detriment of his well being and with great parental displeasure. Someone must have the authority to limit such exposure. The chief nurse on the ward, long experienced in the repeating generations of students, is in the best position to protect the patient from overexposure, invasion of privacy, and even introduction of the ever-present nosocomial infection. This important feature of a teaching environment is too often neglected by failure to establish such authority or by lack of cooperation in recognizing such authority.

A growing addition to the physician trainee is the paramedic trainee. There are pediatric nurse practitioners now being trained and used primarily in office or other ambulatory settings. Surgical associates are also being trained in increasing numbers. In some situations these paramedical personnel work with house staff. Increasingly, the house staff is involved in educational exercises. Many of the service tasks, previously assigned to the house staff, are now being done by this new group. The responsibility for such things as intravenous therapy, dressing changes, cast application and removal, and catheter care may become the paramedics'. Supervision, respect for the position, and parent education are essential as the function of these people expands.

NURSES

The nursing personnel are obviously becoming more proficient and more expert in technical matters, such as monitoring and the use of complex electronic equipment. Their role is becoming more sophisticated as their training increases. The conventional role of the nurse in a domiciliary or custodial role is being taken over by practical nurses and less highly trained individuals and by various paramedical personnel. Nurses are also specializing, as are other members of the medical care team. The clustering of patients by specialty interests lends itself to nurse specialization. Such nurses become even more integral members of the medical care teams. Their role in education of the parents, paramedical personnel, and the patients themselves is expanding and essential to the environment of the pediatric surgical patients.

PARENT EDUCATION

Education and support of the parents, both from a standpoint of their responsibility to their child and from the standpoint of their emotional survival, are vital parts of the pediatric surgical environment. Educating parents is the responsibility of the attending physician, although support can come from the nursing services, the social service worker, volunteers, and others specifically assigned to be the ombudsman for the child and the parent in the busy technical complex environment. These supporting people become as important to the survival of the child and to the understanding of the parent as any other aspect of the child's illness. Parent gatherings where there is group interaction are a very useful way of disseminating information. Skilled leadership is most important. The attention and care that parents can give are very valuable in creating a better environment for the children. It is important that specialized studies be explained, fears about radioactivity be allayed, the need for expensive studies be explained, and uncomfortable or unpleasant treatments be justified to the patients and their families. Group sessions answer many questions, remove much of the anxiety from the foreign environment, and promote the family's confidence in the hospital.

THE CLERGY

The anxiety and spiritual disruption caused by any illness, especially where there exists the threat of death, obviously dictate that there be strong spiritual support in a proper pediatric surgical environment. Many hospitals have chaplains or clergy from various faiths assigned to the hospital. A place for quiet meditation, such as a small chapel, should be provided if possible. An educated clergy can do much to support this aspect of the total hospital environment, by helping the staff and physicians deal with spiritual problems and by helping the family deal with their dilemma, anxieties, and guilt.

SCHOOLING

The more serious the patient's illness, the less important schooling is. There are a certain number of children of school age who have prolonged hospitalization, and these require schooling consistent with their age, length of hospitalization, and degree of illness. Schooling is provided in many cases by part-time or full-time teachers, depending upon the volume, but should be woven into the fabric of total hospital care. This probably applies much more to a chronic disease hospital than to an acute disease hospital. An extension of schooling is occupational therapy and craft work. The availability and intelligent use of the volunteers is essential to this phase of proper care. Relying entirely on volunteers may not be satisfactory, and their coordination, correlation, and training is a full-time job for a paid professional. Feeding of babies, amusement of children, and arts and crafts can all be important support to nursing care and progress toward recovery.

OUTPATIENT PEDIATRIC SURGERY

Some surgical procedures can be accomplished using general anesthesia and do not require overnight hospitalization of the patient. This has long been true and has been practiced in a number of ways. This section will deal with the necessary environment for such ambulatory or outpatient surgical care involving general anesthesia.

The growth of the numbers of such cases has been in response to consumer preference and economic demands. Some of the procedures that require general anesthesia do not need a full hospital support mechanism. Furthermore, crowded operating room schedules, the increased intensity of the ward environment, and the evident increase in nosocomial infections all make the advantages of a very short hospital exposure quite understandable. For some time, complete history and physical examination and all the routines attendant with major surgical procedures have been applied to minor or shorter procedures that do not require prolonged convalescence. This therapeutic "overkill" in accomplishing such procedures as herniorrhaphy or circumcision, can easily be done without.

The requirements of the child who needs minor surgery and his family are quite different from those of a patient needing major surgery. To prevent exposure to hospital infections and the anxieties and intensity of the hospital ward, a separate location should be established for the admissions, preparation, and even the actual surgery for the shorter procedures. The outpatients are not exposed to more acutely ill children, and the hospitalized children who have a prolonged convalescence are not exposed to the child who comes and goes in one day, upsetting the morale of the ward by his appearance and possibly bringing infection from the outside into the ward environment.

A recent development in Phoenix, Arizona, has pointed out the ultimate in this move involving both adults and children with a "Surgicenter" where the entire building is set up for surgery under general anesthesia, short-term recovery, and no overnight hospitalization.[2] Modifications of this concept have been developed in many centers. Children come in with a proper history by their referring physician, have the basic minimum of laboratory work performed, i.e. a hemoglobin determination and urinalysis (though this could even be done in anticipation of the event), a quick screening and evaluation by the anesthesiologist to be sure that there is no immediate infection or contraindication to a general anesthesia, and proper preanesthetic medications can be given in a suitable holding area with the family in attendance. Since the smaller the child, the more important it is to prevent multiple exposures as far as infection is concerned, admission to an isolated environment for examination, preparation, and recovery is essential.

It is most important to choose an anesthetic agent from which recovery will be prompt, the postoperative complications rare, and the need for prolonged observation minimized. Likewise, the type of case and the scope of the operation must be tailored to suit short-term observation and the ability of the family to take care of the child at home following the procedure.

In summary, for proper utilization of this modality, a different set of routines must be established and a different supporting personnel employed than one would have in the conventional hospital setting. It is assumed that before the operation, the conventional complete history is taken and physical examination given in the doctor's office under more relaxed circumstances, to reveal any contraindications. Facilities and space should be available for preoperative examination. Parent education must be complete so that the child has an empty stomach and the full significance of the fasting period has been impressed upon the family. Quite obviously, one must be most careful in providing the equipment and personnel necessary for safe recovery from anesthesia. Time must be taken to explain to parents what they are to expect in the postoperative period at home.

Occasionally, due to postoperative complications, an outpatient must be admitted into the hospital. The hospital design should include facilities to do this easily.

The development of the outpatient concept may require construction of special facilities, such as operating rooms and recovery space, but will relieve congestion in the major operating rooms and in the demand for hospital beds, allowing for better utilization of the personnel, equipment, and space to the advantage of both the patient and the hospital. It should be noted that the cost per diem of those who remain in the intensive area, without the dilution of the less intensely ill patients, will be increased for each person hospitalized, but will decrease the overall cost of hospitalization to the entire community. It is necessary that this fact be impressed on government agencies that are becoming increasingly important in the support of medical care and costs.

Separate from the unit for outpatient operative care, is an observation area for emergency problems such as abdominal pain, head injury, acute dehydration, and recovery from minor trauma, conditions that can be treated in a "short-stay unit." Many of the acute problems are resolved under close observation; some patients will have to be admitted.

Such a unit has been in use for more than a year at the King's County–Downstate Medical Center in Brooklyn. Fifty-eight percent of the patients are discharged from the unit in less than twenty-four hours, decreasing the number of admissions and hospital days.

For many of the same reasons that outpatient surgery is useful, the short-stay unit is of value: the opportunity for abbreviated workup, the reduction of transient traffic in the more intense care units in the hospital, and the prevention of exposure to infection.

The short-stay unit must be staffed twenty-four hours a day. It should be built with a comfortable waiting area for parents as emergencies are especially anxiety-producing. The parent can aid in the observation period with the help of the professional staff.

There is an obvious need to separate children from adults, not only in the general hospital world, but also in the emergency room. Such problems as alcohol, trauma, and psychosis that frequent the adult emergency area are best kept separated from the pediatric care area. This unit will obviously serve both medical and surgical pediatric patients.

An added advantage in continuity of observation is that the physicians and assistants who make the first observation in the emergency room have a chance to confirm their suspicions of an acute or non-acute state before chancing observation at home or involving another entire care team in the problem. Also, the boredom of acute care and triage can be diluted for the emergency care team. Never observing the progress, even short term, of acute illness is a deterrent to intelligent and interested care.

CONCLUSION

Environment is obviously neither just physical nor just human, but a combination of both. The ideal pediatric surgical environment cannot be established without constant interplay between people and places, the hospital and the patient, the trainer and the trainee. No physical plant is ever ideal; no program is ever perfect. Intelligent and well-founded change will, however, lead toward these ideals.

REFERENCES

1. Pickett, L.K.: The hospital environment for the pediatric surgical patient. *Pediat Clin N Amer* 16:531–542, 1969.
2. Cloud, D.T., et al: The surgicenter: A fresh concept in outpatient pediatric surgery. *J Pediat Surg* 7:206–212, 1972.

4

The Seriously Ill or Dying Child: Supporting the Patient and Family

C. Everett Koop, M.D., Sc.D.

No one enters the medical profession skillful in handling the problems that are generated in the hospital, in the family, and in the community by the seriously ill or dying child. The physician who understands well his role in the treatment of disease and the postponement of death for as long a time as possible, frequently does not understand his role in making the serious illness of a child, his impending death, or his actual death as bearable as possible for all of those concerned. Those affected frequently comprise a wider circle than seems to be the case at first glance. The doctor can never escape the tragedy that these circumstances bring to the family of the patient, but is often not aware of the impact of a dying child upon hospital personnel, the community, and the child himself.

The opinions expressed here are those of a surgeon who has spent more than a quarter of a century dealing with sick children and with pediatricians. The surgeon who devotes his major effort to the care of children feels comfortable with children of any age and with their parents. On the other hand, the surgeon who by choice or by assignment focuses his attention on the technical aspects of surgical endeavor may never learn how to develop an intimate relationship with a seriously ill patient and his family. This situation is not ideal for the patient, and it is particularly unfortunate for the patient's family. The crossroad of pediatric and surgical care is at the bedside of the seriously ill child with a surgical problem. The family has the right to expect and to receive a package of services, varying from the delivery of competent surgical technical care to the support of the family in a crisis of anxiety, or from skillful medical management to family counseling and proph-esying. The surgeon familiar with children is in an ideal position to provide many of these services, but if the surgeon is not that familiar with children, it will be the pediatrician who must bridge the gap.

The seriously ill child often recovers and is discharged from the hospital. The successful outcome alone does much to smooth out the emotional rough spots of a long and trying hospitalization for the fam-ily and is reward enough for the hospital personnel. When the seriously ill child dies, however, the rough spots remain abrasive, a sufficient reason in itself for the physician to want to prevent their occurrence when possible and to correct them when necessary.

While it is true that no one enjoys having to manage the emotional problems surrounding the dying child, it is possible for the one who serves as guide through difficult times to derive some satisfaction when the family is salvaged, the community is able to get on without bitter-ness toward the hospital or the medical profession, and the hospital staff is able to return to the routines of care knowing that they have played a positive role in an unpleasant situation.

TYPES OF PATIENTS

From the surgeon's point of view, there are four general classes of pa-tients whose emotional management requires almost as much planning as does specific therapy: the neonatal surgical patient, the child who faces possible death because of an accident, the acutely ill surgical patient, and the chronically ill child whose eventual death seems in-evitable.

The Neonatal Surgical Patient

The neonatal surgical patient is usually one for whom an operative pro-cedure has been undertaken for the correction of a congenital anomaly incompatible with life. The fact that the family has not known the pa-tient as an individual does not lessen the tensions around such an event and the fact that the surgeon does not usually know the parents as a family increases the stress considerably. The mother particularly faces a difficult situation: she may not have seen her newborn infant because it has been whisked away from her to another part of the hos-pital or perhaps even to a hospital in a distant city to have a major surgical procedure. The diagnosis which may have been given to the mother is usually an ominous one and one with which she has had no experience, such as an omphalocele, diaphragmatic hernia, or imperforate anus. Not only does the mother feel deprived of her infant and all of the joys that accompany the arrival of a new baby, but she is frequently told of the child's defect under less than ideal circumstances. The surgeon who will operate upon her child and who has had previous experience with similar situations is, unfortunately, rarely the member of the medical team to talk with the mother preoperatively. When she wakes from her analgesia or anesthesia, the whole situation smacks of unreality. Her husband, on whom she would like to lean at this particular time, may be aiding in the transport of the infant to a medical center and when he does return, she is often overwhelmed by the seriousness of the situation and the speed with which his outlook has changed. It is no wonder that the mother feels a sense of despair and that her hostility is directed toward those unknown members of the medical team who have deprived her of her infant, even though at the same time she knows that their motives are the best and their involvement in the situation unavoidable.

The surgeon's obligation begins with a full explanation to the father, who should be kept on hand until the close of the emergency operative procedure. In the discussion, the surgeon would do well to repeat such statements as "Reassure your wife that . . ." or "Be sure that you do assure Mrs. J. that we will do thus and so" and especially, "I will call your wife tomorrow and give her a first-hand report on where things stand, unless you think you would rather do it." If the father chooses the latter course, the surgeon should be available for back-up explanation. Some facility in the hospital should be activated (social service, nursing staff, or house staff) to provide current information when it is requested.

If the surgical procedure contemplated is not one that must be undertaken forthwith, and if there is no medical contraindication in reference to the mother, a conversation between the surgeon and the mother either in person, in which case the father can be on hand, or at least by telephone, is profitable. It has frequently been my experience that when explanations are left to someone other than the surgeon, the risk and gravity of the procedure are minimized or misrepresented, particularly in cases where the cosmetic result is important, such as surgery for cleft lip. The obstetrician, out of misplaced sympathy for the mother, may advise her not to visit her infant, even though, under ordinary circumstances, the mother would be expected to be up and around and caring for her child. Obviously, the surgeon and his hospital are placed at a disadvantage when the mother stays away, and I believe it is also a disservice to the mother. She should understand the gravity of the situation, so that if the outcome is not favorable, she will have known what the odds are from the beginning and will not be disillusioned into thinking her child did not receive proper care. She is better able to face reality if she is able to see and touch her infant.

Anyone who has watched a mother deprived of her newborn child immediately after delivery make her first acquaintance with the young-ster (particularly if it is her firstborn) knows what a tremendous reward she receives from seeing and handling her child. Her natural hostility disappears; she becomes an understanding participant in the care of her child and a cooperative member of the team seeking a successful outcome.

There is one recurring problem around the care of the neonatal surgical emergency for which there is no pat answer: whether or not to operate when a congenital anomaly incompatible with life but amenable to surgical correction occurs in association with Mongolism or a variety of congenital anomalies concomitantly, the correction of which will result in a severely handicapped child physically, emotion-ally, and perhaps mentally. To state all sides of this issue would take a volume larger than this one and yet there would be no conclusion that was not based upon the moral, ethical, and religious upbringing of the individual physician. If the conclusion is a moral one, morality cannot be legislated.

The physician who says "I will operate in order to save a life under any circumstance" can be accused of "playing God" just as much as the physician who says "I will not operate to save a life if that life will not be reasonably competent." This is not the place to present both sides of the argument nor even to express my own personal practice, but it must be discussed to a certain extent if problems of guilt are to be avoided.

Any surgeon who has dealt with a large volume of congenital anomalies incompatible with life is aware of the fact that many parents assume that the arrival of a defective child is in some way retribution. Whether the parents believe this comes from God or from some other system of justice is not pertinent to this discussion. Surgeons who deal with neonatal emergencies are also familiar with the queries of parents after the death of a hopelessly defective child. Commonly these queries are directed toward what other possible means might have been used to save the life of the child. These attitudes being as frequent as they are, I don't believe that a physician ever has the right to put the deci-sion to withhold life-saving surgery on the shoulders of a parent.

After the neonatal surgical operative procedure has been ac-complished, there must be some protocol for liaison between the family and the medical team. Those in charge of the situation fre-quently forget that with a rapidly changing house staff and with shift-ing nursing personnel well-established protocols break down. Fre-quent reassessment of the efficiency of the channel of communication between parent and hospital must be made. Whether the hospital end of this channel is the nursing service, the house staff, the social service department, or a specific individual assigned the task is not as impor-tant as the establishment of the line of communication. Some of the responsibility at the hospital end can be alleviated by stating to the parents that if they do not hear from the hospital, progress is as expected, but that any variation will be reported immediately. Early on it is well to introduce the family to the possible occurrence of multiple congenital defects so that when a cardiac lesion turns up several days after birth it does not come with the same shock that it might have without prior announcement. The rapport that can be established between parent and physician before such announcement is much easier to achieve than it is after the occurrence of a stressing complication.

The Accident Patient

The child who is in dire straits and who faces imminent death because of an accident presents special problems in emotional management of the family. No accident is planned, and in addition to all of those things which are built into the atmosphere of stress surrounding any instance of serious illness and impending death is the element of shock and disbelief. Frequently, more than one member of the family has been involved in the accident; indeed, one may already be dead. The surgeon in these circumstances has little time to prepare the family for anything. He must be as truthful as possible without removing all hope, and his frequent attendance upon the patient or the constant care of his deputy will support the family as much as any overture in their time of acute crisis.

The importance of the environment of the accident room cannot be overemphasized. It is here that the hospital's efficiency and competence is tested, and it is here that the rapport with the family of a child who might die is established. This is where hospitals' reputations are made or broken, to say nothing of malpractice suits.

Prompt attention to the accident victim is essential and there should be minimum delay between a decision and its being carried out. Honest disagreements concerning therapy on the part of attending physicians should not be discussed in front of the family. Preferably, the family is separated from the child and placed in comfortable adjacent surroundings, but it is foolish to insist upon this if a parent adamantly refuses to leave his stricken child. In these days with increasing numbers of paramedical personnel it is important to caution them against loose talk about the patient, on the one hand, or misinforming parents about the patient's progress, on the other.

The Acutely Ill Surgical Patient

The family of the youngster who has become suddenly and seriously ill with a surgical illness usually has not had no warning of an impending catastrophe and therefore falls in the field of management somewhere between the families of accident patients and chronically ill children. Firm relationships with the family have been established as was not possible in the case of the neonatal surgical patient, and the mother is mobile as well as concerned. The acutely ill surgical patient may represent a delay in diagnosis, an error in diagnosis, or previous medical or surgical mismanagement. The frustration of the medical team confronted with the care of such a patient is understandable, but nothing is to be gained by sharing these frustrations with the family or by criticizing previous medical care. An honest assessment of the situation as it is is what the family needs and avoids the guilt which they may assume in reference to previous care that was less than ideal.

WORKING WITH THE FAMILY IN CHRONIC ILLNESS

The surgical patient who becomes chronically ill often dies. It is around the care of this chronically ill child, whose death seems inevitable, that much of our concern must be centered. His is the family that could be said to lose its child twice, once when the diagnosis is made and the prognosis is explained, and again when the child actually dies. These two dreadful occasions for the family are not easy for any member of the medical team to handle, but the grief of the parents can be assuaged to a great degree and a sense of satisfaction the physician can feel when they are adequately handled. It is in the interval between the diagnosis and death that the physician has the opportunity to build a relationship with the family and the child that will hold together at the time of actual death and even thereafter.

The process of relating to the family and to the child should begin even before the diagnosis is made, at the very first contact with the surgeon. It is at this first encounter that the surgeon must project his integrity, capacity for compassion, and understanding in such a way that the family will be assured during the time of diagnostic studies that when the eventual diagnosis is known, the surgeon will not only be honest in his dealings with them, but will, to the best of his ability, help them to understand and bear their situation. This does not mean that the surgeon must share all of his doubts with the family before an exact diagnosis is reached. Even though there may be relief at times, it is cruel to put a family through the possibility of facing a hopeless prognosis before the surgical procedure that "proves it," even though the diagnosis seems unavoidable in the surgeon's mind. The parents of patients become more knowledgeable about medical and scientific matters as the months go by. It is not uncommon for them to ask a number of searching, "what if" questions. This is the time to say to the family: "If I told you of all the possibilities that exist in a case like that of your child I would have to introduce you to a number of unpleasant things that never will come to pass."

When the unpleasant news must finally be broken, the family is usually keyed to a high pitch because they have been waiting for the

results of the biopsy, the exploratory procedure, or the series of diagnostic tests. When the moment finally comes for the surgeon to inform
the family, attention to a number of seemingly unimportant details will
pay great dividends in days to come. First of all, the news should be
given to a family in the best of all possible surroundings, such as a room
designed for that purpose, the surgeon's office, or a quiet lounge. The
discussion should not be held on the ward, in the corridor, in the outpatient clinic, in the lobby of the hospital, or in any place where a
family cannot let their emotions out without embarrassment. Secondly,
if at all possible, both parents should be together at this time, but if
anyone else is to be present, the surgeon should be certain that it is a
stable member of the family who will supply support, rather than an
unstable member who will add to the emotional strain that the family
is about to face. Under no circumstances should this be an announcement to a "gathering of the clan."

I have used the word surgeon here not only because I am one, but
also because I think this is the surgeon's responsibility. All too frequently, the surgeon who handles his adult patients magnificently turns
his juvenile patients and their families over to the pediatrician, who,
although attuned to problems of children and their families, is not always able to answer questions about the surgical procedure itself. It
has been my experience that families do not generally like having residents or medical students listening in at the time when the surgeon is
telling the family news of grave prognosis. On the other hand, if another physician such as the family doctor or the family's pediatrician is
to be carrying part of the family counseling, it would be of great benefit to have such a physician hear the surgeon's initial description of the
surgical situation, the diagnosis, and the prognosis so that at least at
the outset a unified presentation can be made to the family.

The actual wording of the announcement will have to fit the physician's personality, but it should be gentle rather than abrupt, com-
passionate while factual, and free of confusing scientific terms and
double talk that leave the family uncertain and permit the physician to
escape to more pleasant tasks.

The situation in which a family has waited for several tension-
filled hours, only to have the surgeon return from the operating room
and reveal that the diagnosis is a malignant tumor which carries a high
mortality, is sometimes more than the family can immediately take in.
I have found it invaluable to announce first of all that the youngster is
in the recovery room and that the operation is over and that all concerned with his care are satisfied with his condition. I then proceed to
say that, as we suspected, the diagnosis was confirmed. This indicates
to the family that the diagnosis was not an overwhelming surprise and
they therefore have reason to believe that since we found what was expected, we knew how to take care of it. I usually keep talking about
relatively unimportant things while the family absorbs the first shock
of this revelation and then begin to describe the immediate steps that

we will take to bring about as satisfactory a solution as possible to the terrible problem that we all face. At about this time, I remind the family that this is a lot to take in at one sitting and that I will repeat it all to them in a day or so and am always available to answer questions that come to their mind. No matter what the prognosis, it should be made clear that no matter what the outcome, everything will be done to support the patient.

The physician should also be aware of the fact that there are families who hear only what they want to hear. It is usually possible to get some inkling of this, and the physician can check it out by asking the family questions. If he finds that he is indeed dealing with a family that is screening out all of the factual information that is unpleasant, then he must spell it out exceedingly carefully and perhaps do so in the presence of another member of the family, who is able to understand and emotionally interpret it. It is not uncommon in cases where there are several physicians involved in the care of a patient to have the family ask their questions of the "wrong" physician. They ask the surgical questions of the chemotherapist, they ask the surgeon the hematological questions, and they ask the hematologist the chemotherapy questions. The slightest variation in the opinion of two or more physicians caring for a child is upsetting to most families, but is enlarged out of proportion by others, and the loss of their confidence is inevitable. For this reason, it makes extremely good sense for doctor X not to assume that he knows what doctor Y has just said or plans to do. No physician loses face by referring the question to the individual directly concerned with the answer.

As the reality of the situation is grasped by the family, the first questions asked usually center around the amount of suffering and the duration of life. The question of suffering can always be answered with assurance of a positive nature, but it is best to hedge the timing of death, not only because it is unknown, but because so many therapeutic factors may alter the situation.

One can usually tell whether this is a time when the family would like to be alone, or whether they would prefer to have the continuing support of a stranger who is obviously trying to be a friend. This is the time when the surgeon must be all things to all men. A kindly gesture such as an arm around the father or holding the hands of both parents as they sit facing you may seem embarrassing at times, but is frequently remembered in days to come as an outstanding act of support. Some families indicate that they would like to talk further at this time; others are too shocked to absorb much more until another day. At some time there are a number of things that I think have to be gotten across that are important to the future.

It used to be said in World War II that there were no atheists in foxholes. I have found that there are very few atheists among the parents of dying children. This is a time when religious faith can see a family through the trying circumstances. I think it is well to work closely with the family's clergyman, if this is their wish. Very commonly the minister will accompany the family upon its second or third visit to the hospital after learning of the child's diagnosis.

Again in line with being all things to all men, at a time like this, I can only speak from the standpoint of my own faith, and when I am asked such questions as "Why did God do this to my child?" or "What have we done to be punished like this?" or when I hear statements such as "All we can do is hope and pray," I attempt to meet the family on some compatible ground that will not be argumentative, but might be reassuring. I have found that most commonly, people who ask these questions are reassured by the fact that the God they question is sovereign and does not act capriciously. I am certain that it helps many times for the family to hear me say that if I did not believe in the sovereignty of God, I would find it most difficult, if not impossible, to be caring for their child. If the family requests you to talk to their minister, do so. If they want you to talk to their relatives now that the first awful crisis is past, this is reasonable. If they ask you to pray with them, pray with them. About the only thing you cannot do, much as you might want to, is cry with them. Hospital chaplains can be invaluable at times, yet parents appreciate nonprofessional help from their doctors.

There probably has never been a parent-child relationship in which, under stress, the parent could not find a cause for guilt. These guilt feelings very commonly become exaggerated at the time of the grave illness or death of a child. So frequently do parents, particularly mothers, consider the affliction of their child to be punishment from God that it is commonly openly expressed. No matter what one's theological doctrine on punishment might be, parents benefit by the statement that such an affliction of a child and punishment of a parent would be evil, and that no evil comes from the hand of God.

It is inevitable in a medical center, particularly one well staffed with physicians, residents, and fellows, that all of the statements made about a child's illness will not conform to the statements made by the physician in charge. It is well to point out that if any questions arise because of variations in opinion and advice, that the surgeon's door is always open and that he will try to answer questions. At the same time, it is well to train a house staff we have to be of one mind and one goal in these situations. High on the list of priorities is the admonition never to make a promise that cannot be fulfilled.

THE FAMILY AND THE COMMUNITY

Since the family will face a number of problems in its relationship with friends and the community, it is a good idea to discuss what these problems might be before they present themselves. Parents obviously cannot help but share their tragic news with friends and relatives. Almost inevitably, some well-meaning individual is certain that he understands the situation better than the child's doctors or has such faith in his own physician that he will not rest until the family has had either a change of management or at least another opinion. I usually discuss this eventuality frankly with the family, not because I fear another opinion, but because I am concerned about the family's emotional stability. I tell them that I expect that many well-meaning friends will assume the role of amateur physician or even of expert in their child's diagnosis.

I also tell families that many people have been duped by cancer quacks and fraudulent cancer remedies and assure them that bonafide therapy is never the property of one man or one clinic, but is available to all reputable physicians. In reference to the question of consultation, I make it clear that if there were anything unique that could be offered their child elsewhere, I would see that the referral was made and even find a way to ease the economic burden if that were a problem. Indeed, all of us who deal with dying children occasionally do make such referrals, either for the medical benefit they afford or the emotional support of the family. I usually suggest to the family that the way to avoid confusion is for them to inform me of any advice that sounds reasonable and logical to them. If I know anything about it I will discuss it with them; if I do not, I will investigate and report back promptly. Miraculous cures have been sought by religious people for years. In days gone by this was usually in the Roman Catholic confession, but recently charismatic movements in Protestantism have attracted people to faith healers. The support that a family obtains through their religious faith is immeasurable in some instances and should never be downgraded. On the other hand, some so-called faith healing is made contingent upon the amount of faith engendered by the family. This means that if a miraculous cure does not take place, the family is convinced that their faith is shabby and they have the problem of guilt added to the emotional problem of the seriously ill child.

If this matter comes up, I tell families that I do believe in miracles but have never seen what I would call a miracle in reference to their child's problem. Another way it can be stated is that all healing is miraculous. Naturally, advice against seeking a miraculous cure comes better from someone with strong religious convictions than from one who is obviously on the other side of the fence.

ANSWERING PARENTS' QUESTIONS

There are a number of questions that parents inevitably ask. The first is usually, "When can he go home?" and the second question is frequently, "Can he go back to school?" if the youngster is of school age. Parents will want to know how long they can expect their child to live and whether or not he will suffer.

· These questions should be faced head-on and answered from the physician's experience to the advantage of the particular family. Frequently, the physician must say that the youngster will appear to be so well for a time that the parents will doubt the diagnosis and prognosis. The question of school must be answered on an individual basis, but in general, if a child feels well, it is probably best for him to go to school. Even if his life expectancy is limited, it is very difficult for a family to have what amounts to a "death watch" around a seemingly well child. When he begins to falter and school becomes difficult physically, mentally, or emotionally, he probably should stay at home. In some instances, half-day schooling is good for morale all around.

The promise to alleviate suffering can always be made—but it should then be kept. There are a number of pain-killers and sedatives for the night that should be made available, even if these are narcotics for pain that cannot otherwise be controlled. Families should not be promised this sort of help unless the surgeon and his medical colleagues are determined to deliver on the promise. It is surprising to find occasionally that when a child faces terminal illness at home and is under the care of his family physician there is a tendency to withhold pain killers because they are narcotics. Addiction to a narcotic would seem to be the last concern in terminal cases.

The most difficult question, the one concerning the time of death, cannot be definitely answered, but there are some pitfalls to avoid. Do not be specific; the course of disease is too variable. Do not encourage Christmas in October for the child who may die in November. It takes its toll on the family, the community, and frequently on the child, out of all proportion to the associated reward.

Parents are helped by the statement that the physician will keep no secrets from them and that when he is reasonably assured concerning timing, that information will be shared.

In any circumstances where there is even the most remote possibility of a genetic factor in the illness of the seriously ill or dying child, the family should have the assurance that genetic counseling will be made available to them as soon as they wish it.

DEALING WITH THE SICK AND DYING CHILD HIMSELF

As in any relationship with children, something akin to honesty is probably best. Few children really ask if they are dying; some ask if they are ever going to get better. To the latter question, I frequently say something like, "Of course you're going to get better, but it is also true that I think you will probably feel worse before you start to feel better."

If the physician is one who banters with his patient, such is the way to relate to the child throughout his illness, but avoid the bantering if it is reserved only for the severely ill child out of embarrassment. Youngsters can detect a phony.

I am convinced that many more children have known they were dying than shared that information with me. Some knew it and kept it from their family; with a few I have discussed death, at their request. I have not seen a child upset by this. With many, I have talked about close calls—after the fact. One can only gently feel his way along this uncharted path, and be guided by the child.

THE HOSPITAL FAMILY

In an institution where there is an aggregation of patients of poor prognosis, such as a chemotherapy ward for cancer, a neurosurgical ward for brain tumors, an intensive care unit where the mortality rate is higher than elsewhere in the hospital, there is a recognizable chain of events which repeats itself. Student nurses inevitably look forward to pediatrics because of their mental image of holding a rosy-cheeked baby in their laps for feeding. Instead of this, they are frequently ushered into a pediatric environment consisting of unconscious neurosurgical patients, ecchymotic leukemics, and neuroblastoma patients with bulging eyes. The high concentration of these, particularly in any one area, leads to depression, emotional upset, or frank hysterics, and occasionally to the inability to continue an assignment. Charge nurses, familiar with this "syndrome" are, as a rule, very capable in handling it, but after they have handled a certain number of these situations, they too begin to feel the depression and frustration of the high mortality rate, and they too lean on someone else, who in turn leans on someone else.

In most hospitals where these situations are encountered there is someone who has been around long enough to see the situation in some perspective. If that individual's sense of prophylaxis is as good as his sense of therapy, he can frequently avoid such breakdown. Nurses commonly are deprived of the privilege of seeing the children cured of tumors and are greatly heartened by a seminar or tumor clinic where the triumphs of the oncology service are displayed rather than the defeats. Contact with parents of children who have recovered from malignant tumors or other serious illness is supportive to nursing staff and parents of seriously ill children alike.

PALLIATION WITHOUT CURE

The prolongation of life without the alleviation of underlying disease is a constant temptation. If a patient with a chronic illness or a terminal illness is being treated in an academic institution where there are a number of inquisitive minds as well as some new things to be tried, the temptation is even greater. Nevertheless, even though the patients we are discussing are children, there are times when they should be permitted to die as quietly as possible and in as dignified a manner as possible.

The child with advanced liver cirrhosis who is bleeding profusely from his gastrointestinal tract in spite of having had a definitive portal-systemic shunt is an example. The terminal neuroblastoma youngster with extensive bone metastases and anemia is another.

Many of the terminal illnesses of surgical children are associated with cancer. In these days of combined therapy consisting of surgery, radiation, and chemotherapy we have several modalities of therapy which can prolong life, but in a terminal case can hardly be expected to effect a cure. In the process of prolonging life, we sometimes produce undesirable situations, including pain and the necessity for a transfusion of blood or blood components. Regardless of where one stands philosophically about doing everything for the patient on such an occasion or withholding all therapy, the physician must be on guard so that he never puts a family in the position of being able to say after they have lost a child: "We didn't do all that we could for our youngster." The close relationship which develops between a physician and the family of a chronically ill child permits him to mold a good deal of the family's thinking. Many times it is possible well in advance of the day of decision to acquaint the family with the fact that there may be a time when it is better to withhold a given form of therapy than to administer it. Seldom does the family fail to go along with such thinking if they are properly introduced to it in advance. For example, the youngster with cancer in its terminal phase may be quite subdued, quite comfortable, and of minimal emotional hazard to his family while his hemoglobin is, say 6 gm per 100 ml. If such a patient is transfused to say 11 gm, all of his sensoria are activated; he now perceives his pain more acutely, he is fretful, and his family is put through an additional period of stress.

HEREDITARY DISEASE

The family whose child is dying of hereditary disease must be handled with special care. Not only do the parents carry the guilt of transmission, but they have great questions about future pregnancies and the possible occurrence of similar conditions in other children. Genetic counseling should be provided for parents whose children have died from such things as accidental causes in the presence of hemophilia, cystic fibrosis and perhaps meconium ileus, or neurofibromatosis. Parents should be encouraged to talk about their own feelings in this regard. There are few family situations more pitiful than the silent father with obvious Von Recklinghausen's disease whose child is dying of neurofibrosarcoma in the presence of the same malady. His guilt about his child's condition and his self-reproach before his wife can frequently be talked out satisfactorily, so that these problems are not added to the impending grief of the loss of the child.

THE TERMINAL PHASE OF ILLNESS

As the terminal phase of chronic illness approaches, the physician frequently has the choice of choosing a hospital or the family's home for the final days. There are no flat rules for deciding this. Some people feel that a youngster should not die in a home where there are other children. I have known this to work out very satisfactorily, where the family understands the situation extremely well, and to even salvaging a happy family relationship—perhaps because of it rather than in spite of it.

If the physician thinks he and the family can manage a youngster's chronic illness as it approaches its terminal phase in the patient's home, it is absolutely essential that a house call be made so that the physician can assess the situation at first hand. Some mothers want a dying child at home for emotional reasons which blind her to the fact that the facilities available to her for the comfortable care of the child and the protection of the patient's siblings are just nonexistent. The physician should check on the various members of the household and assess, if possible, their ability to withstand the stresses that will be built around his patient's terminal illness.

Even if a youngster is cared for at home, the family should always know that there will be a place in the hospital for quiet refuge if needed as the end approaches. This facility should be for the family's convenience rather than for the patient's treatment. If such a facility is eventually used, the family should be permitted free access to the youngster's room. It should be a room not shared by others, if possible. It should be at a quiet end of a hospital corridor, and the usual disturbing observations of pulse, temperature, and blood pressure should be eliminated. The child's comfort should be the primary goal of the hospital team, and if this is followed, the family's needs will be automatically taken care of for the moment.

AUTOPSY PERMISSION

The ability of the physician to obtain permission for an autopsy is dependent largely upon the rapport he has established beforehand, and I think that under most circumstances success is more likely if this is handled by the physician in charge rather than by a member of his house staff, unless that individual has had a particular role to play in which he has acted as his chief's surrogate.

As with the breaking of the news of impending death, autopsy permission is the business of the mother and father and not of the entire family. It is well to obtain it early, rather than after relatives have talked to the grieved parents and convinced them that "their child has suffered enough."

If the parents have consented to an autopsy, they are entitled to know what the major findings are, and this should become part of the physician's obligation. I make it a point to write a letter to the family of each child who has died, assuring them that they did all that was possible in providing care for their youngster, pointing out the inevitability of his death with our present state of knowledge, and assuring them of my availability should any questions arise. Some weeks later, I send them an undetailed, but nevertheless informative, summary of the autopsy findings.

Do not avoid the family of the child who has died. There is nothing more disheartening to parents than to have lived through a trying time and given permission for an autopsy, only to realize that the physician who cared for their youngster feels he has come to the end of his obligation. Particularly with children, relatives ask questions long after death. It is frequently very difficult for a family to come back to the same hospital and to the same doctor's office where they once heard the first inkling of the fact that their youngster was going to die. The physician should be aware of this, and if it is impossible for him to meet in another building, he should at least find a different area in his hospital or other office accommodations to meet with parents and answer their late questions.

The willingness of a family to come back to the scene of their previous tragedy is about the highest compliment that can be paid to the hospital and the medical team that cared for the dying child.

5

Genetic Counseling in Pediatric Surgery

Miriam G. Wilson, M.D.

If the surgeon were only concerned with the technical aspects of surgical procedures, he would find little use for genetic information. In the broader application of pediatric surgery, the surgeon finds himself in situations where genetic diagnosis and counseling are important components of medical management. The examples of genetic disorders presented in this chapter were chosen for their particular relevance to pediatric surgery.

The aim of genetic counseling is to provide information about the nature of a genetic disorder and the risk of recurrence. Genetic counseling is sought most often after the birth of a child with congenital anomalies or with a genetic disorder. Occasionally an adult couple planning marriage and children seeks counseling when there is a familial disorder. Less often, genetic information is requested by first cousins who wish to marry and by adoption agencies for assistance in placement. In some instances, questions are raised about the possible effects on chromosomes and later progeny due to drug or radiation exposure.

The basic requirements for genetic counseling are the following:

(1) accurate diagnosis; (2) family pedigree; (3) knowledge of medical genetics, including mode of inheritance of the disorder, theoretical and empiric risk probabilities, the variability of the phenotype (expressivity), failure of manifestation (nonpenetrance), new mutations, and genetic and environmental copies or mimics of the disorder; and (4) full communication of genetic information to the family at risk. An important aspect of counseling is the provision of psychological support for individuals facing the difficult situation of congenital defects or hereditary disease in their family.

Genetic disorders may be classified into one of three categories: those with a single-gene origin, those with complex inheritance involving many genes (polygenic), and chromosome abnormalities. Disorders of single-gene origin (Mendelian disorders) are autosomal dominant, autosomal recessive, or X-linked traits. The total number of individuals with these disorders is small. The genetics is clear-cut; thus, precise information about recurrence risks can frequently be given. In the instance of recessive inheritance involving genes on autosomes (nonsex chromosomes), a double gene dose, i.e. an identical mutant gene from each parent, is required for manifestation of the disorder. The affected individual is homozygous for the gene. When a gene in the heterozygous form is expressed in the phenotype, the phenotype is referred to as dominant. An individual who is homozygous for a given gene can produce only gametes with that gene. In the heterozygous individual, the chance for each gene (allele) of a given pair to be included in a gamete is 50 percent.

Mendelian Inheritance in Man by Victor McKusick is a useful and periodically updated catalogue of autosomal dominant, autosomal recessive, and X-linked phenotypes.[1] A list of 866 disorders generally accepted as Mendelian and an additional 1010 which may be Mendelian are found in the third edition (1971). The total of accepted or presumptive Mendelian disorders is 1876 which is 331 more than those listed in the second edition, representing a noteworthy 20-percent increase within the intervening three years.

SINGLE-GENE DISORDERS

Autosomal Dominant Disorders

Autosomal dominant disorders are determined by a single autosomal mutant gene, usually in a heterozygous state. Homozygosity, which is seldom observed for rare disorders, may be associated with increased severity of the disorder. In general, dominant conditions tend to be structural abnormalities such as skeletal malformations and connective tissue disorders. Many are not severe and do not adversely affect the individual's life or reproduction. The inheritance pattern is unambiguous in the instance of many dominant phenotypes with full penetrance and little variation in severity. Fifty percent of the children of affected parents are affected, the sexes are affected equally, a nonaffected individual does not have affected children, and male-to-male transmission occurs (Figure 5–1). The family pedigree is characterized by a vertical pattern in that the line of transmission clearly extends through affected individuals in each generation without skipping any generation. One example is brachydactyly, which was the first condition described in the literature as an autosomal dominant phenotype. Pedigrees of split-hand deformity with involvement of feet, Holt-Oram syndrome, ulnar polydactyly with well-formed extra digit, and some forms of familial syndactyly tend to show full penetrance, and skipping of generations infrequently occurs.

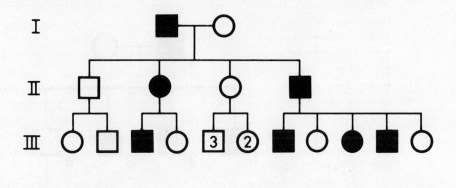

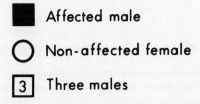

Figure 5–1
Pedigree of autosomal dominant disorder. Approximately one-half of children of affected parent are affected. Transmission of the disorder is independent of sex.

The main problems in genetic counseling in autosomal dominant disorders are variation in severity, reduced penetrance, delayed onset, new mutations, and genetic or environmental mimics or copies. Osteogenesis imperfecta, Marfan's syndrome, familial polyposis of the colon, neurofibromatosis, and tuberous sclerosis may show a wide range of manifestations and severity. This variation of the phenotype is referred to as expressivity. A mildly affected individual may not be detected and, therefore, the risk to his children not appreciated. A wide range of expressivity makes it more difficult for a family to decide about having children since predictability of the severity of the disorder is an important consideration.

In some instances, the disorder is not detectable by presently available tests. This failure of manifestation, also referred to as non-penetrance, gives rise to family pedigrees of dominant traits with skipped generations. Dominant disorders characteristically showing nonpenetrance are Marfan's syndrome, hemolytic anemia due to hereditary spherocytosis, neurofibromatosis, and retinoblastoma, which is considered in detail later. A pedigree of a family with Marfan's syndrome is illustrated in Figure 5–2. In a case such as this, counseling an apparently normal individual (II 4) at risk for the disorder is difficult, since he may be carrying the gene and transmit it to half of his children.

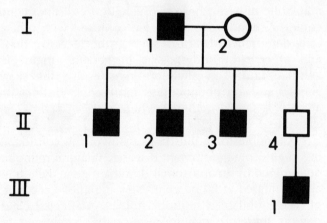

Figure 5–2
Pedigree of family with Marfan's syndrome. A father (I,1) and three children (II,1–3) are affected although the manifestations involve the musculoskeletal system and the eye in I,1 and the cardiovascular system in his sons (II,1–3). A gene with such different and apparently unrelated effects is referred to as pleiotropic. Although a fourth son had no apparent sign of the disorder and married a normal and unrelated woman, their son (III,1) had cardiovascular disease attributable to Marfan's. II,4 presumably carried the dominant gene without manifestation of the disorder (nonpenetrance), or the disorder was so mild it was not detected.

Under usual circumstances, a dominant gene * associated with a severe disorder is expected to decrease in the population as a result of selection. Some very severe autosomal dominant disorders, such as Huntington's chorea and myotonic dystrophy, show a delayed onset, often after the affected individual has had children. Rarely do these diseases arise from new mutations. Dominant genes with severe effects and associated with "reproductive lethality" or "near lethality" are

* For convenience, a gene is referred to as "dominant" or "recessive"; however, these terms properly characterize the phenotype and not the gene.

maintained in the population by fresh mutation. Individuals affected with some dominant conditions such as acrocephalosyndactyly (Apert's syndrome), tuberous sclerosis, or achondroplasia seldom reproduce; therefore, most cases occur as a result of new mutation in a previously normal family. A new mutation presumably arises in a parental gamete prior to fertilization. The identical mutation is unlikely to arise in other gametes of the parent; thus, the risk of another child similarly affected is low. The children of the affected individual, however, have a 50-percent risk to inherit the disorder.

Counseling is difficult when other diseases cannot be readily distinguished from a genetic disorder. A genetic mimic or genocopy is a similar disorder caused by a different genetic constitution (genotype) from that of the disorder under consideration. A similar disorder caused by nongenetic or environmental factors is a phenocopy. Marfan's syndrome resembles homocystinuria, an autosomal recessive metabolic disease; these two genetically distinct conditions are genocopies. Achondroplasia may be confused with other types of genetically determined dwarfism such as the recessive diastrophic dwarfism and other chondrodysplasias of genetic origin. Thorough clinical and laboratory investigation may resolve the diagnosis. However, genocopies and phenocopies represent a distinct problem in evaluation of a family pedigree where precise medical information is not available.

Retinoblastoma illustrates many of the considerations in counseling in autosomal dominant diseases. Bilateral retinoblastoma usually is determined by an autosomal dominant gene. Penetrance is incomplete and estimated at 80 percent. New mutations account for the majority of cases of bilateral retinoblastoma. An affected child born to normal parents, therefore, may represent either a new mutation or a failure of penetrance in one of the parents who is heterozygous for this gene. The risk for subsequent affected sibs is now if the tumor results from a new mutation; the risk is high (50 percent $\times$ 80 percent penetrance) if the disorder is transmitted from a parent.

Counseling in unilateral retinoblastoma is even more difficult, since only about 10 percent of all cases are a result of an autosomal dominant gene. The other 90 percent are not hereditary and represent phenocopies. Inherited retinoblastoma may be manifested as either unilateral or bilateral. Therefore, unilateral retinoblastoma may occur in children of parents with bilateral disease, and parents with unilateral retinoblastoma may have children with bilateral involvement. In the absence of a family history, the genetic form of unilateral retinoblastoma cannot be distinguished from phenocopies. Unilateral retinoblastoma in a family with a negative history is estimated to be inheritable from the affected individual in about four to five percent of the instances.[2] The limitations of this empiric risk figure are obvious: when a parent is an unexpressed heterozygote, the chance that a subsequent sib will be affected is 50 percent diminished slightly by failure of penetrance); when the tumor is a result of a new mutation, the risk for an affected sib is not increased over that of the general population, although the risk of inheritance from the affected individual is high; if the tumor represents a phenocopy, the risk of recurrence for a sib and the risk for inheritance are low, the same as that of the general population.

Retinoblastoma is somewhat more complicated genetically because of the changing pattern of the disorder over the past several decades. Affected individuals now commonly have children because of improved survival by modern surgical and radiation treatment. As a consequence, the incidence of the disorder has increased and the proportion of cases due to new mutation has decreased.[3] The increased survival of affected individuals has provided the opportunity to observe the variability of the phenotype. Affected individuals, presumably those with the "genetic form" of retinoblastoma, appear to have an increased risk of malignancy elsewhere, even in tissues that have not been irradiated and in individuals treated by surgery alone.[4]

Autosomal Recessive Disorders

Autosomal recessive conditions tend to be metabolic disorders rather than gross structural defects, which are more characteristically autosomal dominant. Affected individuals are homozygous for the same mutant gene, having received one gene from each parent. Ordinarily, heterozygosity of parents is first detected following the birth of an affected child. Since many of these disorders are severe, reproductivity is decreased and a parent is seldom homozygous for the mutant gene. Heterozygous parents have a 25-percent chance of having a homozygous affected child, a 50-percent chance of having a child who is a heterozygous carrier like the parents, and a 25-percent chance of having normal, noncarrier children. The usual pedigree pattern is horizontal since affected individuals are likely to be found within a sibship (Figure 5–3). Assuming random mating, the chance of other relatives being affected is low. Consanguinity, on the other hand, increases the chance that parents will be carrying the same recessive gene. When a rare recessive trait appears, consanguinity is likely to be found in the pedigree. Examples of diseases that are ordinarily inherited as autosomal recessive are adrenogenital syndrome, phenylketonuria, galactosemia, Ellis–Van Creveld syndrome, Gaucher's disease (types I and II), cystic fibrosis, sickle-cell anemia, Tay-Sachs disease, Hurler's syndrome (mucopolysaccharidosis type I), mucopolysaccharidosis types III through VI, a severe form of osteogenesis imperfecta, homocystinuria, and suxamethonium sensitivity. Occasionally, an exact diagnosis cannot be made. For example, the autosomal recessive microcephaly may not be distinguishable from microcephaly following maternal irradiation or congenital rubella (phenocopies). In the instance of many metabolic disorders, laboratory tests are required for a correct diagnosis.

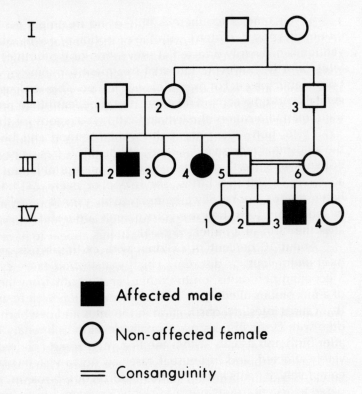

■ Affected male

○ Non-affected female

═ Consanguinity

Figure 5–3
Pedigree of autosomal recessive disorder. Consanguinity has resulted in parents (III,5 and III,6) both heterozygous for the same mutant gene. One parent in generation I; II,1,2 and 3, and III, 5 and 6 are inferred to be carriers.

Once the diagnosis is made, however, the observed recurrence risks for another affected sib correspond to the theoretical risks, and, as a rule, genetic counseling can be precise. Furthermore, some of these disorders can now be diagnosed by amniocentesis early in pregnancy. Parents who are known carriers for genetic disorders that can be diagnosed from analysis of amniotic cell cultures may elect diagnostic amniocentesis. If the fetus is found to be affected, a therapeutic abortion can be done. Some of the recessive conditions that can be diagnosed by amniocentesis are Hurler's syndrome, Tay-Sachs disease, galactosemia, and Pompe's disease (glycogen-storage disease II). The list of metabolic disorders diagnosable by amniotic cell culture is expanding so rapidly that review articles [5,6] require frequent updating. Selected programs for the detection of heterozygosity in populations known to be at risk—for example, Tay-Sachs in the Ashkenazic Jewish population and sickle-cell hemoglobin in blacks—will enable the identification of heterozygosity in parents before the birth of an affected child. Determination of heterozygosity and diagnostic amniocentesis will lead to further prevention of births of individuals affected with severe genetic disease.

At this time, since there is little or no treatment for genetic conditions diagnosed in utero, with the exception of erythroblastosis, intervention is ordinarily directed at prevention of the birth of the affected fetus. Shortly, however, antenatal treatment for some of these conditions is anticipated. For example, once it is possible to diagnose adrenogenital syndrome early in fetal life, it may be feasible to prevent the in-utero masculinization of a female fetus homozygous for this condition.

Cystic fibrosis is one of the most common and best known of the autosomal recessive disorders, although the basic enzyme defect is not known. Since the incidence in Caucasian populations is estimated at about 1:2500 live births, about one of every 25 individuals is a heterozygous carrier. Since heterozygosity cannot be reliably detected by laboratory tests, heterozygous parents are ordinarily first identified after the birth of an affected child.

About 10 percent of children with cystic fibrosis are born with meconium ileus, a disorder which usually indicates cystic fibrosis. Meconium peritonitis, on the other hand, results from the perforation of a meconium-filled intestine and may occur as well in any condition that causes intestinal obstruction in the fetus and newborn infant. Children with cystic fibrosis occasionally develop pulmonary disease soon after birth and usually within the first year. Some children are less severely affected, and in unusual cases an organ-system may be spared completely. Parents known to be heterozygous, however, must be prepared to accept the significant risk of 25 percent for each pregnancy of producing a child who is chronically ill with repeated pulmonary infections, gradually developing pulmonary insufficiency, growth failure, and a shortened lifespan which rarely extends into the second decade. There is no specific treatment available, and the disorder cannot be diagnosed by amniocentesis.

X-linked Disorders

X-linked disorders are transmitted by a gene located on an X chromosome. Therefore, the essential feature of these disorders is that an affected male cannot transmit the disorder to his sons (who have received his Y chromosome).

Most of these conditions are recessive. Examples are hemophilia A (classical), hemophilia B (Christmas disease), glucose-6-phosphate dehydrogenase deficiency, Duchenne muscular dystrophy, Hunter's syndrome (mucopolysaccharidosis type II), and Lesch-Nyhan syndrome. Ordinarily, only males manifest the disease; the females are nonaffected carriers. One-half of the sons of carrier mothers are affected and one-half of the daughters are carriers (Figure 5–4). All the daughters of an affected male are carriers; all his sons are normal. Affected males in a family are related through females, described by an oblique inheritance pattern resembling the move of a chess knight.

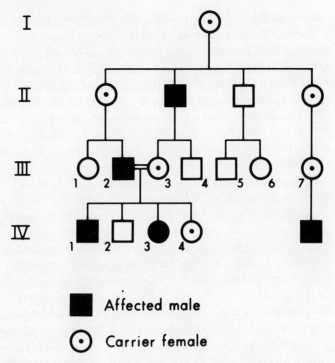

Affected male

Carrier female

Figure 5–4
Pedigree of X-linked recessive disorder. Note that consanguinity between III,2 and 3 results in an affected female child (IV,3). Affected male (IV,1) has inherited the X-linked mutant gene from his carrier mother.

Occasionally a female is affected. For example, a daughter of a carrier mother and an affected father has a 50-percent chance of being affected. This is more likely to result from consanguinity if the trait is rare (refer to Figure 5-4). A female with Turner's syndrome may manifest an X-linked disorder since she has only one X chromosome, as does the normal male. A heterozygous female may be affected with an X-linked disorder because of the possibility that, by chance, the X chromosome carrying the "normal" gene was inactivated in most of her cells, as a result of random inactivation according to the Lyon hypothesis.

The primary counseling problem in X-linked disorders is to determine if an affected individual, when he is the first affected in a family, represents a new mutation or has inherited the disorder from a carrier mother.

Comments previously made regarding prenatal diagnosis of autosomal recessive disease also apply to many of the X-linked disorders. Hunter's syndrome, Lesch-Nyhan syndrome, and glucose-6-phosphate dehydrogenase deficiency can be diagnosed prenatally. The close gene linkage between the loci for hemophilia A and glucose-6-phosphate dehydrogenase may soon permit the prenatal diagnosis of hemophilia.[7]

Occasionally, parents where the mother is a known carrier of a severe X-linked recessive disease that cannot be diagnosed prenatally will request amniocentesis for the diagnosis of the fetal sex, electing to abort the males who have a 50-percent chance of being affected with the disease. Abortion on the basis of diagnosis of sex rather than diagnosis of the disorder has the obvious disadvantage that normal males are aborted as well as affected males, without selection against carrier females.

POLYGENIC INHERITANCE

Many relatively common congenital anomalies are known to have a significant genetic component which is complex and difficult to define. Congenital defects such as anencephaly and other major central nervous system anomalies, cleft lip with or without cleft palate, cleft palate alone, pyloric stenosis, congenital hip dysplasia, and club foot occur with increased frequency in close relatives of affected individuals. The observed frequencies, however, do not conform to expected Mendelian ratios. A reasonable assumption is that the genetic component includes a number of genes at different loci interacting with environmental factors to contribute to the manifestation of the disorder. Such inheritance is polygenic. Since the inheritance is not known precisely, there are no theoretical risk figures. Empiric risks, largely derived from Northern European populations, are available for some of these disorders[8] (Table 5–1). In general, the recurrence risk for a subsequently affected sib increases from about one in 1000 (general population incidence) into the range of three to five percent for any one of the listed congeni-

Table 5–1
Recurrence Risk for Common Congenital Malformations

	Overall Population Incidence (per 1000)	One Affected Sib, Parents Normal (per 1000)
Spina bifida, meningomyelocele and anencephaly	1–2	50–60
Cleft lip, with or without cleft palate	1	30–50
Cleft palate	0.5–1	20–50
Congenital hip dislocation (males only)	2	50
Talipes equinovarus	1	30

(Adapted from Carter, C.O., *Brit Med Bull* 25:52, 1969[8])

tal abnormalities. Particularly important to recognize, however, is that empiric risk figures represent averages obtained from a heterogeneous group of families with high, low, or intermediate risk. The empiric risks substantiate a genetic component for the disorder, but have limited value for individual family counseling. If there is no family history and only one affected child in a small family, the magnitude of risk cannot be determined for a given set of normal parents who wish to know whether they are at high or low risk, rather than the average for the group.

The relatively common congenital anomaly of pyloric stenosis is estimated in North European populations to occur in about one to three of every 1000 live births. It is found less frequently in South Europeans and non-Europeans. Boys are affected about five times as frequently as girls. The vulnerability of firstborn children so far is not adequately explained and may result from the fact that if the firstborn is affected, families refrain from having any more children, in which case the firstborn is an only child (and the statistics only give the *appearance* of vulnerability for firstborn).

Pyloric stenosis is known to occur more frequently in siblings of an affected child than in the general population. The chance for a monozygotic twin to have pyloric stenosis if the other twin is affected is increased over the concordance in dizygotic twins, which is about the risk for nontwin sibs. Since Rammstedt's surgical procedure (1912) lowered the mortality due to pyloric stenosis, the incidence of pyloric stenosis in the children of affected individuals is now known [9] (Table 5–2). An affected mother has a much greater chance of transmitting the

Table 5–2
Risk for Pyloric Stenosis in Children of Affected Parent

	Sons	Daughters
Affected Fathers	6%	2%
Affected Mothers	19%	7%

(Adapted from Carter, C.O., *Brit Med Bull* 17:251, 1961[9])

disorder to her children than an affected father. About 14 percent of children of affected mothers had pyloric stenosis, in comparison to only about four percent of children of affected fathers. Similarly, the first-degree relatives of an affected female are at significantly greater risk than first-degree relatives of an affected male. Since females are generally resistant to the disorder, an affected female may be considered, theoretically, to have a greater number of genes contributing to the disorder than an affected male. As a consequence, a relative of an affected female has a greater proportion of the genes than the relative of an affected male and is, therefore, more likely to develop the disorder.

A similar situation is observed in congenital hip dysplasia, which is about six times more frequent in females than males. Relatives of affected males show a higher incidence of congenital hip dysplasia than do relatives of affected females.

CHROMOSOME ABNORMALITIES

Genetic disorders of Mendelian and polygenic inheritance are accompanied by a normal chromosome pattern since the gene mutations responsible for the disorders exist at a submicroscopic level and cannot be detected by our present methods. In contrast, chromosome abnormalities are identified by microscopic examination and represent abnormalities in the number or structure of chromosomes.

In 1956, Tjio and Levan demonstrated that man has 46 chromosomes.[10] These consist of 22 pairs of autosomes and one pair of sex chromosomes (XX in the female and XY in the male). In 1959, Down's syndrome (mongolism) was found to be associated with an extra small chromosome. In the same year, a patient with Turner's syndrome was found to have a karyotype of 45 chromosomes; missing was an X chromosome. Since that time other chromosome abnormalities have been described, but Down's syndrome and the sex chromosome abnormalities are the most common and the most important clinically.

Cells for chromosome analysis are usually obtained from peripheral blood. Heparinized blood is cultured with the use of special techniques to stimulate lymphocyte division and to increase the visibility of chromosomes. The chromosomes are stained, photographed through a light microscope, cut out from an enlarged photographic print, and arranged in pairs in order of descending length. This final arrangement, known as a karyotype, conforms to an internationally set standard.[11] More recently, in Chicago, a notation for cytogenetic description was generally accepted.[12] Normal male (46,XY) and female (46,XX) karyotypes are illustrated in Figure 5–5. Another laboratory procedure is autoradiography, in which chromosomes are identified and homologues paired in accord with their DNA-replication pattern as determined by tritiated thymidine uptake. This time-consuming process gives useful information in selected cases, such as the identification of a late-replicating X chromosome. Recently developed are special laboratory staining techniques, such as quinacrine fluorescence and Giemsa-banding, which are used for identification of individual chromosomes and for study of chromosome structure. The quinacrine fluorescence technique is particularly valuable for identification of the Y and other fluorescing chromosomes, and Giemsa-banding for chromosome structure.

Chromosome abnormalities occur in about five percent of all zygotes, of which the majority result in fetal death. One to two percent of all live births show chromosome abnormalities, about equally di-

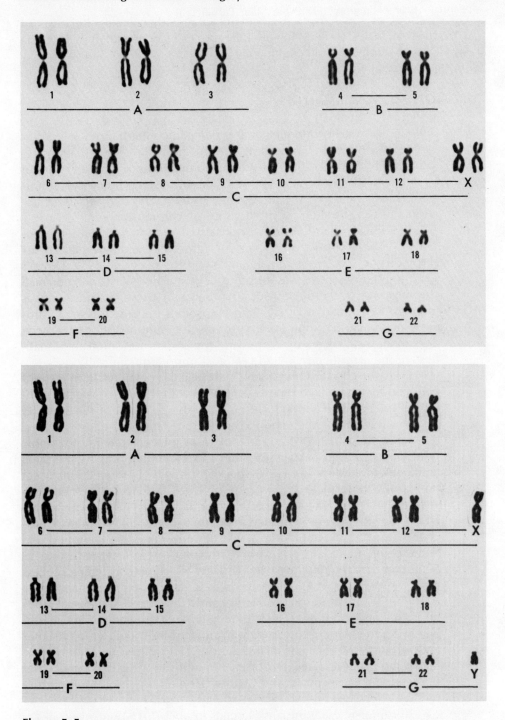

Figure 5–5
Normal female (top) and male (bottom) karyotypes. Solid lines between numbers indicate the chromosomes that require special procedures for identification.

Table 5–3

Congenital Chromosomal Syndromes in Man (Partial List)

	Syndrome	Estimated Frequency in Live Births
Autosome Abnormalities		
With additional chromosomal material:		
Trisomy 13 (Trisomy D) (occas. translocation-trisomy)	Patau's	1:7000–1:8000
Trisomy 18 (Trisomy E) (rarely translocation-trisomy)	Edwards'	1:4000–1:5000
Trisomy 21 (Trisomy G) (translocation-trisomy in about 3% of Down's syndrome)	Down's	1:600
With deleted chromosomal material:		
Monosomy: reported for G-group chromosome, not proved	"antimongolism"	
Deleted short arm 4 (4p-)	Wolf or Wolf-Hirschhorn	
" " " 5 (5p-)	Cri du chat	
" long arm 13 (13q-)		Unknown, believed to be rare
" short arm 18 (18p-)		
" long arm 18 (18q-)	Lejeune	
" long arm 21 (21q-)	"antimongolism"	
Ring chromosomes of 4, 5, 13, 18, 21, and 22		
Other: Simple duplications, isochromosomes, and inversions		
Sex Chromosome Abnormalities		
With additional chromosomal material:		
47,XXX	Triplo-X	1:1000 female births
48,XXXX	Tetra-X	Rare
49,XXXXX	Penta-X	Rare
47,XXY (48,XXXY; 48,XXYY; others) (mosaicism is relatively common)	Klinefelter's	1:400 male births
49,XXXXY		Rare
47,XYY	YY syndrome	1:500–1:1000 male births
With deleted chromosomal material:		
45,X (mosaicism is common)	Turner's syndrome	1:2500 female births
X isochromosome, ring, partial deletion of short or long arm	Turner's syndrome and variants	Unknown
Other: 45,X/46,XY and 45,X/46,XY/47, XYY mosaicism		Unknown

vided between the autosomes and sex chromosomes. A partial list of chromosome abnormalities is found in Table 5–3.

Chromosome abnormalities are associated with congenital defects and impaired growth and development. Abnormalities of the sex chromosomes are characterized by deviant growth, abnormal sexual development, and infertility or diminished fertility. The loss of a sex chromosome results in short stature, as in Turner's syndrome (45,X), which is characterized in addition by sexual infantilism, streak gonads, and congenital anomalies (Turner's stigmata). The male counterpart, a 45,Y constitution, has not been encountered in a living child or abortus, and is apparently not viable even in a young fetus. An extra X or Y chromosome, especially the Y, confers additional height. Thus, men with the YY syndrome (47,XYY) are tall, and those with Klinefelter's (47,XXY) tend to be tall.

Sexual development is ordinarily affected in individuals with sex chromosome abnormalities, but there are some exceptions. Individuals with chromosomal mosaicism in which a normal cell line is present may show apparently normal sexual phenotypes. Triplo-X females (47,XXX) as a group are less fertile and are at greater risk for intellectual impairment than normal XX females, but the phenotype is not consistent. There may be minimal or no impairment. XYY males are apparently fertile; they are probably at increased risk for psychosocial abnormalities. Both triplo-X females and XYY males have had children who (with few exceptions) have had the normal number of sex chromosomes.

The phenotype associated with a given sex chromosome abnormality is variable. Individuals with Turner's syndrome may show only short stature and hypogonadism. Others show a varying number of congenital anomalies such as webbed neck, pigmented nevi, shield chest, coarctation of the aorta, cubitus valgus, transient congenital lymphedema, short fourth metacarpals, and other skeletal and facial abnormalities. Mental retardation is usually not found in Turner's syndrome and may not be present in Klinefelter's, although the prevalence of mental retardation is increased in these syndromes compared to the general population. The only consistent feature of Klinefelter's syndrome is hypogonadism and resultant infertility.

Since in many sex chromosome abnormalities, prediction of the phenotype from the karyotype alone is difficult or impossible, the current follow-up studies of individuals with sex chromosome abnormalities detected by surveys of newborn infants are of immense importance. The partial inactivation of X chromosomes in excess of one and the apparently small genetic component attributable to the Y chromosome presumably account for the mild phenotypic effects in many sex chromosome abnormalities.

Chromosomal mosaicism is more frequently encountered in sex chromosome disorders than in autosome disorders and undoubtedly contributes to the phenotypic variability. For example, the fertility of several women with Turner's syndrome may be accounted for by mosaicism in which a normal 46,XX cell line is present with a cell line missing an X chromosome. When Turner's syndrome is associated with 45,X/46,XX or 45,X/46,XY mosaicism, stature may be normal. An important feature of 45,X/46,XY mosaicism is the frequency with which gonadoblastomas are found in the dysplastic gonadal tissue. Gonadal exploration and gonadectomy should be done in patients with Y mosaicism.

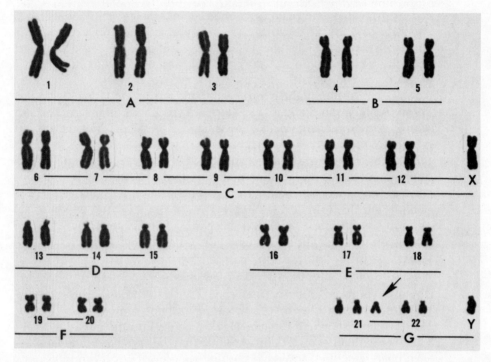

Figure 5–6
Karyotype of male with trisomy G(21). The arrow indicates the three number 21 chromosomes.

There are much simpler procedures than complete chromosome analysis that are useful screening tests for the number of X and Y chromosomes. For optimal medical management, all newborn infants should have at least a sex chromatin examination from buccal smears as a screening test for the number of X chromosomes. Quinacrine fluorescence for the Y body, which can be done directly using peripheral blood smears, may also be used as a screening test in the newborn. This procedure has more errors of interpretation because of brightly fluorescing portions of other chromosomes and the failure to detect the normal Y's that are small. Once chromosome analysis is automated and, therefore, less expensive, newborn infants will probably be routinely tested by this means.

Down's syndrome, occurring in about one of every 600 live births, is the most common autosomal abnormality. The peculiar facial appearance is remarkably similar from patient to patient. Individuals are mentally retarded with an I.Q. in the range of 30–40, usually short, clumsy, hypotonic in infancy, and endowed with a placid disposition. About one-quarter have congenital heart defects, the endocardial cushion defect or atrioventricularis communis being the most common of these. The lifespan is only about 8–10 years on the average, and a large proportion of deaths occur in infancy because of congenital heart disease and respiratory infections.

Down's syndrome in a newly born infant is ordinarily recognized by clinical features, although in some infants the diagnosis is not readily apparent and is made with the help of the chromosome analysis. The association of Down's syndrome and congenital duodenal atresia or stenosis is well recognized. Certainly a newly born infant with a high small intestinal obstruction should be examined carefully for Down's syndrome. Infants with Down's syndrome also appear to have a higher risk than other infants for gastrointestinal abnormalities such as imperforate anus, Hirschsprung's disease, tracheoesophageal fistula and esophageal atresia, annular pancreas, and pyloric stenosis.

The majority (about 96 percent) of individuals with Down's syndrome have a karyotype with an extra chromosome in the G group, by tradition considered to be number 21 (Figure 5–6). The extra chromosome ordinarily results from a failure of normal division of chromosomes, usually at meiosis. This failure to divide properly is referred to as nondisjunction. In almost all instances, the parents of a child with Down's syndrome due to trisomy G(21) show normal chromosome analyses. Rarely, a phenotypically normal parent is mosaic for trisomy 21, in which instance, if the mosaicism extends into the gonadal tissue, a gamete with an extra 21 chromosome may be formed. Some families have been described in which chromosome errors of the nondisjunctional type, such as Down's, Turner's, and Klinefelter's syndromes, are found in a number of family members, even though there is no evidence of mosaicism. These families may have a genetic predisposition for nondisjunctional chromosome abnormalities.

About two or three percent of individuals with Down's syndrome show a karyotype with the extra number 21 chromosome attached or translocated to another chromosome. Most commonly, the translocation is an attachment of a number 21 and a chromosome of the D group. A child with typical Down's syndrome and his karyotype, showing a DG translocation, are illustrated in Figure 5–7. Occasionally a parent, usually the mother, is a carrier of the translocated chromosome which may be transmitted to an affected child who has also received a parental number 21 pair. The parent shows no ill effects because the total amount of chromosome material is normal (Figure 5–8). Such an individual is referred to as a balanced translocation carrier.

Techniques have now been developed for diagnosis of chromo-

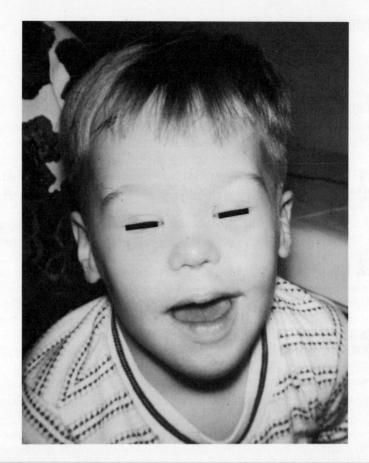

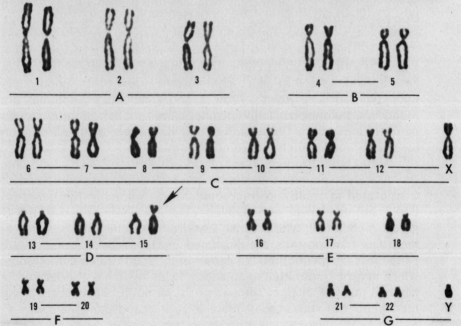

Figure 5–7
Boy with Down's syndrome due to DG translocation and his karyotype. This child shows typical Down's syndrome. The arrow indicates the DG translocation chromosome.

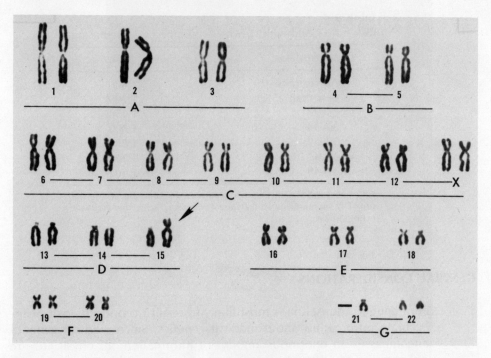

Figure 5–8
Karotype of female with balanced DG translocation (mother of child in Fig. 5–7). The arrow indicates the DG translocation chromosome. Note the missing chromosome in the G group.

some abnormalities during fetal life. These techniques involve the culture of fetal cells obtained by amniocentesis at about 16–17 weeks gestation (dated from the last menstrual period) and analysis of the chromosomes. Fetal diagnosis may be indicated when a couple has a significant risk of producing a child with a chromosome abnormality that will be apparent in chromosome analysis. Amniocentesis for chromosome analysis may be considered in pregnancies where the mother is older than 40 (and possibly older than 35) because of the known association of Down's syndrome and maternal age (Table 5–4).

Amniocentesis is also a consideration when a parent is a known carrier of a structural chromosome abnormality. Such parents are at increased risk to have affected children, although the risk for some structural abnormalities does not appear to be so high as expected on theoretical grounds.[13] A mother who is a carrier for a DG translocation has a theoretical risk of about 30 percent of having a child with Down's syndrome, but the empirical risk is about 10 to 15 percent. This risk is further diminished if the father is the carrier rather than the mother. The most common balanced chromosome constitution in the general population is a DD translocation. The risk for unbalanced progeny resulting in a D trisomy phenotype (Patau's syndrome) is probably less than one percent, which is considerably less than the theoretical risk. Amniocentesis may also be considered in the infrequent instances where a parent has a chromosome disorder or is mosaic for an abnormal cell line.

Table 5–4

Risk for a Child with Down's Syndrome by Maternal Age

Maternal Age	Risk
All mothers	1:600
Less than 25	1:2000
25–29	1:1500
30–34	1:800
35–39	1:250
40–44	1:100
45–49	1:50

After one child with Down's syndrome (trisomy 21), the risk is probably increased over that due to maternal age; the magnitude is not known.

GENERAL CONSIDERATIONS

Poor genetic counseling is most likely to result from insufficient or inaccurate information about medical genetics. Since medical genetics encompasses an enormous amount of information, all physicians are not genetic specialists. A physician who is not confident of the genetics of a condition can refer the family to a genetic center rather than undertake the counseling himself. In a number of situations, however, a physician who is not a genetic specialist may give his families useful information regarding the heritable aspects of a disorder, as, for example, in the case of a family with an autosomal recessive disorder ascertained by the birth of an affected child where the diagnosis is known for certain. The recurrence risk of an affected homozygous child is known to be 25 percent for each pregnancy. Even here, though, considerations of prenatal diagnosis and detection of heterozygosity are relevant and may indicate consultation with a genetic specialist.

In America, as in Great Britain, the customary policy of genetic counselors is to transmit genetic information and discuss the implications with families, but not to give specific advice. This policy is based on the belief that the individual family, when informed, is best able to make the decision regarding children and, indeed, the decision is properly theirs to make. The genetic counselor is obligated to be certain that the family is fully informed. This involves an understandable explanation of hereditary disorders at the family's level of genetic knowledge, the avoidance of terms that may be interpreted as judgmental or fixing "blame" on one or the other parent or parent's family, and the perception to determine whether the family understands.

A couple may need assistance to interpret mathematical probabilities and to apply these probabilities to their own situation. Families are sometimes helped to understand risks by the counselor's statement of what is considered a high risk in genetics, such as 25 percent or higher, in comparison to a moderate risk of 10 to 25 percent, and a low risk of one percent or less. It is helpful to state the risk for a normal as well as for an affected child, as, for example, in the instance of an autosomal recessive disorder, where there is a 75-percent chance of having a normal child, as well as a 25-percent chance of having an affected homozygous child.

A couple with one or more healthy children may decide to have no more children even when faced with a recurrence figure only slightly higher than that of the total population. Another couple without children may chance a significant risk of 25 percent in the instance of autosomal recessive disorders in order to have their own normal child, while another couple in the same circumstance will choose adoption. Within the last decade society's emphasis on planned reproduction and limited population growth has caused many couples to accept childlessness as a normal and occasionally welcome state.

In addition to the risk of recurrence, other considerations in a couple's decision regarding children are the severity of the disorder and expected results from treatment. For example, a couple may accept a significant risk of a disorder that is not severe or varies in expressivity so that it may appear in a mild form. They may chance the birth of a child when the disorder can be diagnosed early and treated with an expected good outcome. On the other hand, very severe genetic disorders causing fetal or early neonatal death may be risked, and moderately severe disorders compatible with life, not risked. At present, an important consideration for many families is the availability of prenatal diagnosis by early amniocentesis so that an affected fetus can be aborted. Since amniocentesis has become available, many families who would have otherwise curtailed their family have proceeded to have children.

In general, individuals without special training in genetics tend to overemphasize its predictive value and weigh too heavily the genetic significance of disease found in a family. In many instances, the genetic counselor is able to reassure the family that the risk is not so great as they believed. Relatively few diseases have moderate or high risk of recurrence.

REFERENCES

1. McKusick, V.A.: *Mendelian Inheritance in Man,* ed 3. Baltimore: Johns Hopkins Press, 1971.
2. Nielsen, M., and Goldschmidt, E.: Retinoblastoma among offspring of adult survivors in Denmark. *Acta Ophthal* 46:736–741, 1968.
3. Schappert-Kimmijser, J., Hemmes, G.D., and Nijland, R.: The heredity of retinoblastoma. *Ophthalmologica* 151:197–213, 1966.
4. Jensen, R.D., and Miller, R.W.: Retinoblastoma: Epidemiologic characteristics. *New Eng J Med* 285:307–311, 1971.

5. Milunsky, A., et al,: Prenatal genetic diagnosis. *New Eng J Med* 283:1370–1381, 1441–1447, 1498–1504, 1970.
6. Nadler, H.L., and Gerbie, A.B.: Role of amniocentesis in the intrauterine detection of genetic disorders. *New Eng J Med* 282:596–599, 1970.
7. Boyer, S.H., and Graham, J.B.: Linkage between the X chromosome loci for glucose-6-phosphate dehydrogenase electrophoretic variation and hemophilia A. *Amer J Hum Genet* 17:320–324, 1965.
8. Carter, C.O.: Genetics of common disorders. *Brit Med Bull* 25:52–57, 1969.
9. Carter, C.O.: The inheritance of congenital pyloric stenosis. *Brit Med Bull* 17:251–254, 1961.
10. Tjio, J.H., and Levan, A.: The chromosome number of man. *Hereditas* 42:1–6, 1956.
11. Denver Conference: A proposed standard system of nomenclature of human mitotic chromosomes. *Lancet* 1:1063–1065, 1960.
12. Chicago Conference: Standardization in human cytogenetics. Birth Defects: Original Article Series, II:2 (The National Foundation, New York) 1966.
13. Hamerton, J.L.: Robertsonian translocations in man: Evidence for prezygotic selection. *Cytogenetics* 7:260–276, 1968.

Section II

Critical Care

6

The Preoperative Medical Evaluation

Donald A. Lackey, M.D.

Ideally, the preoperative medical evaluation should be a part of continuing pediatric care. The child who has had his entire emotional and physical growth and development supervised by a single responsible physician and his staff has his pertinent medical data readily available for analysis and discussion. This permits the surgeon and the anesthesiologist to take a thoughtful and well-coordinated approach to the problems of the patient and his family, regardless of how acute the circumstances might be.

However, all too often, the admission to the hospital for surgery is the first opportunity for the initiation of comprehensive pediatric care. This, then, is the justification for the following discussion. A need exists to point out most of the specific items necessary for the physician to consider as he performs a preoperative medical evaluation of his pediatric patient.

A "child-oriented" medical center will permit the evaluation to be carried out with great facility. The physical surroundings should be appealing and not frightening to a child, and the hospital personnel (physicians, nurses, aides, and ancillary personnel) should have an approach and attitude which is empathetic and sympathetic to the patient and his family. The hospital environment is discussed in detail in Chapter 3, but is mentioned now because the preoperative medical evaluation is carried out as the first item after admission and, if properly handled, can set the stage well for what follows.

Whether surgery is contemplated electively or in an acute situation, a meticulous history, a detailed physical examination, and the intelligent use of the laboratory remain the basis for excellent care. However, some special modifications must be made when the need for surgical intervention occurs in the neonate, the chronically ill child, or the child involved in trauma.

HISTORY

Aside from the information directly pertaining to the surgical condition, several other important aspects of the history must be elicited. Recent exposure to infectious disease, especially respiratory illness, is extremely important. It is distressing to be obliged to treat postoperative pneumonia following an elective operative procedure because little attention was paid to the history of recent exposure to or early symptoms of upper respiratory infection. Elective surgery should be delayed until the appropriate period of incubation has passed. This is true for all contagious disease, but particularly for varicella which can present a severe threat to patients already on hospital wards.

Of prime importance to the surgeon and anesthesiologist is the patient's pharmacological history, particularly in regard to the current use of medications. Adrenal steroids, antibiotics, antihypertensive agents, salicylates, antiepileptic medications, and psychopharmaceuticals are used very often in pediatric practice. Children who have received seven-to-ten days of adrenal steroid therapy within an 18-month period prior to surgery should receive hydrocortisone, 50 mg per day in four divided doses, starting on the day prior to operation and continuing for two days following. During the procedure, 100 mg can be administered intravenously. Children on regular daily steroid therapy should have their doses brought up to at least these levels. The plethora of drugs available for use in children presents a significant, potential hazard to the patient about to undergo anesthesia. An excellent example of this is the fact that there is now a large number of children who are using a single drug or a combination of drugs for the management of minimal cerebral dysfunction (hyperkinetic behavior syndrome, dyslexia, and other learning disorders), whose pharmacologic effects must be considered during anesthesia.

An important aspect of the pharmacologic history is hypersensitivity to drugs. Although they are often difficult to document, attention must be paid to the history of allergy or suspicious allergic reactions. The preoperative or postoperative periods are not the times to prove or disprove the presence of hypersensitivity to drugs being utilized.

Although the laboratory has improved our ability to document specific coagulation defects, from a practical point of view, the detailed history of family members involved in bleeding disorders or a history of bleeding problems with previous surgeries (circumcision, dental procedures) or the history of unusual bleeding associated with trauma is still very useful in helping to decide whether one should conduct further investigations (see Chapter 17).

In a general way, the past history of the child should also be reviewed. Familial illnesses, past illnesses, food and pollen allergy, immunizations, and the dietary history may reveal important data for consideration.

PHYSICAL EXAMINATION

The physical examination, aside from that of the surgical problem, serves two purposes: to substantiate any suggestion of a medical condition alluded to in the history; and to discover or uncover a previously unanticipated condition.

The presence of congenital abnormalities should warn the surgeon of possible anatomical variations and alert the anesthesiologist to possible alterations in cardiorespiratory physiology if the anomaly happens to fall within that system. Serious orthopedic abnormalities might make proper positioning for surgery difficult, and possible metabolic abnormalities which accompany anomalous states (e.g. adrenogenital syndrome) must be identified to assist the anesthesiologist in having complete control of his patient's condition.

Congenital heart disease or acquired lesions of the heart (rheumatic heart disease) must be evaluated to establish the evidence for normal cardiac output. The presence of impending congestive heart failure must be evaluated thoroughly and careful consideration given to the timing of needed digitalis therapy. Antibiotic prophylaxis may be considered in the patient with significant cardiac disease particularly if the surgery entails involvement in a potential bacteriologically "dirty" area.

An elevation in blood pressure or an unusual heart rate or rhythm should be noted and attempts made to determine the significance of the finding. Table 6–1 contains some helpful physiologic data.

Table 6–1

Age	Weight (kg)	Pulse (quiet)	Respirations (quiet)	Blood Pressure (mm Hg)	Hemoglobin (gm%)	Blood Volume (ml)
Newborn	3.4	125	40	70/50	16–20	275
3 mo	6	120	30	80/50	12	450
1 yr	10.3	110	25–30	90/60	10–12	750
5 yr	20	100	20–25	90/60	10–12	1500
10 yr	32	90	20	100/65	12–14	2400

Any suggestion of hepatic or renal abnormality or dysfunction should be investigated as soon as possible because of the need for these organ systems to function well during the metabolism of the anesthetic and analgesic agents commonly used during the entire surgical period. Adequate renal function in order to maintain proper fluid and acid base balance is, of course, especially desirable during the postoperative period.

The upper and lower airway should be carefully evaluated in order to provide the anesthesiologist with enough information to conduct a safe, uncomplicated anesthesia and allow recovery to proceed without the stress of additional serious respiratory problems. The nares should be evaluated for patency. The tongue and dental structures should be intact and the presence of a large tonsillar or adenoidal mass noted. Rales, rhonchi, and wheezing should be noted and investigated.

LABORATORY

Any condition discovered or suggested by the careful history and physical examination must be intelligently pursued, documented, and treated. Routinely, a hemoglobin determination is obtained and lower values of 10 to 12 gm% are acceptable. This figure has probably been set empirically because many have allowed a level of 8 mg% during an urgent situation without untoward results. (Compare with Chapter 17.) Careful studies in oxygen physiology during the anesthetized state at various hemoglobin levels and at various ages have not been carried out in enough detail to make definite statements in this matter. However, there is no question of the concern over infants and children with lower than 10 grams of hemoglobin in regard to their possible poor nutritional or chronically debilitated states.

If the history and physical examination suggest the need for further evaluation of the cardiopulmonary structures, a chest film, and perhaps an ECG, should be done. There is no need for these procedures on a routine basis for elective surgery particularly if general health care has been carefully supervised. Usually an x-ray examination of the chest is mandatory for children who are being evaluated for an acute abdominal condition.

The yield from a single careful urinalysis will probably not be great, but there remains no better way to screen renal function and perhaps discover urinary tract lesions. For most general surgical procedures, the tuberculin test, "metabolic screens," and specific immunizations are not necessary unless the current hospitalization represents the first opportunity for the initiation of comprehensive health care.

When the need for more thorough investigation is suggested by the history and physical examination in regard to possible coagulopathies, the Ivy bleeding time, platelet count, prothrombin time, and partial thromboplastin time will serve to delineate any specific coagulation defects. (See Chapter 17.) In some institutions, the blood type is determined before any surgery so that in the situation where unexpected blood loss has occurred, time will be saved in preparing emergency blood replacement.

THE ACUTELY ILL CHILD

Few surgical lesions require immediate operation. Therefore, when delay for supportive treatment lessens the risk to the patient, operation is postponed. However, there are instances where the specific items discussed above must be investigated in an expeditious manner. Whenever possible, the physician should decrease excessive fever, convert dehydration, compensate for acidosis, and restore a depleted blood volume before surgery. These general principles apply both to the acute situation and to the preoperative care of the chronically ill child.

In cases of trauma or shock, immediate attention should be paid to the establishment and maintenance of an adequate airway, an adequate blood pressure, an adequate blood volume, and an adequate urine flow. The patient involved in trauma must be screened carefully for multiple or hidden injuries, particular attention being paid to cerebrocranial injury.

Specifically, injuries to the kidneys and bladder can be evaluated by monitoring urine flow and studying the urine for blood cells. Injury to the kidneys with retroperitoneal hemorrhage or extravasation of urine from the renal pelvis, ureters, or bladder should be evaluated by intravenous pyelography or cystography. Splenic, hepatic, or renal rupture can be evaluated by serial hematocrits to document blood loss or by four quadrant paracentesis. Rupture of a hollow viscus can be detected by properly obtained abdominal films for free air. Skull films, bone survey, and frequent evaluation of the nervous system serve to complete accurate recording of possible neurological or orthopedic complications.

The need for short-term endotracheal intubation or if necessary tracheostomy must be considered in the comatose child. Both procedures need similar, particular attention to details in terms of proper placement of tube, patency of airway, careful and frequent suction, and the evaluation of the possible need for assisted ventilation. Whenever a surgical procedure is to be done in an acute situation, careful anesthesia demands decompression of the stomach and evacuation of gastric contents to prevent vomiting and aspiration and perhaps to prevent prolonged ileus.

The most common acute surgical problem other than trauma will be that of the acute surgical abdomen. Appendicitis, intussusception, and other obstructive conditions are the most common. Careful history, repeated physical examination, and assistance from the laboratory can usually establish the diagnosis. Complete urinalysis, plain and upright abdominal films, plus a complete blood count should help exclude the medical conditions which can confuse the surgical diagnosis. These conditions commonly include urinary tract infection, pneumonia, mesenteric adenitis, diabetes mellitus, and rheumatic fever. More specialized radiologic procedures will be necessary if ulcer disease, intussusception, or other obstructive diseases are being considered.

The determination of the fluid and electrolyte status and the assurance of adequate maintenance therapy during the various stages of operative care are particularly important during acute surgical problems, but must be a part of all preoperative evaluations. An estimate of fluid losses can be made by noting the important points in the history (total intake, fever, urinary and gastrointestinal output, and weight loss) and the completion of a detailed physical examination for signs of fluid loss. (Once again, gastrointestinal decompression becomes important.) A loss of five percent of body weight in fluid is the smallest which can be detected clinically. Children with a moderate amount of dehydration are assumed to have lost about 10 percent of their body weight. Children who are moribund and in shock approach a fluid loss of 20 percent of their body weight.

Preoperative restoration of such losses to the furthest extent possible and the frequent reevaluation (perhaps every eight hours) during the postoperative period are essential. Care must be taken while administering replacement and maintenance fluids that overexpansion of the extracellular fluid compartment does not take place. When losses are especially great, 48 hours may be taken for correction.

At our institution, it is the common practice to calculate maintenance requirements on the basis of surface area. (Compare with Chapters 9 and 18.) It has been pointed out that fluid intake per unit of surface area is constant from about one week of age through adolescence and adult life. A figure between 1500 and 2000 ml per square meter provides an adequate intake for all individuals except the infant less than one week of age. (See page 89.) Direct determination of surface area is usually difficult so that nomograms are available for reference from which surface area can be read if height and weight are known. The normal daily requirement (per square meter) of sodium is 35 to 50 mEq and of potassium 30 to 40 mEq. Because measurement of urinary output is so important, utilizing the figure of 1000 to 1500 ml/m^2 per day of urine volume completes this approach.

THE CHRONICALLY ILL CHILD

The following conditions are seen frequently enough to warrant consideration as chronic states in childhood:

1. Renal disease
2. Cardiopulmonary disease

3. Malabsorptive gastrointestinal disease
4. Inflammatory gastrointestinal disease
5. Chronic nutritional deprivation
6. Chronic infectious disease states
7. Endocrine disease
8. Central nervous system disease
9. Malignancy
10. Collagen disease

The general concepts previously discussed apply to this category of surgical patient, but various depletion states which can cross through all of the above conditions must be considered as well.

The degree of hypovolemia which is often present can be difficult to ascertain with accuracy, but isotope or dye dilution studies could be carried out for more definite documentation. Since protein depletion nearly always occurs, serum protein determination becomes almost mandatory. Despite the need for documentation with the laboratory, deficiency states should always be assumed and the following guidelines used for treatment:

1. Whole blood transfusions to bring hemoglobin to 10–12 gm%.
2. Plasma and/or albumin to bring total protein to 5 gm% and albumin to 3 gm%.
3. One hundred total calories per kilogram per 24 hours is given when very long term or unrelenting caloric deprivation requies replacement parenterally.

Chronic renal disease can be controlled fairly easily during the short term of surgical care. Careful fluid management utilizing a low maintenance or oliguric regimen and correction of acidosis is obviously needed. Should uremia, oliguria, and hyperkalemia intervene, peritoneal dialysis or hemodialysis can be utilized to restore homeostasis.

A child with congenital heart disease must have congestive heart failure entirely in control before surgery, and the child chronically involved with pulmonary disease must be insured of excellent pulmonary toilet which includes physical therapy, postural drainage, and appropriate mist therapy. Excessive secretions must be controlled particularly when the real hazard of postoperative atelectasis is considered. Cultures of sputum for appropriate choice of antibiotics, when indicated, is important. Before contemplating surgeries of great magnitude, pulmonary function studies including circulation time and central venous pressure might be indicated to insure quality anesthesiology control.

Children with various endocrine diseases need careful management in terms of support and control. For example, the patient with diabetes mellitus demands expert insulin and glucose monitoring during periods of fasting, surgery, and the postoperative state which is discussed in detail elsewhere in this volume. (See Chapter 18.)

Children with malignancy, serologically rich collagen disease, or immunologically active gastrointestinal inflammatory disease need individual attention for many reasons, but one primary aspect is the potential difficulty in cross matching blood for needed replacement.

THE NEWBORN

The newborn infant, particularly the premature infant, is subject to a variety of stresses and can manifest unusual or unexpected responses to them. These often make preoperative evaluation difficult and can complicate the postoperative period. The newborn infant's history is that of his mother and often supplies the clue for diagnosis (e.g. polyhydramnios and high intestinal obstruction). Excellent communication between the obstetrical service and the physician responsible for the infant, therefore, remains very important.

The careful physical examination often reveals more than the obvious major or minor congenital abnormality. A few examples here might serve to illustrate the point. The patency of the nares must be insured. If in doubt, a number 5 or 8 French feeding catheter can safely be passed in patients older than 5 minutes of age. This catheter should be passed gently further, into the stomach. This rules out esophageal atresia and permits an estimation of the volume of gastric content. The flat or scaphoid abdomen suggests diaphragmatic hernia, particularly if any degree of respiratory distress is present. After careful inspection of the perineal area for ambiguous genitalia or anorectal anomalies, a careful rectal examination or passage into the rectum of the same catheter will insure patency and probably provoke the passage of a meconium stool which should then be examined.

Careful attention must be paid to the complaints or suggestions by nursery personnel regarding the possible onset of early symptoms of surgical problems. Prompt evaluation of jaundice, cyanosis, abdominal distention, vomiting (particularly if projectile or stained with bile or blood), and constipation will often be fruitful in securing an early surgical diagnosis.

The improved mortality and morbidity rate of surgery in the neonate is due to two major developments: first, a vast improvement in technical skill and modification of techniques by the pediatric and neonatal surgeon; and, secondly, a better understanding of the needs of the newborn infant and the construction of centers properly equipped to give intensive care to these infants.

The following general aspects of neonatal intensive care apply in a very significant manner to the evaluation of an infant with a surgical problem.

Temperature Control

The result of cooling and attempts at thermogenesis on the part of the newborn can result in hypoxia, acidosis, and hypoglycemia, all of which can make preoperative evaluation difficult or add to the severity of the surgical conditions which most commonly affect the newborn. A thermoneutral environment should be maintained (32°–34°C) after warming to a core temperature of 36°–37°C. The temperature should be monitored closely and large drops in ambient temperatures in areas such as the ambulance, operating suite, or recovery room anticipated. (See Chapter 8.)

Metabolic and Physiologic Evaluation

Careful evaluation and correction of aberrations in pH, pCO_2, pO_2, glucose, and calcium become exceedingly important, particularly for the newborn with a surgical condition. During the first few days of life, the umbilical artery provides a relatively safe route for sampling to determine the result of oxygen therapy, acid-base correction, and glucose and calcium levels. Infusion of blood, fluids, electrolytes, glucose, and protein can be accomplished with relative safety through this vessel for several days. Aortic blood pressure can be monitored via the same vessel by utilization of a strain gauge transducer, thus guarding against preoperative shock.

Studying the character of the urine, the amount of urinary output, and the taking of daily weights are important considerations particularly during the postoperative period. Caloric needs in the period immediately after birth are probably 50 to 60 calories/kg per day. When growth requirements are included, the total increases to between 100 and 150 calories/kg per day. Fluid management requires considerable clinical judgment in regard to the individual variations in renal maturity and the effects of unusual pathological or physiological states. In general, fluid requirements gradually increase from 65 to 150 cc/kg per day during the first seven to ten days of life. If the surface area method for maintenance fluid determination is used then during the first week of life, the full term and premature infant needs between 750 and 1000 ml/m^2. After seven to ten days, renal function begins to correspond to that of older infants so that 1500 to 2000 ml/m^2 may be used. (Compare with Chapter 9.)

Evaluation of the degree of and the causes for hyperbilirubinemia in the preoperative state is of concern because of the anesthetic and analgesic agents which may be competing for albumin binding sites. If a significant amount of unbound, unconjugated bilirubin is released into the tissues, kernicterus could result. On the other hand, this same process might impair the efficiency of the agents being used or allow the untoward effects of these agents to become prominent.

Coagulation Problems

Here the newborn presents a strange paradox. There is no question that there are decreased levels of some clotting factors of whole blood of newborn infants, especially premature infants. However, it can also be stated with some degree of certainty that the whole blood of the newborn infant is probably hypercoagulable. One, therefore, must be certain that vitamin K has been administered to the newborn preoperatively (0.5 to 1.0 mg of vitamin K_1 oxide) and strict attention paid to the early signs of coagulation problems particularly if respiratory distress, infection, or shock are part of the infant's status.

Cardiorespiratory Evaluation

The newborn infant presents a particular challenge in the evaluation of his cardiopulmonary status. The continued changes in physiology during the transition period from fetal to neonatal life are many and are often confused with the early signs of serious lesions. (See Chapter 12.) Monitors of several types for respiratory rate, apnea, and cardiac rate are available, and these combined with the frequent use of a stethoscope are mandatory in determining the cardiopulmonary status of an infant during the preoperative and postoperative period.

Infection

The generally increased susceptibility of newborns to infection in association with the nature of the surgical problems to which he is most often exposed seriously threaten his bacteriologic status. As well, the manipulations alluded to above often increase the hazards of infection. Careful physical examination, attention to subtle changes in the clinical status, and frequent cultures should be utilized as a major part of the evaluation of the newborn in the period of time surrounding surgery.

Decompression of Gastrointestinal Tract

The nature of the majority of surgical lesions which affect the newborn almost always require decompression of the stomach. This is emphasized here again as many problems can be stabilized and prevented by this simple technique.

SUMMARY

A preoperative medical evaluation of excellent quality has as its basis the expeditiously performed history and physical examination. The evaluation must be precise, thorough, and designed to permit the acquisition of data necessary to insure optimum anesthesia control and reduce postoperative complications. The chronically ill child, the child with an acute surgical problem, the child involved in trauma, and the neonatal patient require special modifications of the history and physical approach to the preoperative evaluation.

REFERENCES

1. Kinney, J.M., Egdahl, R.H., and Zuridema, G.D.: *Manual of Preoperative and Postoperative Care,* ed 2. Committee of the American College of Surgeons, Philadelphia: W.B. Saunders, 1971.
2. St. Geme, J.W., Jr.: Preoperative evaluation. *Pediat Clin N Amer* 16:573–580, 1961.
3. Owen, G.M., Ed.: *Problems in Neonatal Surgery.* Columbus: The Forty-Ninth Ross Conference on Pediatric Research, Ross Laboratories, 1965.
4. Dennison, W.M.: *Surgery in Infancy and Childhood,* ed 2. Edinburgh and London: E. & S. Livingston, 1967.
5. Kaplan, S.A.: Fluid therapy in pediatrics. In Gellis and Kagan: *Current Pediatric Therapy #5.* Philadelphia: W.B. Saunders Company, 1971, pp. 718–725.
6. Swenson, O.: *Pediatric Surgery I and II,* ed 3. New York: Appleton-Century Crofts, 1969.

7

The Responsibilities
of the
Anesthesiologist
in Pre- and
Postoperative Care

Robert M. Smith, M.D.

The child who is exposed to hospitalization and surgery faces two very distinct types of problems: those associated with his physical condition, which are usually cared for in exhaustive detail; and those having to do with his emotional needs, which frequently are granted slight notice.

It is gratifying to see that the editor of this volume has already directed an unusual amount of attention toward the child as a whole person. Several of the major factors that cause emotional stress in the hospitalized child, such as separation from parents and apprehension of the unknown, have been discussed, and the roles of parent, pediatrician, and surgeon have been described. (See Chapter 1.)

Although the anesthesiologist usually is the last to encounter the child, it is he who must take the child through what is often the most upsetting experience of the hospital stay, the induction of anesthesia.[1,2,3]

The fact that the anesthesiologist has the last opportunity to prepare the child for the stress of operation gives him a chance to reinforce the work of others or attempt to correct any remaining misconceptions. It is also the responsibility of the anesthesiologist to ensure the maintenance of the best possible physical condition of the child through the operative period.

PREOPERATIVE EVALUATION

Under usual circumstances the anesthesiologist visits the child the afternoon or evening before operation.[4,5] If a child is known to have unusual fear of anesthesia, possible ventilation inadequacy, or other problems, the anesthesiologist should be forewarned and be allowed additional time to overcome them.

Before seeking out the patient, the anesthesiologist gets all he can out of the child's chart, thereby avoiding the repetition of many questions and much poking and prodding.[6] Chief complaint, contributing factors, site and extent of the lesion involved, and any effects on normal anatomical or physiologic conditions should be appraised. The anesthesiologist must know the surgeon's plan of attack, the desired position for operation, expected duration, blood loss, organs involved, and postoperative therapy required. The choice of the anesthetic which will best serve the surgeon and be safest for the patient will depend upon many factors such as whether the patient will be supine or prone (when endotracheal intubation will be necessary), whether nerve stimulation will be used to locate muscle bundles (which will rule out use of muscle relaxants), whether a child is to be discharged after operation (which will rule out long-acting agents like Ketamine), whether the child has had recent respiratory infection or croup (contraindicating endotracheal intubation), and so on.

The medical history may be brief for a normal child, but no positive finding should be overlooked. The severity and extent of the child's disease should be clearly understood by the anesthesiologist, for many times he must weigh the need of operation against such contraindications as a fresh cold or severe cardiac disease (or both). Surgeon and pediatrician will not have overlooked this problem, but will have different viewpoints, and will be less able to judge the anesthetic risk.

Obviously, any disease process or abnormality should be noted prior to anesthesia, but cardiorespiratory problems are of special concern.[7] Infants and children seem especially harassed by a multitude of anomalies and lesions that threaten the airway.[8] Some anomalies are immediately evident, such as a large hemangioma of the tongue or cystic hygroma, but choanal atresia or a vascular ring may be unrecognized for several months after birth. History of recurrent bouts of croup is a real danger sign, especially if tracheostomy has previously been necessary, since even a well-healed tracheostomy usually leaves a narrowed area in the trachea. Asthma, recurrent respiratory disease, cystic fibrosis or scoliotic or other thoracic deformity may cause serious complications during or following operation and should be considered in planning the course of anesthesia.

Among other features of importance in the child's history, the anesthesiologist should note his birth history, any delay in onset of respiration, convulsions, and other signs of central nervous system damage, and hepatic or renal disease. Sensitivity to drugs is important, especially if they are sedative or anesthetic agents. Familial cholinesterase abnormality will result in prolonged apnea following use of succinylcholine, and, of course, exposure to halogenated anesthetics may set the stage for fatal response on succeeding use of these agents. This reaction is so very rare that one might be justified in disregarding it purely on the basis of statistics, but it is certainly better to be aware of this hazard. The usual course of events entails an initial anesthesia with halothane or methoxyflurane,[9] after which there is some fever, plus upper abdominal tenderness, jaundice, eosinophilia, and laboratory evidence of hepatic injury. On the second or third exposure to one of these agents (not necessarily the same each time), the affected patients show fulminating hepatic response, usually fatal. Thus far, several hundred adults are believed to have died from this lesion, but only seven children,[10] out of the many millions who have received the agents. Furthermore, since this "sensitivity"[11] has almost always been evident following one or two exposures to these agents, a child who has survived three such anesthetics probably will never show this complication. It is widely believed that in these children it is relatively safe to use halothane repeatedly. Children have received the agent 30–40 times without incident.

At present, the use of methoxyflurane is regarded with considerable disfavor because of renal toxicity.[12,13] In addition to the usual concern over hazards such as diabetes or anemia, we have learned that the development of high fever during anesthesia may be due to a familial metabolic defect.[14,15] Consequently, history of such an incident in the patient or any relative must be regarded as a real danger sign. Since many cases of malignant hyperthermia have been reported, with fatal outcome, a history suggestive of this syndrome should call for careful investigation and the avoidance of two agents frequently associated with its occurrence, succinylcholine and halothane.

Still another peril recently recognized is the use of succinylcholine in any patients who have suffered extensive tissue damage, either as burns or direct trauma, or due to muscle denervation. In these patients, succinylcholine is again contraindicated, since its use induces rapid release of potassium from damaged muscle cells, resulting in a high incidence of cardiac arrest.

Having assured himself that there is no record of such obvious or obscure problems nor recent exposure to diseases, the anesthesiologist can next peruse the recorded physical examination and laboratory findings. Here he evaluates the general condition of the patient as evidenced by body size and development, notes details of the surgical lesion as described by the surgeon and any abnormal supplemental findings of heart, lungs, or neuromuscular system. Significant abnormal

findings here are usually an indication for further examination or consultation by experts in pediatric cardiology or other specialties whose
reports should be recorded for review at this time.

The traditional requirements for laboratory work prior to operation call for hemoglobin of 10 gm%, or over, and normal urine examination. The minimum acceptable hemoglobin level is the most
frequent cause of dissent between surgeon and anesthesiologist. An
unbending rule is necessary only when irrational individuals are concerned, for many variables enter the picture. A 6-month-old child with
incarcerated hernia and hemoglobin of 9.5 gm% seems a reasonable
exception to the rule, but somewhere the line must be drawn, perhaps
at 9 gm%, where transfusion or shift from general to local anesthesia
might be preferable.

Concern over sickle cell anemia has grown with the increasing
black population. (See Chapter 17.) A sickle cell examination should be
obtained on any black person on admission to hospital. Furthermore,
use of surgical tourniquets is definitely contraindicated in black patients
unless the sickle cell defect has been proved to be absent.

Other laboratory figures of special value are hematocrit in cyanotic children (over 65 percent signifying increased danger of thrombosis), serum potassium in cardiac patients (hypokalemia) or renal disease
(hyperkalemia), electrolytes in any metabolic imbalance, blood gas
studies in acid base disturbances, and others.

X-ray findings are often helpful in evaluation of patient risk, but
those of an enlarged heart are particularly significant, and the ones
that the wise anesthesiologist examines for himself.

For obvious ethical considerations, the anesthesiologist makes certain that proper written consent for anesthesia and operation has been
obtained.

INTERVIEWING THE PATIENT AND PARENTS

The anesthesiologist finally doublechecks the child's first name and
seeks him out. With luck, he might find a quietly sleeping infant, a
composed child who has been gently informed of his problem a few
days previously, or an intelligent adolescent who has already picked up
enough medical lore through school and television to put him well
in tune with the situation. Under such ideal circumstances, the anesthesiologist finds small need for an excessive outlay of effort. He dis-
turbs these patients as little as possible and refrains from waking a
sleeping infant who is known to be sick or fatigued from crying. He
speaks to older children to briefly acquaint them with the sound of his
voice and give them a final word of reassurance before their anesthesia,
and then he doublechecks heart, lungs, upper airway, and teeth.

Instead of finding the happy situations described above, the anesthesiologist is more likely to find a screaming, dehydrated infant with a runny nose, a fearful 6-year-old whose parents have promised her she would only have her picture taken, a cyanotic 13-year-old boy in the late stages of cystic fibrosis with the expectation of death in his eyes, or a "pee wee" hockey star facing amputation for sarcoma. The care required for these may include several days of physical and emotional preparation, or postponement of operation. Visits by a special staff psychiatrist have been of great help for children prior to amputation.

Obviously, the approach must be suited to the individual situation. Some shy, apprehensive children need only encouragement and reassurance. Others must be convinced of the anesthesiologist's reliability, especially if they have been duped by parents or doctors at a previous time. Deception must be avoided in dealing with patients of any age. Although many parents fail to tell their children the truth about a coming operation, they are often relieved to have physician or nurse do it for them and escape being the bearer of unwelcome news themselves. Parents may suffer considerably more apprehension than small children, and the anesthesiologist often has an opportunity to fill in details that are of considerable comfort on the eve of operation. Parents should be questioned by the anesthesiologist too, for they often sense changes in a child's physical condition that the admitting physician has missed, especially in reference to respiratory disease, and are most likely to know when the child last ate.

A receptive child should be given some warning of what he will encounter. This can be initiated prior to hospitalization with the use of booklets designed for this purpose. The anesthesiologist can fill in necessary details and answer questions. It is unwise to go to extremes by describing things that the child is unlikely to see.

Preoperative medication of patients is traditional, and innumerable drugs and combinations have been employed.[16,17] Since weight, age, and other physical measurements give no measure of a child's emotional makeup, most medication has been somewhat less than perfect. At present, pediatric anesthesiologists seem to favor reduction or elimination of sedatives. When such medication is used, the predictable combination of pentobarbital (Nembutal), morphine, and atropine is still the most popular.

The final determination of agent and dose varies considerably with the child's age, his physical condition, the operation to be performed, and other factors. For many years, the following regime proved reliable.

1. The use of atropine for all patients to receive general anesthesia, starting at birth, and given by subcutaneous injection, 0.1 mg/10 lbs (maximum 0.6 mg) 45 minutes before anesthesia.
2. Pentobarbital (Nembutal), for children over 6 months old,

given by rectum (2.5 mg/lb) to children under 8 years old, and by mouth (1.5 mg/lb) in older children, 90 minutes or more before operation (maximum 120 mg).

3. Morphine sulfate for children over one year of age, given subcutaneously 0.1 mg/lb 45 minutes prior to anesthesia (maximum 10 mg).

The aim recently has been to avoid preanesthetic injections. This has been possible by retaining the above use of pentobarbital, omitting morphine, and delaying the injection of atropine until after initiation of anesthesia, then giving it either by intramuscular or intravenous route. If children are obviously highly emotional, pentobarbital is given at bedtime, again in the morning, and the child reevaluated prior to transportation to the operating room. If they are unusually disturbed in the operating room, rectal thiopental 10–15 mg/lb is used, thiopental is given intravenously, or Ketamine is employed. Forceful mask induction is especially to be avoided.

Rather than relying upon drugs to induce quiescence or sleep prior to anesthesia, the anesthesiologist, in many instances, can achieve a more satisfactory result by spending a few extra minutes with children, asking them about their brothers, sisters, pets, or favorite games or television programs. The next day in the operating room, he will be able to continue this dialogue about subjects with which the child is familiar. This will do much to overcome apprehension and the feeling of strangeness. Whenever possible, the child should be encouraged to take the lead in such storytelling, for this more effectively captures his attention. It is also reassuring to have children bring a favorite toy or blanket with them when they are anesthetized.

PREPARATION FOR EMERGENCY PROCEDURES

In unscheduled, and the rare, truly urgent operation, special precautions are observed to avoid pitfalls of expediency. The greatest problem involved in anesthesia is vomiting and aspiration of food eaten shortly before the injury or onset of illness. Food may remain undigested for many hours under stressing situations. Information concerning the child's food intake is important, but usually unreliable, unless there is evidence that the child refused food due to anorexia, as usually occurs in appendicitis.

The child with peritonitis and a high fever requires definitive preparation aimed first at restoring fluid and acid-base balance, then at combatting infection and controlling fever. Antipyretics are permissible, but attempts at cooling an awake child by alcohol, ice, or other external methods are definitely to be avoided, since they greatly increase oxygen demands. After hydration is satisfactorily restored, these children may be anesthetized to control their shivering response, then, prior, to operation, external cooling will rapidly reduce their temperature to an acceptable level (below 102°F).

Other critical situations include the bleeding tonsil, aspirated foreign body, injuries to the eyeball, and many more too numerous to be discussed individually, but which certainly demand special consideration. Above all, one should realize that few such procedures call for haste or omission of basic therapeutic principles.

INTRAOPERATIVE COURSE

The progress through operation is not our concern here, other than to mention that the chance of an anesthetic death is extremely small for a normal healthy child. "Anesthetic death" means any death occurring during or after operation that can be attributed either to the action of an anesthetic agent or to the fault of the anesthesiologist.[18] Children have been said to be poorer risks than adults, but there is little to substantiate this, a normal child having somewhat greater tolerance for many drugs, and better recuperative power than older individuals. Operative deaths in the past have all too frequently been caused by lack of understanding and experience of the personnel involved. Available statistics do not tell the whole story. The greater mortality in the neonate is heavily weighted by the high incidence of prematurity and complicating anomalies. Data compiled at Children's Hospital of Boston show no anesthetic deaths in 10,000 procedures on normal, healthy children, but a total of 11 deaths in children having moderate or severe complicating disorders.[6] Other sources give figures approximating 3.3 deaths in 10,000 pediatric operations, against 2.7 deaths in 10,000 procedures on adults.[19]

The incidence of cardiac arrest during operation is probably more frequent among infants and children also, partly due to children's more rapid response to many intraoperative stimuli and the more frequent occurrence of respiratory obstruction and depression. Recovery is more prompt in young patients, however, and death following cardiac arrest due to these causes is usually avoidable.

POSTANESTHETIC RECOVERY

Recovery from anesthesia begins in the operating room immediately after inhalation agents have been stopped and/or injected anesthetics have passed their peak effects. With short-acting agents, patients may awaken completely while still on the operating table. In general, the anesthetic recovery period entails the first one to three hours after operation. This is a period of many potential hazards, and it is almost mandatory to provide a specially equipped area close to the operating room,[20] manned by skilled personnel competent in the care of unconscious patients.[21] It is also advisable to have this area under the supervision of a physician expert in emergency procedures who is always immediately available. In many situations an anesthesiologist is best suited to this responsibility, and he is also the one who judges when patients are ready for discharge to their own rooms.

Maintenance of a free respiratory exchange is the first requirement during recovery, and all anesthetized patients must be under continual supervision to prevent airway obstruction due to blocking tongue, blood, secretions, or vomitus. Position, suctioning, and stimulation of breathing are important in all such situations.

Postanesthetic stridor frequently occurs in children and may be caused by preexisting irritation of airway, motion of endotracheal tube, irritants in the tube, or excessive tube size. Often no cause can be found. Treatment should be started promptly, to prevent progression of this dangerous condition, when reintubation or tracheostomy could be indicated. Treatment consists of intravenous (or intramuscular) use of dexamethasone and mist tent.[22] If symptoms become more severe, racemic epinephrine should be given by intermittent positive pressure breathing.[23] Although the incidence of croup remains relatively high, no patient has required reintubation or tracheostomy during the last 5 years under our care.

Depression of respiration also occurs frequently and may be due to an overdose of premedicant agents, the prolonged effect of anesthetics, or underlying pathology. Decreased metabolism, as in hypothermia, will also cause increased depressant effect of anesthetic agents. Prolonged apnea following succinylcholine can be caused by deficient plasma cholinesterase, following d-tubocurare, by use of antibiotics, mycins, and following thiopental in patients with porphyria. Muscle stimulators may be used to help determine the cause of prolonged muscle weakness.

The child's awakening after halothane is fairly prompt, but often associated with some excitement which is heightened by the addition of pain. Morphine given via intravenous infusion has an immediately soothing effect. Ketamine may cause prolonged sleep if other sedatives have been added, but may be of special concern because of the hallucinations and other unpleasant sensations experienced during recovery, especially if children are aroused prematurely.[24,25] Nurses are cautioned to avoid unnecessary stimulation of these patients and to refrain from any attempts to hasten their awakening. Children seem less bothered by pain than adults, but stiff casts, orchidopexy, pneumoencephalography, and other procedures often cause real discomfort and require effective control.

Prolonged unconsciousness may follow an inadvertent overdose of inhalation agents, but in small infants is occasionally due to intracerebral hemorrhage.[26] Cerebral depression may also be caused by overhydration, air embolism, intraoperative hypoxia, hypothermia, or septicemia. Cardiovascular complications are relatively infrequent in early recovery from pediatric operations, except for hypovolemic hypotension following open heart procedures and similar major operations.

The temperature of children during anesthetic recovery tends to be low.[27] In small infants, it may be extremely so and lead to severe respiratory depression. Older children are seldom endangered by this, more often showing moderate temperature elevations. Prior to awakening, they may be cooled by alcohol sponging or ice packs, but when shivering occurs this should be discontinued. Aspirin (300–600 mg) or thorazine (0.1 mg/kg) may be given after patients have awakened.

Renal shutdown is rare in children, but has occurred following severe hypoxia or hypovolemic episodes. Liver damage following halogenated agents has been discussed. Signs seldom appear until 2 or 3 days after operation, when patients may appear jaundiced, complain of tender epigastrium, and show a moderate temperature elevation.

Care during the immediate postanesthetic period should consist of a 1-to-1 or 1-to-2 nurse/patient coverage, with continuous observation of ventilation until return of gag reflex, and recording of temperature, pulse, and blood pressure at 10-minute intervals for at least an hour. Special attention must be paid to all unusual conditions such as bleeding after oral surgery, chest tube drainage, and such. Intravenous fluids and blood, as indicated, will be continued and may require special attention in an active, uncontrolled child.

Special monitoring devices in the recovery room are not of great practical importance in children. Those designed for use in several patients at once have virtually no application.

In individual cases, especially those with known cardiac or respiratory lesions, electrocardiogram, pacemaker, and ventilatory monitors may be of value. Mechanical ventilators should always be available for either temporary or continual use during recovery.[28] They are routinely employed following open heart procedures and many of the more extensive spinal fusions.

Patients who require continued ventilator therapy will need monitoring of blood gases for the necessary precision of ventilator adjustment.[29]

Discharge from the recovery room is determined by the physician in charge. It is advisable to allow discharge of normal patients after a minimum of one hour, if they have awakened and regained full control of reflexes. Any complicating factors must be weighed individually.

In the case of outpatient surgery (see Chapter 3), children often require longer periods of observation, especially if there has been question of airway irritation. Since endotracheal intubation may be complicated by early postoperative croup, intubation is avoided if possible, but if children have been intubated, they are kept under observation for three hours before being allowed to go home with their parents.[30]

REFERENCES

1. Jackson, K., et al: Behavior changes indicating emotional trauma in tonsillecto-mized children. *Pediatrics* 12:23–28, 1953.
2. Eckenhoff, J.E., Kneale, D.H., and Dripps, R.D.: The incidence and etiology of post-anesthetic excitement. *Anesthesiology* 22:667–673, 1961.
3. Mellish, R.W.P.: Preparation of a child for hospitalization and surgery. *Ped Clin N Amer* 16:543–553, 1969.
4. Smith, R.M.: Children, hospitals and parents. *Anesthesiology* 25:461–465, 1964.
5. Egbert, L.D., Lamdin, S.J., and Hackett, T.P.: Psychological problems of surgical patients. In Eckenhoff, J.E.: *Science and Practice in Anesthesia.* Philadelphia: J.B. Lippincott, 1965.
6. Smith, R.M.: *Anesthesia for Infants and Children,* ed 3. St. Louis: C.V. Mosby, 1968.
7. Downes, J.J., and Nicodemus, H.: Preparation for and recovery from anesthesia. *Ped Clin N Amer* 16:601–611, 1969.
8. Downes, J.J., et al: Acute respiratory failure in infants with bronchiolitis. *Anesthesiology* 29:426–434, 1968.
9. Brenner, A.I., and Kaplan, M.M.: Recurrent hepatitis due to methoxyflurane anesthesia. *New Eng J Med* 284:961–962, 1971.
10. Carney, F.M.T., and Van Dyke, R.A.: Halothane hepatitis: A critical review. *Anesth Analg* 51:135–160, 1972.
11. Klatskin, G., and Kimberg, D.V.: Recurrent hepatitis attributable to halothane sensitization in an anesthetist. *New Eng J Med* 280:515–522, 1969.
12. Holaday, D.A., Rudofsky, S., and Trevhaft, P.S.: The metabolic degradation of methoxyflurane anesthesia. II Fluoride concentration in nephrotoxicity. *JAMA* 214:91–95, 1971.
13. Crandell, W.B., Pappas, S.G., and MacDonald, A.: Nephrotoxicity associated with methoxyflurane anesthesia. *Anesthesiology* 27:591–607, 1966.
14. Denborough, M.A., et al: Anesthetic deaths in a family. *Brit J Anaesth* 34:395–396, 1962.
15. Britt, B.A., and Kalow, W.: Malignant hyperthermia: Etiology unknown. *Canad Anaesth Soc J* 17:316–330, 1970.
16. Rackow, H., and Salnitre, E.: Modern concepts in pediatric anesthesiology. *Anesthesiology* 30:208–234, 1969.
17. Keller, M.L., Sussman, S., and Rochberg, S.: Comparative evaluation of combined preoperative medications for pediatric surgery. *Anesth Analg* 47:199–206, 1968.
18. Beecher, H.K., and Todd, D.D.: A study of the deaths associated with anesthesia and surgery. *Ann Surg* 140:2–34, 1954.
19. Graff, T.D., et al: Baltimore anesthesia study committee: Factors in pediatric anesthesia mortality. *Anesth Analg* 43:407–414, 1964.
20. Schweizer, O.: The recovery and intensive care unit: A clinical laboratory. *Anesthesiology* 32:246–254, 1970.
21. Wiklund, P.E.: Design of a recovery room and intensive care unit. *Anesthesiology* 26:667–674, 1965.
22. Eden, A.N., and Larkin, V.D.: Corticosteroid treatment of croup. *Pediatrics* 33:768–769, 1964.
23. Adair, J.C., et al: Ten-year experience with IPPB treatment of acute laryngo tracheobronchitis. *Anesth Analg* 50:649–654, 1971.
24. Corssen, G., et al.: Computerized evaluation of psychic effects of Ketamine. *Anesth Analg* 50:397–401, 1971.
25. Reier, C.E.: Ketamine—Dissociative agent or hallucinogen?, Letter to the Editor. *New Eng J Med* 284:791–792, 1971.
26. Gilles, F.H., et al: Fibrinolytic activity in the ganglionic eminence of the prema-ture human brain. *Biol Neonate* 18:426–432, 1971.

27. Roe, C.F., Santulli, T.V., and Blair, C.S.: Heat loss in infants during general anesthesia. *J Pediat Surg* 1:266–275, 1966.
28. Crocker, D., and Young, J.: Principles and practice of inhalation therapy. Chicago: Yearbook Medical Publishing, 1970.
29. Gregory, G.A.: Ventilatory support of infants and children. American Society of Anesthesiologists 1971 Annual Refresher Course Lectures 206:1–4, 1971.
30. Ahlgren, E.W., Bennett, E.J., and Stephen, C.R.: Outpatient pediatric anesthesiology: A case series. *Anesth Analg* 50:402–408, 1971

8

Temperature Monitoring and Regulation

Robert M. Smith, M.D.

Emphasis is justly being placed upon the importance of body temperature during the operative period in pediatric surgery. The high incidence and severe consequences of both hypothermia and hyperthermia [1,2] have aroused widespread concern and stimulated considerable enthusiasm for monitoring body temperature and attempting to regulate it.

Because of numerous recent developments in both theoretical and technical aspects of temperature control,[3] there appears to be confusion over the general application of available information. This confusion is seen in the choice of monitoring techniques, in the evaluation of data, and especially in the approach to temperature regulation. Failure to recognize obvious clinical syndromes, on the one hand, and overzealous and poorly regulated use of temperature-controlling devices, on the other, have resulted in too many catastrophes. Outstanding examples of such incidents are those in which patients' temperatures have been allowed to reach 108°F unnoticed, and others in which patients have been severely burned due to faulty use of heating devices.[4,5]

Several underlying conditions contribute to the increased incidence of temperature-related complications in pediatric surgery. It is common knowledge that children, and especially infants, are subject to greater variation in body temperature than are adults and that infants, due to their greater body surface area and increased tissue conductivity, have a marked tendency to become hypothermic.[6,7] The newborn infant begins to lose body heat the moment he is born and usually suffers a loss of 2° to 4°F in the interval between his delivery and arrival in the nursery.[3,8] Premature infants have greater difficulty maintaining temperature stability, and their problems may be compounded by interaction of hypoglycemia, metabolic acidosis, and respiratory distress syndrome.[9]

The effect of hypothermia upon the neonate was in question until recently, it having been held possible that intentional cooling of depressed neonates might reduce their oxygen requirement and improve overall survival. Conclusive proof by Silverman [10,11] that infants maintained at temperatures above 95°F have a better survival rate established the dictum that cooling was to be avoided in infants under all conditions. Subsequent investigation by numerous workers has disclosed the mechanism of nonshivering thermogenesis, which further explains the harmful effect of exposure of infants to cold. Other significant complications associated with hypothermia are increased blood viscosity, cardiorespiratory depression, and delayed metabolic breakdown of drugs.

Studies of the routes of heat loss by exposed naked infants have demonstrated that radiation accounts for approximately two-thirds of the loss under normal conditions [12] and, consequently, have suggested proper avenues of correction.[8,13] Many other factors contribute to the hazards of the neonate, most of them pointing in the direction of hypothermia.

Older children undergoing operation have a greater tendency to develop hyperthermic complications. Rapid temperature elevation and overzealous and poorly regulated use of temperature-controlling deconvulsions were seen with ether and often terminated fatally. Many factors may cause intraoperative temperature elevation, among them transfusion reaction, exacerbation of preexisting infection, and drug reaction. Children undergoing pyeloplasty and other genitourinary procedures may develop septicemia with alarming speed. There is tremendous concern at present over a newly recognized syndrome labelled "malignant" hyperthermia,[1,2] characterized by sudden unexpected intraoperative rise in temperature, occurring in both children and adults, frequently seen in siblings, and carrying a high mortality rate unless recognized promptly and treated intelligently. Surgeons should be aware of this syndrome, and pay attention to any details suggesting such reactions in previous experiences of the patient or his relatives. Several instances are on record in which surgeon and anesthetist disregarded clear-cut stories of sibling death, and proceeded to precipitate another. Obviously, hyperthermia is our main concern in older children, however, excessive cooling does occur, though much less frequently. It is seen in extensive operations, especially in procedures involving massive blood replacement.

In the postoperative recovery room, in intensive care units, and in nursing divisions, we are faced with a variety of temperature-regulation problems which actually may be more difficult to manage than those in the operating room. Their difficulty lies in the fact that, first, they are often of prolonged duration, and secondly, one has less choice in methods of treatment. For example, if a child has a fever of 103°F in the operating room, he can be treated by application of ice or cold fluids to his body and his temperature drops rapidly. Since this type of surface cooling makes conscious patients shiver actively, it is ill-advised, and other less effective alternatives must be substituted. Unfortunately, these patients may be critically ill, whether with pneumonia, status asthmaticus, or some neurological lesion, and speed is important. This problem, which is one of our oldest, remains unsolved.

The mechanisms of temperature control have been extensively described, as have various approaches to the situations mentioned above. These have been noted here merely to illustrate the present need for measuring and governing body temperature.

METHODS OF MONITORING TEMPERATURE

The term "monitor," as currently used in the practice of medicine, is employed either as a noun to describe any one of a variety of devices of increasing cost and complexity which measure and indicate or record some physiologic variable such as pulse or temperature, or as a verb, implying continuous watching or observation. In both cases it appears that the term has been altered somewhat from its original implication, that is, not only of measuring or observing, but of *guarding*. This is a significant point, because it brings out a real weakness encountered with increasing frequency, that of measuring or observing without meaningful application of the results. If our medical monitors were to live up to their names, they would either include a warning device or have a feedback system that would correct abnormal deviations automatically. Such systems are not in general use, although they have been initiated to a certain extent, especially in temperature control.

The above digression has relevance here because, as has been shown by Adamsons [6,7] and others,[10,14] a single temperature reading or even a series of readings from any single area of the body may have little significance unless this information is related to measurement at other parts of the body or surrounding objects.

Monitoring by Observation of Clinical Signs

In order to monitor body temperature, we might expect to start with the use of the clinical thermometer. To begin with a device even as simple as this one, we would be disregarding a number of obvious leads which may be of great value. To one who has been made aware of the dangers of body cooling, the mere sight of a newborn infant lying uncovered and exposed upon an operating table or treatment stand should cause alarm.

Signs of Hypothermia

The clinical signs of hypothermia in infants are not so obvious as those of hyperthermia in older patients, but several indications may exist which, without recourse to a thermometer, should alert one to the possible existence of excessive cooling as in the exposure of infants at operation.

Most pediatricians are aware of situations that involve increased danger of exposure and hence require more scrupulous observation and care. These include the immediate postnatal period and transportation, not only the infrequent moving between hospital and home (see Chapter 2), but much more common moves between various hospital facilities such as admitting department, operating room, x-ray room, and treatment room. Since the hazards of cooling during such trips are obvious, and the means to avoid them are available, failure to regard them must be attributed to poor supervision or carelessness.

One of the most obvious signs of hypothermia is the temperature change of the patient's skin. Cold hands or feet should be noticed, but do not always denote severe change. However, when the body or head feels appreciably cooler than normal, the changes should be recognized and corrective measures initiated.

Direct observation of an infant who has become hypothermic gives relatively little proof of his plight, but there are several clues that should alert one to the danger. The child's skin may become more pallid, and his extremities often become cyanotic. The child's peripheral vasculature becomes constricted, and with vasoconstriction the circulation is reduced. The infant may increase his muscular activity at first, but with increasing cooling may become flaccid. This is seen especially in the anesthetized infant, where the usual degree of flaccidity may be increased by greater solubility of anesthetics in cool blood. With marked cooling, pupils will show greater dilation. Shivering is obviously a useful sign in older children, but rarely occurs in small infants. Shivering is blocked in patients of all ages during general anesthesia.

Several clinical situations should arouse immediate concern. During resuscitative procedures, when protective covers are usually thrown clear to allow accessibility of all areas of the body to the procedures of respiratory ventilation, cardiac massage, intravenous medication and samplings, and attachment of electrodes, the child may become so cold after five minutes that his chances of revival are considerably diminished.

In the operating suite, one occasionally finds that the room temperature has been so drastically reduced to comply with the wishes of the surgeon that circulating nurses have draped blankets over their shoulders for protection. One should immediately check to see that the anesthetized child has been equally protected.

Occasionally, operating rooms are so cold that vapor can be seen rising from the surface of the exposed bowel or lung. Here again, steps should be taken to correct the temperature and specific action initiated to meet the danger of severe hypothermia.

Signs of Hyperthermia

Early detection of hyperthermia is of extreme importance. To overlook developing fever until the temperature is 106°–108°F is usually due to inadequate attention. Signs of hyperthermia are gross and abundant. All body surfaces become obviously overheated, especially those of the head, which is most frequently under the direct observation of the anesthesiologist. There is also flushing of the skin, often accompanied by labored respiration, tachycardia, and increased blood pressure. Sweating is less marked in young children, but increased skin moisture is usually evident even in infancy.

The onset of malignant hyperthermia is often preceded by an unusually prolonged rigidity following the use of succinylcholine,[15,16,17] and occasionally when only halothane has been used. Undoubtedly, a most obvious and alarming sign of hyperpyrexia is a seizure of any form during anesthesia. In cardiac arrest of undetermined origin, hyperthermia must always be considered as a possible primary or secondary factor.

Surgeons also may notice signs of hyperthermia. Although complaints about increased bleeding are heard too frequently to cause immediate alarm, they must always be investigated. At extremely high temperatures, the body tissues will feel so hot that the surgeon may remark on it when he puts his hand in the chest or abdomen. This usually denotes a serious situation that demands immediate action.

Clinical Signs in the Recovery Room

As patients awaken from anesthesia, the pattern of temperature control may be markedly altered and the signs correspondingly confusing. They frequently exhibit a variety of shaking motions that resemble both convulsions and severe shivering. In the infant, these appear to be neither, but rather an irregular return of muscular control. In slightly older children and adults, true shivering of an intense degree is frequently seen following anesthesia with thiopental or halothane.

This shivering may occur with minimal loss of body heat and probably denotes an altered temperature threshold for shivering due in part to the depression of catechol release that is associated with these anesthetics.

Monitoring by Measurement of Temperature

Measurement of Environmental Conditions

Each nursing division or ward and every individual operating room should be fitted with a wall thermometer and hygrometer. It is also essential that each operating room have individual temperature control, and that it can be adjusted between 65° and 85°F within fifteen minutes. In many operating facilities, temperature adjustment is so slow that an infant is badly chilled at the start of the operation, and then, after the child is safely covered with drapes, the room becomes overheated, to the intense discomfort and irritation of the surgical team.

Air conditioning is usually provided in all operating rooms and undoubtedly will be in all modern nursing wards. Airflow meters should be available in the hospital to check the rate of airflow, which is measured in linear feet per minute (lf/m).

Indications for Measurement of Body Temperature

To insist that every patient has his temperature measured by a constantly monitoring instrument is as unreasonable as demanding a traffic officer at every street corner. There are many operations during which such monitors are mandatory, but we are not ready to legislate the necessity for such devices for all, certainly while monitoring devices themselves still carry an appreciable risk. The incidence of significant temperature change in uncomplicated operations taking less time than 30 minutes is extremely low. If we anticipate and prevent cooling in healthy infants, it seems reasonable to omit thermometry during such minor procedures as circumcision and myringotomy, and also during herniorrhaphy and pyloromyotomy, when performed expeditiously.

Not enough attention has been placed on the patient's preoperative temperature. Surgeon and anesthesiologist should have accurate knowledge of any abnormality in the child's temperature during the 48 hours prior to operation, and especially in the immediately preoperative period. Body temperature below 97°F or over 100°F should be investigated before anesthesia is undertaken.

One can't quarrel with those who wish to measure temperature during all operations, provided they watch the monitor and act when action is indicated. The mere use of the thermometer, like other monitors, provides no guarantee of safety. Monitoring enthusiasts have been known to establish the monitor carefully and then never look at it.

Others watch it carefully as it registers 100°, 101°, 102°F and do nothing or take action which is entirely inadequate.

Several situations present increased risk of temperature change, and here temperature monitoring becomes mandatory. Situations that suggest increased danger of hyperthermia include patients whose temperature is elevated before operation (most frequently those having appendicitis), as well as those with latent sources of infection, such as the patient having low-grade genitourinary infection. Other candidates are children who have been held without fluids for more than four hours, those receiving blood, and those operated upon in a warm room or under excessively warm operating lights. Finally, any patient whose history arouses suspicion of malignant hyperthermia must be most carefully and continuously scrutinized.

Choice of Site for Temperature Monitoring

The chief sites presently used for monitoring body temperature are the rectum, esophagus, nose, axilla, and tympanic membrane.[18,19] The ideal site is the area that provides greatest accuracy, with the fewest disadvantages. These factors vary. The esophagus, tympanic membrane, and rectum are considered the most accurate noninvasive sites under favorable circumstances. However, the esophageal temperature will be altered by proximity to the end of the endotracheal tube in adjacent trachea, or by irrigation of a nasogastric tube, and tympanic and rectal temperatures can be affected by presence of wax or feces, respectively. A probe inserted along the floor of the nose is perhaps the most reliable of all. Each of these sites has some factor of trauma, however. A stiff probe easily causes nasal bleeding, and perforation of esophagus and rectum have both been known to occur.

An unusual type of injury has occurred several times in our experience when a rectal probe was used in patients who were lying on a cautery plate. Each of these patients sustained a painful linear burn of the perineum where the probe was in contact with the skin. This is believed to be due to an induction or reinforced electrical current following the line of the probe.[4] It is now believed important to use another site for the probe, at the greatest possible distance from any cautery plate, or to make sure that the probe cannot contact the patient's skin.

The axilla has become the standard site for temperature monitoring in several pediatric centers, including our own. If the bead-tipped probe, or, preferably, the flat metallic probe is used, it is virtually impossible to injure the patient. The accuracy of this site is surprisingly high. The probe is positioned as near to the axillary artery as possible, and held in place by tape or, preferably, a shielded EKG pad (Figures 8–1 and 8–2). The only mandatory feature here is that the arm must be kept at the patient's side, the axilla closed. We have found that there is an initial difference between esophageal and axillary temperatures of

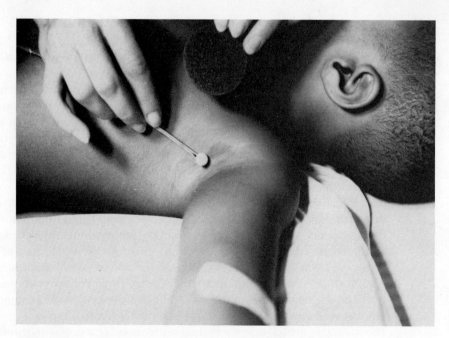

Figure 8–1
The axillary probe is placed directly over the axillary artery.

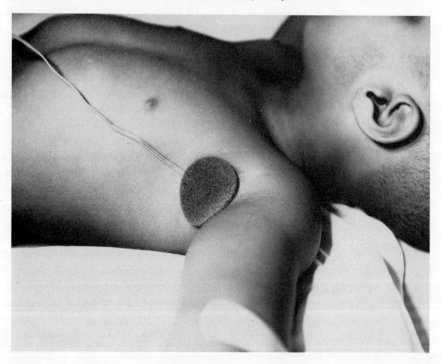

Figure 8–2
A firm pad holds the axillary probe in place. (The arm should then be held close to patient's side.)

approximately 1°F, which is reduced to less than 0.5°F within 30 minutes in average children. In small infants, we have been impressed by practically identical measurements at axilla and rectum taken throughout operation. At present, the axilla seems a reasonable site for monitoring in nearly all procedures, with the possible exception of open-heart procedures, during which both rectal and nasal temperatures have been monitored for maximum accuracy.

Thermometers

In caring for the sick, whether in the home or the hospital, measurement of body temperature has been accomplished most widely by the so-called "clinical," mercury-in-glass thermometer, which was introduced by Allbutt in 1870. Although this familiar object is generally shunned by anesthesiologists, it has the unique combination of extremely low cost and high accuracy. A price of 35 cents per thermometer renders it almost a disposable item by present medical standards. Unless obviously shattered, it never misfunctions, as do almost all other types of thermometers. In fact, the accuracy of each common clinical thermometer is such that any one of them can (and should) be taken to standardize any of the electric thermometers that are so popular in operating rooms today. In many of the United States, each clinical thermometer is inspected before sale and must be accurate to 0.2°F.

The clinical thermometer is four inches in length with a ¼-inch rounded bulb. It is calibrated in degrees Fahrenheit, 94° to 106°, and is designed for rectal use in infants and children. A variation upon this is the thermometer designed for premature infants, which is similar in construction, but calibrated from 84° to 108°F in order to allow for the lower temperatures sometimes found in these weaker infants. A third type, designed for sublingual use, has an elongated (1-inch), mercury bulb to allow more surface contact with the tongue and more prompt response.

Clinical thermometers are usually made as "nonretreating" thermometers, which means that near the base the mercury tube is angulated and constricted. When warmed, the mercury expands and pushes past the constriction, but on cooling, the mercury above the constriction does not "retreat" past the constriction until forcibly shaken. Therefore, it continues to indicate the highest temperature measured.

Obviously, the glass thermometer has a major disadvantage in its fragility, and it is definitely not recommended as a standard monitoring instrument. However, its availability and reliability are such that it still proves useful in limited situations, and, as a basic instrument, should be kept available at all times.

At present, the glass clinical thermometer has several uses during the operative period. It is used for final preanesthetic check within 30 minutes of anesthesia. One should be used to standardize any electronic thermometer and thermistor. During anesthesia, when an electric thermometer registers significant rise or fall of temperature, it is highly advisable to *check with a glass thermometer before taking active measures to warm or cool the patient.* Since battery-run devices may easily be 2° or 3°F in error, one could be led into definitely inappropriate measures that might aggravate the situation, as well as invite the usual hazards common to temperature-controlling measures (see below).

The standard clinical thermometer may reasonably be used during anesthesia if it is not left in sites where it could be broken or hidden from continuous observation of the anesthesiologist. During neurosurgical procedures, it may be inserted rectally for intermittent use, but should not be left in place. During inhalation anesthesia given by mask, a glass thermometer often may be safely placed in the patient's axilla with the upright thermometer in easy view of the anesthesiologist. During endotracheal anesthesia, the thermometer can be inserted in the patient's nostril. For all such uses, the blunt-tipped or rectal thermometer should be used, not the slender-tipped, oral model. If a nonbreakable material could be substituted for the glass, it would solve many of our problems. Such an instrument is in developmental stage, but has not reached a practical form. As a safety measure, one can apply a narrow strip of scotch tape along the length of the thermometer. As yet, no thermometer has broken in our experience.

During anesthesia, the temperature of children over 3 or 4 years of age is more apt to rise than fall. The nonretreating clinical thermometer giving continuous, accurate display of the maximum temperature, then, serves its purpose quite adequately. With small infants, however, where there is greater danger of rapidly falling temperature, the nonretreat type of thermometer is less suitable, for it does not show decreasing temperatures unless shaken. For this situation, a glass thermometer in which the mercury *does* retreat is more useful.

For operating room use, by far the greatest call at present is for electronic thermometers, powered either by batteries or electricity. Several varieties, produced by a host of manufacturers, are now available, most of them constructed as resistance-measuring devices built on the principle of the Wheatstone bridge, with a sensing element consisting of a seven-foot wire bearing a thermistor tip. The thermistor is a thermally sensitive resistor made from compressed metal oxide powders and fused into a terminal bead, appropriate for use in rectum or esophagus. Elongated metal probes, needle probes, and flattened oval probes are also fashioned for special sites. Instruments built in this way include those made by Dupaco, Medtronic, Yellow Springs, Ivac, and others.

Measurement of temperature by thermocouple is also used for clinical monitoring. A thermocouple consists of a pair of wires of different composition welded together at one pair of ends. This point of union, called the measuring junction, responds to a change in temperature by generating electromotive force, measurable by a galvanometer. The instrument recently introduced by Radiation Systems, Inc. for tympanic membrane thermometry and another thermometer under construction by Bailey Instruments are built on this principle. The Wheatstone bridge is not a required component here. One advantage of the thermocouple lies in the fact that the sensing unit may be as small as the head of a pin.

The above instruments are battery-powered, and have meter readout design. Thermometers with digital readouts have been constructed, such as that made by Digitec and RdF Corporation. This is basically a resistance thermistor Wheatstone bridge system, to which a potentiometer and electromechanical digital display have been added. (It is expected that the electromechanical type of digital display will soon be displaced by a more reliable electronic digital readout.) The unit is powered by house current rather than battery.

Thus far, the electric instruments have proved less reliable than the simple clinical thermometers. Unless fixed to a solid body such as an anesthesia machine, they are easily traumatized and malfunction varies in direct proportion to maltreatment. Even when they are properly handled, their accuracy decreases with use and age, and most instruments require considerable checking and recalibration. Faulty performance may be due to poor calibration or other disfunctions within the detecting cabinet, or may be due to the probe, and both should be tested before use. For practical use, most electrically powered thermometers appear very similar, each using a detecting cabinet of similar size, with probes which may be interchangeable between several different products.

The probe used most frequently for anesthesia is the pliable plastic cord with terminal sensing bead. These probes can be dangerously stiff, and must be used with care. One has recently appeared for sale which is particularly stiff and pointed and should not be used at all for any body orifice.

Bead-ended probes may be carefully inserted into rectum, nostril, or esophagus and are also used for axillary monitoring. However, the flat, rounded probe is preferable for this and other skin surfaces (Figure 8–3). Needle probes may be used for muscle temperature when special information is desired, but their use is not justified for routine purposes. Most electrically powered thermometers may be connected to recording devices.

In addition to the frequently mentioned need for greater reliability, the addition of an alarm system would be a valuable innovation for these monitors, so that there would be no chance of a dangerous temperature change passing unnoticed. Alarms have been incorporated into bassinet monitoring systems, and are urgently needed in the operating room. Such a device is now under production at Bailey Instruments. It would seem reasonable to set the alarms at 96° and 100°F.

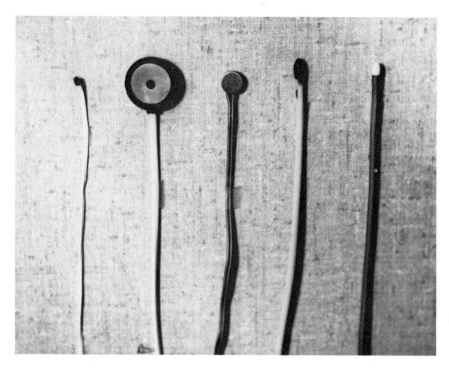

Figure 8–3
Thermistor probes. Left to right: flexible probe for tympanic temperature (Dupaco); flat skin temperature probe (Dupaco); skin probe (Yellow Springs); round tip probes for esophageal, rectal, or nasal route (Dupaco and Yellow Springs).

EVALUATION OF DATA

Problems in temperature regulation, like many others in medicine, may best be managed in a three-step process consisting of measurement, evaluation, and therapy. Methods of measurement and therapy, or control, of body temperature have at least been explored, but the rationale for suiting the type of treatment to the nature of the lesion remains vague. Although specific criteria are not available for all situations, some guidelines may be suggested.

The best start in evaluating temperature change is to make a practice of charting it at frequent, regular intervals during the operative period. It is advisable to have a regular column for this purpose in all charts used for pediatric anesthesia.

Some variability of body temperature must be expected, but standards should be established determining the degree of acceptable variation. It has proved helpful to regard the range between 96° and 100°F as the safe zone during anesthesia. When either limit is passed, suitable steps should be taken.

Several factors must be considered in judging whether a situation is to be taken as a note of warning, or as a signal for immediate interruption of the operation and heroic therapy. Among these are the following:

1. Direction and degree of temperature change. Cooling of patients, though more common, is less to be feared than is overheating. Cooling during anesthesia causes cardiorespiratory depression, reduces enzyme activity, prolongs recovery, and, when carried to an extreme (below 85° to 88°F), may induce ventricular fibrillation. However, irreversible changes do not occur until tissues are frozen. Hyperthermia, on the other hand, acts more rapidly and, in the vicinity of 108°F, causes irreversible brain damage.[20]

2. Rate of temperature change. Obviously, a rapid fall or rise in temperature is more significant than one that occurs over a period of several hours. When the change is abrupt, one should look for such specific causes as the use of cold blood or a faulty heating unit. It should be emphasized that cooling usually occurs as a passive phenomenon with decreasing speed, while the process of hyperthermia appears to feed upon itself and accelerates markedly as it advances.

3. Physical characteristics of patient. The size, age, and vigor of the child, as well as the disease he is suffering from, have important bearing on the significance of temperature changes encountered. Similarly, the operation underway, its expected duration, and blood transfusion requirement are to be considered in planning treatment. If the temperature of a weak, 4-year-old child undergoing removal of a large abdominal tumor falls to 94°F, one could expect that subsequent blood loss, manipulation, and transfusion might result in disaster. However, in a strong 12-year-old undergoing a relatively atraumatic procedure, this degree of heat loss would be of little consequence.

METHODS OF CONTROLLING BODY TEMPERATURE

When temperature changes are discovered or expected in pediatric surgery, there is a widespread tendency to place the child on a temperature-controlling water mattress and go ahead with the operation. Although this technique frequently does succeed, it must be emphasized that one should not depend primarily upon temperature-controlling devices that actively warm or cool patients. Most of these devices, whether water blanket, air blower, or heating lamp, entail definite hazards. It is preferable, whenever possible, to attempt by nonphysical means to correct existing hypothermic or hyperthermic abnormalities or to prevent their occurrence by other methods. Since there are numerous contributing factors, there are many methods available. If these are rationally employed, heating and cooling devices will serve more properly for supplemental use or often will be completely unnecessary.

Preventive Methods

Among the many factors that contribute to undesirable temperature changes in operative patients, one must consider preexisting hypothermia and hyperthermia of the child during surgical preparation, premedication, anesthetic agent and technique, temperature of irrigating fluids, temperature and amount of intravenous fluid and blood, type of wound, and duration of operation.

Atropine, usually administered 40 to 60 minutes before the operation, promotes heat retention. When a child already has a temperature elevation (as with acute appendicitis), it is preferable to delay administration of atropine until actual induction of anesthesia.

As previously noted, environmental factors should be suited to individual needs. The warmth of a child being transported may be ensured by adequate covering, but operating rooms should be under accurate control. After investigating the problem of room temperature for operations on neonates, Martin found 80°F to be optimum for normal neonates and recommended 85°F for premature infants (unpublished data). It would seem reasonable to use this temperature during preparation of the infant and then, for general comfort and efficiency, reduce it slightly after the infant has been draped. Relative humidity must be at least 50 percent, and, if possible, the air conditioning should be run at reduced rate, preferably at an airflow rate of about 20 lf/m.

Protective Covering of Infants

Undoubtedly, the greatest heat loss occurs when an infant lies exposed on the operating table during preparation for operation.[12,21] To prevent cooling at this time and throughout the remainder of the procedure, every attempt should be made to retain the child's own body heat. An effective and safe method of protecting infants is to wrap their limbs in protective covering. Sheet wadding, like that used to line plaster casts, has proved excellent for this purpose as it serves several functions.[22] It protects the tissues from mechanical or thermal trauma, assists in immobilizing the child, and reduces heat loss. Considerable heat loss can occur through the bare scalp of a small infant; consequently, the infant's head should be covered. Stockinette is excellent for this purpose. Better methods of retaining heat by covering the body surface with plastic drapes, or by adding plastic or silver foil outside the protective sheet wadding, are under investigation.

Fluids used during operation may precipitate rapid and even fatal complications. Although irrigating solutions should play only contributing roles, rapid intravenous infusion of cold blood is known to have caused cardiac standstill. Use of warmed blood is believed mandatory when patients receive large amounts of blood rapidly. A guideline to follow is to warm blood if one-third of the blood volume is or may be replaced.

Anesthetic management may play a part in both cause and treatment of thermal complications.[20,23] Halothane and relaxants act to increase heat loss; cyclopropane acts to reduce it. Open, semiopen, and nonrebreathing techniques promote heat loss, especially if gases are not humidified, while closed techniques act to retain body heat and moisture.[12,24] Pulmonary ventilation is of extreme importance in the management of patients during hyperthermic crisis. These patients rapidly develop marked metabolic acidosis, and ventilation should be increased to approximately three times the usual volume to overcome excessive CO_2 production.

Supplemental Warming and Cooling Devices

Probably the first warming device brought into the operating room was the standard hot water bottle. If a temperature of 103°F is not exceeded, the hot water bottle can be effective, but the speed with which this device loses heat and the high incidence of body burns make it definitely unsatisfactory except in an emergency. In such an emergency, for greater safety, invert an instrument tray over two hot water bags, making a small platform on which the neonate lies, warmed by, but out of contact with, the source of heat.

To provide continuous and controllable warmth (or cooling) during anesthesia, water-circulating mattresses have been widely used. The first of these, designed by McQuiston,[31] was a mattress 20 × 30 inches with an inlet through which water at the desired temperature could be added from a suspended irrigation can and an outlet for drainage. This was first used for cooling children during cardiac surgery, but is equally useful for warming infants and children. When in use, it should be covered by at least one thickness of a blanket or its equal. The danger of burning patients is great, since the repeated addition of hot water increases the opportunity for error.[5,25]

Somewhat more versatile is the unit which warms or cools fluid to a designated temperature and pumps it through coils of tubing that are incorporated into blankets of various sizes.[21] This combination has had wide commercial distribution. It is effective and, in some situations, essential, and should be available in every hospital where pediatric surgery is performed.

Because of the rapid developments in this field, it would be unwise to recommend any specific make of heating-cooling device, but certain criteria are important in the choice. They include the following:

1. The machine should contain both heating and cooling units and pump.
2. One thermometer should read the temperature of the fluid in the central unit; another, the temperature of the mattress where it contacts the patient.
3. All construction must be sturdy and shockproof.
4. Mattresses should be varied in size and weight, and should be durable, resistant, and easily repaired if damaged.
5. The machine should be quiet when in action.

As an additional refinement in temperature-controlling machines, a servomechanism may be attached to the unit just described.[26] This "brain" picks up the patient's temperature by a sensing probe to skin or rectum and then adjusts the heating and cooling mechanisms until the patient's temperature reaches the level for which the device has been programmed. Although this appears to represent an advanced step, performance has not been sufficiently reliable for enthusiastic acceptance. It appears less hazardous to operate a water-circulating mattress by manual control and to use an independent thermometer for temperature measurement and personal judgment as the computer.

Although pads and blankets warmed by means of electric coils have been popular in American homes, fear of faulty wiring has prevented their admission to our operating rooms. The British use them and find them effective.[23] One obvious disadvantage is that even if they could be made to be entirely safe, they do not provide cooling as does a water mattress.

Roe and Santulli have more recently investigated the use of an electrically controlled rectal probe for maintaining body heat.[12] This proved effective in dogs, but it would seem inadvisable to attempt to introduce an appreciable amount of heat through such a limited area.

If an infant must be exposed, it is natural to look for methods of keeping him warm that do not require physical contact. Both air blowers and heating lamps have been advocated. An ordinary hair dryer, as used in many American homes, will deliver a jet of air at room temperature or heated to temperatures varying from 103°–140°F. This instrument and variations upon its basic structure have been employed as supplemental devices for use during operative procedures. There are obvious dangers and disadvantages. Standard precautions must be observed with the heating coil, and the air temperature should never exceed 103°F. It is preferable not to direct the airstream toward a sterile surface or into the operating field. Actually, its best use might be for supplemental warmth delivered under draped-off areas. Neurosurgical procedures have provided opportunities for this approach, but the actual use has been limited. In England and Sweden, warm air has been employed, generated by heating units outside of the operating room and blown in via tubular conduits.

Observations that the exposed infant's heat loss is largely due to radiation [27] have resulted in attempts to meet this by use of radiant energy in the form of infrared lamps or similar sources.[8,13,28] Bassinets thus adapted are constructed with a plastic hood containing a heating element. A sensing device on the infant's abdomen activates the heating unit to vary its intensity as needed. Both ends of the bassinet are open to allow access for exchange transfusion or other prolonged therapeutic maneuvers that usually involve exposure of the infant. These bassinets are relatively safe and are recommended for use in nursing divisions and recovery room care, but do not allow sufficient access for use during major surgical procedures.

Infrared lamps and radiant heat sources mounted above open-top bassinets for use in the delivery area and treatment room are now available. When they are used, one must observe strict precautions as to distance between lamp and patient and duration of exposure. The temperature at a point 27 inches away from the lamp is 40°F, but at a point 18 inches away from the lamp it is 140°F! Based on clinical experience, Eastwood's recommendation is for exposure of not more than 15 minutes at a distance of 27 inches (unpublished data).

It must be emphasized that: (1) heating instruments are subject to faulty operation; (2) tolerance of normal tissues to degrees of heat, distance from source, and time of exposure have not been determined; and (3) any tissue that has less than normal circulation will tolerate less thermal trauma than tissues with normal circulation.[5,25,29,30]

Internal Methods of Temperature Control

Measures to be undertaken for hyperpyrexic patients should be suited to each situation. Several examples are outlined at the end of this article. With minor temperature rise, one starts with simple methods of *environmental* cooling, reducing room temperature, increasing air flow, and uncovering the patient, then proceeds with active *external cooling*, which begins with application of ice to exposed areas, especially neck, groins, axillae, and scalp. The ice may be held in plastic bags, or applied directly to the skin, and will not injure the tissues unless pieces of ice stay in contact with the same area for more than 10 minutes or the patient is allowed to lie on them. A most effective cooling method is to soak the sheet under the patient with ice water if it can be done without encroaching upon the operating field. If a cooling mattress is already in place under the patient, it should be used, but it is an inefficient method for real emergencies. It is not advisable to attempt to move a patient onto such a mattress in the middle of an operation.

For hyperthermic children, some enthusiasts advocate stopping the operation and immersing the child in a tub of ice. In some situations, such as an operation to repair a cleft palate, this is possible, but it would be less desirable during thoracotomy or spine fusion, and in general, seems a poor method to rely upon when others are more practical. During laparotomy or thoracotomy, irrigating the viscera would cool the patient more promptly with considerably less confusion.

Internal cooling is by far the most effective method. The stomach and rectum usually offer easy avenues of approach for internal irrigation. When any patient's temperature exceeds 101°F, it is our custom to pass a nasogastric tube for this purpose. A liter of saline is poured into a pan of ice and irrigation is carried on until the temperature falls. Cold intravenous fluids have been advocated, but, if given in sufficient quantities to be effective, could dangerously overload the patient. In real emergencies, chilled saline poured into peritoneal or chest cavities will bring prompt response. For this purpose, several liters of saline or electrolyte solution should be kept refrigerated at all times.

Additional Measures in Extreme Hyperthermia

High fever of any origin causes an increasing degree of metabolic and respiratory acidosis,[9,14] and specific measures to counteract this are essential. Respiratory ventilation should be augmented so that alveolar exchange is at least three times normal. Blood gases should be drawn to determine the progress of the acid-base balance, and sodium bicarbonate should be administered in generous and repeated amounts. The usual dosage recommended is 4 mEq/kg for each 0.1 pH below 7.35 (arterial blood). Since it is important to reduce heat production in every possible way, anesthesia should be continued to prevent the increased activity of awakening. Since halothane is suspected as one of the etiological agents in malignant hyperthermia, this should be discontinued.[1] Probably the best method is to use 50-50 N_2O—O_2, thiopental, and d-tubocurare. D-tubocurare will not release a patient from the spasm of succinylcholine if the patient has true malignant hyperthermia,[15] but the above combination remains indicated in all cases of extreme hyperthermia.

Finally, it should be stated that if any patient develops marked, continuous, generalized muscle contractions at any time during operation, maximum precautions should be instituted at once. If operation had not been started, it is best to postpone it and undertake it later under morphine, nitrous oxide d-tubocurare, or a neuroplegic such as Innovar.[17] If operation is already underway, one should prepare to take all the measures described above, and terminate operation if feasible.

ILLUSTRATIVE CASES

To emphasize suggested steps in temperature control, procedures are outlined in various types of situations.

Case 1. *Premature infant undergoing repair of intestinal obstruction.*
  1. Adjust the operating-room temperature to 85°F, relative humidity to 50 percent, and, if possible, reduce airflow rate to 20 lf/m.
  2. Transport the infant to the operating room in a warm, covered bassinet. Keep him in the bassinet until the surgeons are scrubbed and present inside the operating room.
  3. Wrap the infant's limbs in sheet wadding while he is still in the bassinet.
  4. Prepare a water-circulating mattress, covering the mattress with four thicknesses of sheet. Warm the mattress to 100°F.
  5. Place the covered infant on the operating table for anesthetic induction.
  6. Use an infrared lamp during cutdown and surgical prep.
  7. Uncover only the area required for operation.
  8. Use nonvolatile liquids for skin preparation.
  9. Fix one thermistor in the rectum, another on the skin near the liver.
  10. Chart both temperatures during operation.

Case 2. *Two-year-old facing removal of abdominal tumor and possible hemorrhage.*
  1. Warm the room to 75°F.
  2. Use a water-circulating mattress (manual control) with an esophageal or axillary thermometer probe.
  3. Attach an electrocardiogram to warn of cardiac depression.
  4. Buffer blood and warm it by standing bags in a 100°F bath or by attaching an additional length of tubing to infusion and submerging it in tub of water 90°–100°F.

Case 3. *Six-month-old infant undergoing neurosurgical operation whose temperature falls to 94°F.*
  1. Warm the room to 85°F.
  2. Warm the blood.
  3. Cover the patient with prewarmed blankets.
  4. Blow warmed air under drapes (protect skin).
  5. Humidify the anesthetic gases.
  6. Reduce the gas flow to minimal acceptable flow.
  7. Warm the mattress to 100°F.

Case 4. *Ten-year-old with ruptured appendix with a temperature of 104°F before operation.*
  1. Pass nasogastric tube.

2. Start intravenous infusion (plasma or electrolyte mixture).
3. Start antibiotics.
4. Delay premedication and operation until hydration is confirmed by the passage of normal urine.
5. Reduce the operating-room temperature to 70°F.
6. For the operation, place the infant on a cooling blanket and induce anesthesia with intravenous barbiturate and halothane.
7. Monitor axillary temperature. If it is 102°F or above after induction, sponge the infant with alcohol or ice water until his temperature is under 102°F. Continue to monitor temperature during and after operation.
8. Watch for tremors, muscle rigidity, and respiratory abnormality.

Case 5. *Hyperthermia during operation.*
If rectal temperature exceeds 99°F:
1. Reduce the room temperature.
2. Uncover the patient where possible.
3. Employ semiopen or nonrebreathing anesthetic technique.
4. Increase ventilation to three times basal need.
5. Use a cooling blanket, if one is already in place.
6. Run intravenous fluids at 8–10 ml/kg/hr.
If temperature exceeds 102°F:
1. Notify the surgeon and request all reasonable speed.
2. Apply ice in plastic bags to the patient's limbs, head, neck, and groin, as possible.
3. Pass a nasogastric tube. Irrigate with iced saline.
4. Soak the sheet under the patient with iced fluid.
If temperature exceeds 104°F:
1. Stop the operation and keep the patient asleep with thiopental and d-tubocurare.
2. If the thoracic or abdominal cavity is exposed, irrigate it with cooled, sterile solutions, or with room-temperature solutions, if cool solutions are not available.
3. If the body cavities are not exposed and the patient's temperature is 108°F or above, the abdomen may be opened for the purpose of irrigation. Otherwise, remove the drapes and apply ice all over the body.
4. Give intravenous procaine amide, 1 mg/kg.[32]

Case 6. *Neurosurgical patient 3 days postcraniotomy whose temperature is 105°F.*
1. Aspirin.
2. Fluids.
3. Cooling mattress, temperature 95°F.
4. Thorazine 2mg. IV, p.r.n.

    5.   Expose the skin surface to air and electric fan.

    6.   Sponge patient's body with alcohol to shivering threshold.

Case 7.   *Eight-year-old awakening from 3-hour orthopedic procedure under halothane anesthesia, shivering violently, temperature 97.3°F.*

    1.   Continue intravenous infusion.

    2.   Administer morphine 4 mg. IV, stat, to control shivering.

    3.   Cover him with blankets.

SUMMARY

Although there is an increased incidence of complications related to body temperature in pediatric surgery, the overenthusiastic use of poorly controlled devices has resulted in many injuries.

As a practical guide to measurement and regulation of body temperature, the following points are emphasized: (1) monitor temperature by observing many clinical signs, as well as by thermometer; (2) take preventive measures to control heat loss, rather than rely on heating devices; (3) body tissues are damaged at much lower temperature when circulation is reduced by disease or position; and (4) for rapid cooling during operating-room emergencies, internal methods are more effective than surface methods.

REFERENCES

1. Britt, B.A., and Kalow, W.: Malignant hyperthermia: Aetiology unknown. *Canad Anaesth Soc J* 17:316–330, 1970.

2. Britt, B.A., and Kalow, W.: Malignant hyperthermia: A statistical review. *Canad Anaesth Soc J* 17:293–315, 1970.

3. Aherne, W., and Hull, D.: Site of heat production in the newborn infant. *Proc Roy Soc Med* 57:1172–1173, 1964.

4. Battig, C.G.: Electrosurgical burn injuries and their prevention. *JAMA,* 204:1025–1029, 1968.

5. Crino, M.H., and Nagel, E.L.: Thermal burns caused by warming blankets in the operating room. *Anesthesiology* 29:149–150, 1968.

6. Adamsons, K., Gandy, G.M., and James, L.S.: The influence of thermal factors upon oxygen consumption of the newborn human infant. *J Pediat* 66:495–508, 1965.

7. Adamsons, K., and Towell, M.E.: Thermal homeostasis in the fetus and newborn. *Anesthesiology* 26:531–548, 1965.

8. Agate, F.J., Sr., and Silverman, W.A.: The control of body temperature in the small newborn infant by low-energy infrared radiation. *Pediatrics* 31:725–733, 1963.

9. Challoner, D.R.: Hypermetabolic states. *Lancet,* 2:681–683, 1966.

10. Silverman, W.A., Fertig, J.W., and Berger, A.P.: The influence of the thermal environment upon the survival of newly born premature infants. *Pediatrics* 22:876–886, 1958.

11. Silverman, W.A., Sinclair, S.C., and Scopes, J.W.: Regulation of body temperature in pediatric surgery. *J Pediat Surg* 1:321–329, 1966.
12. Roe, C.F., Santulli, T.V., and Blair, C.S.: Heat loss in infants during general anesthesia and operations. *J Pediat Surg* 1:266–275, 1966.
13. Friedman, F., Adams, F.H., and Emmanouilides, G.: Regulation of body temperature of premature infants with low energy radiant heat. *J Pediatrics* 70:270–273, 1967.
14. Stern, W., Lees, M.H., and Leduc, J.: Environmental temperature, oxygen consumption, and catecholamine excretion in newborn infants. *Pediatrics* 36:367–373, 1965.
15. Cody, J.R.: Muscle rigidity following administration of succinylcholine. *Anesthesiology* 29:159–162, 1968.
16. Harrison, G.G., et al: Anaesthetic-induced malignant hyperthermia and a method for its prediction. *Brit J Anaesth* 41:844–855, 1969.
17. Relton, J.E.S., et al: Generalized muscular hypertonicity associated with general anesthesia: A suggested anaesthetic management. *Can Anaesth Soc J* 14:22–25, 1967.
18. Benzinger, M.: Tympanic thermometry in surgery and anesthesia. *JAMA* 209: 1207–1211, 1969.
19. Benzinger, T.H.: Human thermostat. *Yearbook Science and Technology*. New York: McGraw-Hill, 1963.
20. Hogg, S., and Renwick, W.: Hyperpyrexia during anesthesia. *Canad Anaesth Soc J* 13:429–437, 1966.
21. Stephen, C.R., et al: Body temperature regulation during anesthesia in infants and children. *JAMA* 174:15–79, 1960.
22. Smith, R.M.: *Anesthesia for Infants and Children,* ed 3. St. Louis: C.V. Mosby, 1968.
23. Wilton, T.N.P., and Wilson, F.: *Neonatal Anesthesia.* Philadelphia: F.A. Davis, 1965.
24. Relton, J.E.S., et al: Hyperpyrexia in association with general anesthesia in children. *Canad Anaesth Soc J* 13:419–425, 1966.
25. Scott, S.M.: Thermal blanket injury in the operating room. *Arch Surg* 94:181, 1967.
26. Fuson, R.L., and Stephen, C.R.: Servo temperature control instrument for use in clinical medicine. *Surg Gynec Obstet* 117:636–640, 1963.
27. Oliver, T.K., Jr.: Temperature regulation and heat production in the newborn. *Pediat Clin N Amer* 12:765–779, 1965.
28. Levison, H., Linsae, L., and Swyer, P.R.: A comparison of infra-red and convective heating for newborn infants. *Lancet* 2:1346–1348, 1966.
29. Collins, H.A., Stahlman, M., and Scott, H.W.: Occurrence of subcutaneous fat necrosis in infant following induced hypothermia used as adjuvant in cardiac surgery. *Ann Surg* 138:880–885, 1953.
30. Lebowitz, M.H.: Gangrene of a thumb following use of photoelectric plethysmograph during anesthesia. *Anesthesiology* 32:164–169, 1970.
31. McQuiston, W.O.: Anesthesia in cardiac surgery. *Arch Surg* 61:892–899, 1950.
32. Strobel, G.E., and Bianchi, C.P.: An in-vitro model of anesthetic hypertonic hyperpyrexia-caffeine-induced muscle contractures. *Anesthesiology* 35:465–473, 1971.

9

Fluids, Electrolytes, and Intravenous Nutrition

Robert M. Filler, M.D.

Angelo J. Eraklis, M.D.

John B. Das, M.D.

The purpose of this chapter is to present the principles of intravenous fluid therapy which we have found useful in treating infants and children ill from a variety of surgically correctable causes. Methods of short-term standard parenteral fluid therapy and methods of long-term intravenous nutrition will be discussed.

SHORT-TERM INTRAVENOUS FLUID THERAPY

Methods

Venous Cannulation

The site and method chosen for venous cannulation depend on the size and age of the child, the indications for intravenous therapy, the relative hazards of a particular method, and the experience of the therapist.

For routine intravenous therapy in a child of any age, delivery of fluids through a needle, either a standard needle or a scalp vein needle, is recommended because fewer complications result than when other cannulas are used. In the older child, many veins are suitable for vene-puncture, but in children under 3 months of age, scalp veins are most commonly used. Techniques for inserting a needle into a small scalp vein have been well described, but several points should be empha-sized. Before venepuncture, a large area on the scalp should be shaved so that the skin can be properly prepared and tape can be applied to secure the needle in the vein after the vein is successfully entered. A small electric razor is useful to avoid superficial lacerations com-monly caused by razor blades. Adequate lighting and an assistant re-straining the infant are essential. The most obvious scalp veins, the superficial temporal veins, are not necessarily the best, and often veins which are less tortuous, such as those on the forehead, remain intu-bated for longer periods before infiltration. Care must be taken that the temporal artery is not mistaken for a vein. The plastic wings which are attached to the short, blunt, scalp vein needle aid in fixation which is readily accomplished with half-inch tape. The use of a small protective cover such as an inverted paper cup over the scalp vein needle is also helpful in preventing accidental dislodgement. A single scalp vein often can be used for several days before infiltration occurs, about the same length of time that fluids can be administered through a cutdown. By alternating sites on the scalp, infusions can be maintained for several weeks by this method.

Although the needle technique is satisfactory for most stable clin-ical situations, during major operative procedures, or whenever large volumes of fluid or blood are required rapidly, a softer plastic catheter with a blunt tip which can be inserted a distance into the lumen of the vein is more reliable since infiltration is less likely. Venous cannulation with such a catheter can be accomplished percutaneously or by cut-down technique. When venous cannulation is indicated in the newborn, cutdown is usually necessary, and the saphenous vein at the ankle is the preferred site because anatomic variations of this vein at this loca-tion are almost nonexistent. Cannulation of the saphenous vein is almost always successful, even though the vein cannot be palpated or seen until the skin is incised. In addition, the sizable lumen of the saphenous vein will accept a catheter of adequate diameter in all pa-tients. For example, in most full-term newborns, a number 18 catheter can be used and, even in the smallest premature infants, a number 20 catheter will pass. Saphenous vein cutdown is commonly employed in older patients as well and is a reliable site for cannulation in the pa-tient in shock whose peripheral veins are collapsed and not visible. An acceptable procedure for saphenous vein cutdown is shown in Fig-ure 9–1.

Two basic methods are available for percutaneous cannulation. In one, venepuncture is performed with a hollow needle through which an eight-inch-long plastic catheter is passed into the vein. With this method, the long catheter can be passed centrally into the superior vena cava. In the second method, venepuncture is performed with a

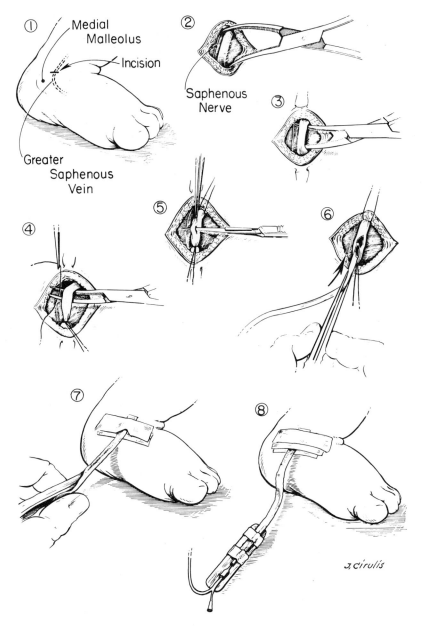

Figure 9–1

A method for saphenous vein cutdown. (1) The saphenous vein is found at the superior, anterior margin of the medial malleolus. (2) Transverse incision is developed by blunt dissection when the vein is not apparent. The hemostat is inserted to the level of the periosteum and the full thickness of subcutaneous tissue in which the vein courses is elevated. Dissection into this pad exposes the vein. (3 and 4) Vein dissected circumferentially and distal end ligated. A retention suture superiorly allows the vein to be stretched. (5) An incision is made on the anterior wall with a no. 11 blade. (6) A catheter, previously beveled, is introduced and the upper suture tied with care to avoid occluding the tubing. The skin incision is closed. Antibiotic ointment and a very small gauze dressing are applied. (7 and 8) Tincture of benzoin is applied to the skin about the ankle and tape placed to fix the catheter. Proper taping avoids the need for a foot board. The intravenous line is attached to the catheter and fixed to a tongue blade to avoid kinking and perforation by the metal adapter.

hollow needle which, except for its exposed distal point, lies within the lumen of a short segment of plastic tubing. After successful venepuncture, the needle is withdrawn, leaving the larger-caliber plastic tube within the lumen of the vein. To secure the position of a plastic catheter, a single strip of half-inch tape should be applied longitudinally to the skin three to four inches proximal to the entry site of the catheter and the shaft of the exposed portion of plastic tubing (Figure 9–1).

In many clinical situations, venous cannulation in an upper extremity is preferable to one in a lower limb. Infusions in the upper extremity veins are indicated when (1) blood flow through the inferior vena cava may be interrupted, as, for example, during resection of a Wilms' tumor or after severe trauma; (2) the position of the foot and

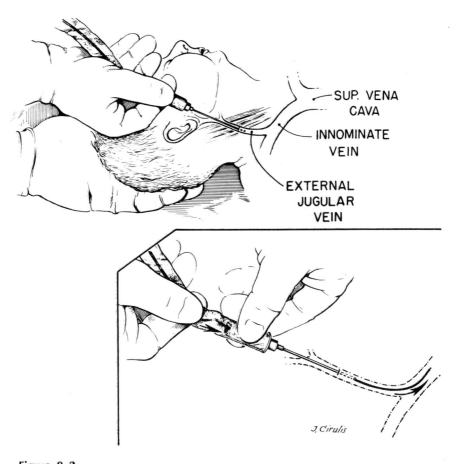

SUP. VENA
CAVA

INNOMINATE
VEIN

EXTERNAL
JUGULAR
VEIN

J. Cirulis

Figure 9–2
Percutaneous intubation of external jugular vein. The infant's head is extended and turned to the opposite side. The head is supported by an assistant in a dependent position to fill the vein. Sometimes compression of the vein at the clavicle will aid in filling. After venepuncture, the plastic catheter is advanced for the distance estimated to place the catheter centrally. The free flow of blood indicates its central location which can be confirmed radiographically.

leg precludes adequate flow through an ankle vein, as for example when an infant is in the lithotomy position; or (3) central venous pressure measurements are necessary. In addition, upper-extremity infusions are used in most older children because upper-extremity veins are less likely to produce symptomatic superficial phlebitis, are easier to cannulate percutaneously, and are large enough to accept a large-bore catheter. The cephalic and basilic veins at the antecubital fossa are the preferred sites for infusion in the upper extremity. Since these vessels are smaller than the saphenous vein, they are often difficult to cannulate in the smallest infants, and cutdown may be necessary. In the very young, the brachial artery may be easily mistaken for a vein, but this error can usually be avoided by limiting dissection to the subcutaneous fat superficial to the deep fascia. Occasionally, even the smallest available intravenous tubing cannot be passed into a vein. In this event, the tip of the plastic tube may be tapered to a smaller size by stretching.

In the event that extremity veins are not available, catheters can be inserted into external jugular veins, often percutaneously. This site of venous cannulation also provides a relatively straight route to the superior vena cava. Jugular vein cannulation is especially useful for central venous pressure monitoring in infants or small children, since attempts to pass venous catheters centrally through the subclavian vein from the arm often fail. The method of insertion of a central venous catheter into the neck of an infant in shown in Figure 9–2.

In some intensive care nurseries, the umbilical artery and vein are used for infusing fluids. We do not use these vessels in our surgical patients because of the potential hazards and interference with the operative field during abdominal surgery.

Infusion Circuit

Since most intravenous fluids are supplied in units of at least 250 ml, inadvertent overinfusion is possible if fluid is delivered directly from such large reservoirs. To avoid this hazard, special infusion sets which place a calibrated burette and drip chamber in the infusion circuit between the fluid reservoir and the patient are used. The burette can be accurately filled from the reservoir to any desired volume. If the reservoir hangs from an intravenous stand above the burette, one must be certain that the tubing connecting these two chambers is securely clamped to prevent undetected filling of the burette from the reservoir. This accident can also be prevented by placing the reservoir bottle below the level of the burette. In children under 5 years of age, 100-ml burettes are used, but when used in infants, they are never filled to more than 50 cc. In older children, 250-ml burettes are satisfactory. When the burette empties, a float valve at the base of the burette closes. This valve prevents air embolism and also tends to prevent blood from backing up into the tubing. An additional feature of these intravenous delivery sets is the drip chamber which has been designed to deliver a drop whose volume approximates $\frac{1}{60}$ ml. A count of the number of drops per minute is therefore a reliable estimate of the number of milliliters infused per hour, a flow rate easily confirmed by monitoring the hourly fluid level in the calibrated burette.

Because of the rapid rate of water turnover and the relatively narrow range of urine-concentrating ability in the infant, it is usually desirable to administer a day's requirement of fluid at a relatively constant rate over a period of twenty-four hours. A continuous infusion will also avoid clotting within the lumen of the needle or catheter. Constant infusion pumps can be used to insure a constant infusion rate, but they should be used cautiously. If the patient is left unattended, infiltration may be associated with massive extravasation of fluid, since the pump can generate infusion pressures far in excess of the resistance of the subcutaneous tissues.

Complications

Extravasation of fluid is the most common complication of intravenous therapy and is more often associated with infusions given through needles than those given through plastic catheters. Such infiltrations are usually not troublesome, and, unless the infusate contains an irritating medication or chemical, large volumes of fluid are quickly absorbed from tissues without sequelae. However, serious problems may arise when extravasated fluid collects in certain locations such as the volar aspect of the wrist, where the superficial veins are in close proximity to the fascia. Infiltration into the closed space beneath the fascia has caused extensive soft-tissue loss and hand paralysis. A policy of never using volar wrist veins for intravenous infusions has been adopted at our institution. Other complications from extravasation have occurred when intravenous fluid has accumulated within the peritoneum, thorax, or pericardium.

Superficial localized phlebitis and venous thrombosis are other common complications of therapy and are characterized by pain, redness, and swelling at the site of venepuncture extending along the vein a variable distance proximally beyond the tip of the cannula. This inflammatory reaction is not usually due to microorganisms, but probably is caused by the irritating properties of the intravenous infusate and/or the cannula. Attempts to prevent this reaction by adding heparin or steroids to the intravenous solution have not been successful. To eliminate this complication, buffering of intravenous fluids which have an acid pH has been suggested. Venous thromboses in extremity veins of children secondary to intravenous therapy may produce swelling, but are almost never associated with pulmonary emboli. To decrease the incidence of sterile inflammation, venous thrombosis, and perforation, silicone rubber catheters are now used whenever possible for cannulation since they are softer and less reactive than ones of polyethylene plastic. Catheters of silicone rubber are not currently available in percutaneous intubation sets, but all sizes are available for insertion by the cutdown technique.

Sepsis is the most serious complication of intravenous fluid therapy. The longer a needle or catheter remains in the vein, the greater is the risk of local and systemic sepsis. The following precautions should be routinely observed even when administering short-term intravenous therapy: remove all hair from the area around the skin entry site; prepare the skin site with a bactericidal and fungicidal solution (povidone-iodine, Betadine); employ strict aseptic technique for cutdowns; use sterile gloves when inserting plastic catheters percutaneously; apply povidone-iodine ointment to the catheter entry site in the skin to kill organisms which might gain entry to the bloodstream along the tract of the catheter; change infusion sites every 72 hours, or more frequently if signs of local inflammation develop; discard intravenous infusion tubing daily; and do not infuse fluid from any bottle which has been in use or unsealed for more than eight hours.

Arterial thrombosis, with resultant tissue necrosis, occasionally occurs when infusions are given into a small artery which has been mistaken for a vein. A test injection of ½ cc of saline into the vessel before starting therapy will detect the error, since the surrounding skin blanches if an artery is injected. Thromboses of major branches of the aorta have been noted following the use of umbilical artery cannulas.

Extremity restraints are often necessary in the younger patients to prevent accidental removal of the venous cannula or uncoupling of the venous circuit. For this purpose, linen tapes may be placed around the wrists or ankles and pinned to the patient's bedsheets or tied to a crib railing. In addition to restraints, it is often helpful to apply a flat board to the extremity into which an intravenous infusion is being given to prevent flexion or extension of a joint which might dislodge a needle or flex and occlude the catheter. These restraints should be used with caution, for if they are applied too tightly over a bony prominence, pressure necrosis of the skin may occur. In addition, an encircling tape which secures a board to an extremity may also constrict the extremity and cause peripheral edema, impaired flow through the venous line, and even arterial occlusion.

Fluids Commonly Used

The standard solutions used for short-term intravenous therapy are noted in Table 9–1. A solution of 5 percent dextrose in ¼ normal saline, containing 38.5 mEq/L of sodium and chloride, and providing 50 grams of dextrose/L is used routinely to supply maintenance requirements for infants and children with normal renal function. In the premature infant, we prefer to use a 10 percent dextrose solution to prevent hypoglycemia. Although 10 percent dextrose in dilute normal saline solutions are not available commercially, a maintenance fluid for prematures can be prepared at the bedside by the addition of 50 cc of 50 percent dextrose (25 grams of dextrose) to 500 cc of 5 percent dextrose in ¼ normal saline solution.

Table 9–1
Useful Intravenous Solutions Commercially Available

Solution	Dextrose gm/L	Na	Cl	K mEq/L	Ca	Lactate
5% Dextrose	50	—	—	—	—	—
10% Dextrose	100	—	—	—	—	—
5% Dextrose in ½ normal saline	50	77	77	—	—	—
5% Dextrose in ⅓ normal saline	50	51.3	51.3	—	—	—
5% Dextrose in ¼ normal saline	50	38.5	38.5	—	—	—
Lactate Ringer's solution	—	130	109	4	3	28
Normal saline	—	154	154	—	—	—

Planning a Treatment Program

Infusions of fluid and electrolytes in surgical patients are calculated from a consideration of requirements for normal urinary function and insensible water loss, repair of preexisting solute, water, and acid-base abnormalities, and replacement of anticipated or actual additional losses. Intravenous therapy is routinely planned on a 24-hour basis, but revision of this plan may be necessary if unpredicted changes in the condition of the child occur. Review of intake and output charts and reevaluation of the status of the small infant are necessary every eight hours and must be performed in all children at least every 12 hours. In the critically ill, even more frequent evaluations are necessary.

Daily Maintenance Requirements
    Many formulas exist for calculating daily requirements of water for adequate renal function and for replacement of insensible water loss in normal infants and children. Perhaps the most physiologic and accurate method is based on body surface area (see Chapter 6) rather than body weight or caloric requirements (see Chapter 18). When calculated from body surface area expressed in square meters, fluid requirements are 1000 ml/m²/day for normal renal function, and 500 ml/m²/day for insensible water losses. Since most clinicians are accustomed to the use of weight rather than surface area to estimate the dose of drugs, fluids, electrolytes, and other body needs, it is often more convenient to calculate maintenance fluid requirements on the basis of body weight (Table 9–2). Except on the first day of life, when there is a surplus of extracellular water, the administration of 75 ml of water per kg of body weight per day (not to exceed 1500 ml/day) will supply sufficient water to meet the requirements for renal solute excretion (50 ml/kg/day) and insensible water loss (25 cc/kg/day) in a child of any age with normal renal function. Water gains from water of oxidation and water losses from a normal intestinal tract do not need to be considered in these calculations. Although there is great variation between patients, 25 cc of water/kg/day generally suffices to replace in-

Table 9–2
Daily Maintenance Requirements for Infants and Children

	Per kg	
Urine output	50 ml	
Insensible water loss	25 ml	
Total water requirement*		75 ml†
Na requirement		4 mEq†
K requirement		2 mEq†

* Not to exceed total volume of 1500 ml.
† 75 ml/kg/day of dextrose in ¼ normal saline solution with 2 mEq.
KCL/100 cc will supply these needs.

sensible water loss in surgical patients. Even in febrile newborns whose relatively large body surface area might lead to excessive evaporative losses from the skin, this volume is sufficient since these patients are routinely nursed in humidified isolettes in which temperature is controlled.

Compared to values given in most pediatric texts, daily maintenance fluid volume of 75 cc/kg is somewhat on the low side for the newborn and on the high side for the older child. However, calculation errors can be minimized by utilizing such a simple standard formula for all children, the administration of less than "ideal" maintenance fluid volumes to infants and greater than "ideal" volumes to the older child is safe and well tolerated.

The only electrolytes required for short-term maintenance therapy are sodium (4 mEq/kg/day) and potassium (2 mEq/kg/day), since body stores of other essential minerals are adequate. The administration of 75 ml/kg solution of 5 percent dextrose in ¼ normal saline solution (Table 9–1) with the addition of 2 to 4 mEq KCL per 100 cc will supply the daily maintenance requirements of water, sodium, and potassium in all children.

Estimation and Repair of Preexisting Water, Electrolyte and Acid-Base Abnormalities

Infants and children admitted for surgery vary widely in their state of hydration depending on their age and the pathology leading to hospitalization. For example, the state of hydration of a 3-day-old infant with low intestinal atresia differs greatly from that of a day-old edematous infant with esophageal atresia from a diabetic mother.

Useful estimates of electrolyte and fluid deficits require evaluation of the clinical history, physical examination, and certain laboratory data. Information relating to the patient's previous oral intake, the duration and character of gastrointestinal losses, and the number of urinations a day, are helpful. On physical examination, the state of hydration can be crudely estimated from skin turgor, the presence or absence of a depressed fontanelle or sunken eyeballs, and weight loss.

A more accurate assessment of water and electrolyte deficit can be made by measuring hematocrit, serum electrolytes, and serum proteins. In addition, a measure of serum and urine osmolarity is especially useful in determining the state of hydration. For example, a normal infant has a serum osmolarity of 280–290 mOsm/L, whereas we have noted an osmolarity of 258 mOsm/L in an edematous infant of a diabetic mother and an osmolarity of 350 mOsm/L in an infant with massive fluid losses from an omphalomesenteric duct. Although urine osmolarity can be variable even with normal hydration, urine osmolarity above 300 mOsm/L usually indicates a modestly dehydrated infant. A urine osmolarity of 600–700 mOsm/l in an infant indicates severe and potentially lethal dehydration because the maximal concentrating ability of the infant kidney is in this range. In the older child whose kidneys can concentrate to 1200–1400 mOsm/L, a urine osmolarity of 600 does not indicate as serious an abnormality.

Even with these clinical and laboratory evaluations, a precise measurement of fluid deficit is not usually possible. To avoid the hazards of undercorrection or overcorrection in an infant or child with any degree of dehydration, it is safe to consider that the total fluid deficit is equal to 10 percent of the patient's weight. Correction is achieved in 48 hours by adding half the calculated deficit to the volume of maintenance fluid administered on the first day of therapy, and the remainder (if necessary) is added on the second.

The electrolyte content of the fluid chosen for correction of the deficit depends on an estimate of the electrolyte content of the fluid lost, serum electrolyte concentrations, and the acid base status. Table 9–3 lists the approximate electrolyte concentrations of body fluids

Table 9–3
Electrolyte Composition of Body Fluids

	Na+	K+ mEq/L	Cl−
Sweat	11–35	4–8	10–35
Gastric	20–80	5–20	100–150
Pancreatic	120–40	5–15	90–120
Bile	120–40	5–15	80–120
Small intestine	100–140	5–15	90–130
Ileostomy	45–135	3–15	20–115
Diarrhea	10–90	10–80	10–110

which are commonly lost in patients with surgical lesions. Be aware that certain other electrolytes not listed in the table may be lost also. For example, deficiencies of magnesium may occur with starvation, malabsorption syndromes, and protracted losses of gastrointestinal fluids. Hypocalcemia may result from long-standing pancreatic or small bowel fistulas as well as from acute pancreatitis, renal failure, and hypoparathyroidism. As a rule, water loss exceeds electrolyte loss. Since the concentration of electrolytes in these body fluids is generally less than the concentration of electrolytes in blood, electrolyte solutions should contain more water and less electrolytes than the patient's serum. In the small infant whose kidneys cannot conserve water as efficiently as those of an older child, a high obligatory water loss leads to an even greater likelihood of hypertonic dehydration, hypernatremia, and a high serum osmolarity. Extreme caution is necessary during correction of electrolyte abnormalities in the infant with hypertonic dehydration, since the use of large quantities of very dilute electrolyte solutions may result in convulsions and brain damage. As a rule, solutions no more dilute than ½ normal saline are safe in all patients with serious water and electrolyte losses.

The many physiologic events which influence the acid-base status at birth assume a greater importance in the infant who must undergo a surgical procedure and a general anesthetic. Significant metabolic acid-base abnormalities have been noted in many children with surgical lesions and are most pronounced in the premature and in infants with intestinal atresia, gastroschisis, and pyloric stenosis.

The pH of blood reflects the summation of its respiratory and metabolic components. The Siggaard-Andersen nomogram based on arterial blood pH and pCO_2 enables the calculation of the base excess and the separation of metabolic from respiratory causes of serum pH abnormalities. It also allows quantitative adjustments in intravenous therapy and ventilatory control before, during, and after surgery. The base excess is defined as zero for blood with a pH of 7.40 at a pCO_2 of 40 mm Hg. A negative base excess indicates a deficit of base or an excess of fixed acid, i.e. metabolic acidosis. Positive base excess indicates an excess of base or a deficit of fixed acid, i.e., metabolic alkalosis. The normal range for base excess is from -2 to $+2$ mEq/L.

In surgical patients, metabolic acidosis may result from a decrease in peripheral tissue perfusion, selective loss of alkali from the intestinal tract, renal disease, inappropriate fluid therapy, and large-volume transfusions of highly acid stored blood.

A rational approach to the therapy of the infant with severe metabolic acidosis must be directed toward correction of the underlying physiologic cause rather than reliance on titration of the extracellular fluid to a normal pH by the infusion of buffers. The pathophysiology of metabolic acidosis often exists at the tissue level. Hypothermia, dehydration, hypovolemia, and hemoconcentration will result in lowered tissue perfusion and accumulation of acid metabolites from anaerobic glycolysis. The high hematocrit of the neonate further exaggerated by dehydration will result in high-viscosity blood which perfuses small vessels poorly. At normal body temperature, blood with a hematocrit of 70 percent may show a threefold increase in viscosity when compared to 60 percent hematocrit blood. A decrease in body temperature further increases blood viscosity and decreases peripheral blood flow. Acidosis on the basis of poor tissue perfusion is best managed by maintenance of normal body temperature and replacement of blood, plasma, fluid, and electrolytes as indicated.

Sodium bicarbonate and Tham are useful to correct acute life-threatening metabolic acidosis, especially during resuscitation for cardiac arrest. A standard 50-cc ampule of $NaHCO_3$ contains 44.6 mEq of bicarbonate (0.8 mEq/ml). The number of milliequivalents of $NaHCO_3$ required to correct acidosis can be calculated by multiplying the base deficit (mEq/L) by the volume in liters of the patient's extracellular fluid. In the newborn, extracellular fluid represents 40 percent of the patient's weight, whereas it accounts for only 25 percent of the weight of an older child. Tham should be reserved for the rapid treatment of severe metabolic acidosis with associated respiratory component (pCO_2 greater than 55 mm Hg). However, Tham is contraindicated whenever renal disease is suspected. For gradual correction of mild acidosis, the infusion of 4.2 cc/kg of ⅙M sodium lactate solution will increase serum bicarbonate concentration by 1 mEq/L.

In surgical patients, metabolic alkalosis is most commonly due to either excessive gastric losses, inappropriate fluid replacement therapy, or the transfusion of large volumes of citrated blood. The selective loss of hydrogen chloride and potassium from the stomach, usually seen with pyloric stenosis, will lead to a hypochloremic hypokalemic alkalosis. The large potassium loss from the stomach (and kidney during the early period of alkalosis) eventually results in "paradoxical" aciduria, further accentuating the alkalotic state. In addition to the replacement of sodium chloride, the repair of this defect requires the administration of large quantities of KCL. As a rule, the addition of 4 mEq of KCL to each 100 cc of fluid used for maintenance and replacement will suffice. Metabolic alkalosis may also develop in patients who require long-term gastric suction and in whom gastric losses are replaced with electrolyte solutions which do not contain adequate quantities of potassium and chloride.

Several hours after the transfusion of large volumes of citrated blood during surgery or for major trauma, metabolic alkalosis is frequently observed. The citrate infused is rapidly metabolized by the liver, leaving an excess of sodium bicarbonate to be excreted by the kidney. The alkalosis persists because renal excretion of sodium in the post-traumatic state is decreased by increased adrenocortical activity. Alkalosis from this cause may be compounded by hyperventilation. Infusion of acid ions is not recommended to correct this type of alkalosis, although KCL is given when it is complicated by hypokalemia.

The progress in repairing the preexisting fluid, electrolyte, and acid-base abnormalities can be assessed by a measure of body weight, urinary output, the clinical status of the child, and the laboratory tests already described. A urine output of 50 cc/kg/day (or 5 voidings a day in a newborn) generally implies adequate hydration. It is desirable to restore the system of a depleted child to optimal fluid, electrolyte, and acid-base balance prior to the induction of anesthesia, to avoid hypotension and cardiac arrhythmias. However, surgery is often necessary prior to a complete replacement of all calculated deficits. Improvement in the vital signs, adequate urinary output, and a return to normal of the serum electrolyte concentrations generally indicate sufficient improvement to proceed safely with surgery.

Repair of Additional Intraoperative and Postoperative Fluid Losses

In addition to the fluids and electrolytes needed for maintenance and repair of preexisting deficits, extra quantities are often necessary to replace sensible losses which occur during surgery and in the immediate postoperative period.

During the course of an uncomplicated operative procedure, only the fraction of the total daily fluid requirement which correlates with the length of the operation need be given. However, during major intraabdominal or thoracic procedures, additional fluid apart from blood is necessary because of sequestration of extracellular fluid into the peritoneum, pleural cavity, bowel wall, or wound and increased insensible losses from lungs, exposed viscera, and body cavities. For each hour of surgery, the administration of 5–10 ml/kg of a balanced salt solution (Ringer's lactate), plasma, or 5 percent albumin in saline will suffice to replace these additional losses.

Gastric drainage is probably the most common cause of extra fluid losses in postoperative surgical patients. Despite the wide range of electrolyte concentrations in gastric aspirates, as noted in Table 3, replacement of gastric losses with equal volumes of 5 percent dextrose in ½ normal saline with 2–4 mEq/KCL/100 ml will usually be satisfactory. Occasionally, it is wise to determine the exact electrolyte content of the aspirate.

Replacement of fluid lost through drains is often necessary. Serous drainage, such as that which occurs from the pleural cavity or peritoneum is usually replaced with plasma or a 5 percent albumin solution. Drainage from the biliary or intestinal tract is replaced by a fluid with the appropriate electrolyte content (Tables 9–1 and 9–3). The exact volume of fluid loss is known when it occurs through a chest tube or any other tube connected to a closed container. However, losses must be estimated when drainage accumulates in wound dressings. Careful weighing of dressings before and after placement on the wound will aid in this estimation.

ILLUSTRATIVE CASE REPORTS

Case 1.   *Management of infant with esophageal atresia; no preexisting deficits.*

A 3-kg infant was diagnosed as having an esophageal atresia, Type C, at 18 hours of age. A sump tube was placed in the proximal esophageal pouch and the infant transferred. At 24 hours of age, he was taken to the operating room where a saphenous vein cutdown at the ankle was made. A gastrostomy and a primary repair of the defect were carried out. Sixty cc of Ringer's lactate (10 ml/kg/hr) was given during the two-hour operation. Intravenous therapy for the first 24 hours postoperatively was

MAINTENANCE REQUIREMENT (75 ml/kg)	225 ml
GASTROSTOMY LOSS	50 ml
	275 ml
REPLACEMENT FLUID 5% D/W in ¼ normal saline	275 ml
2 mEq KCL/100 ml	

Because 1-day-old infants have excess utilizable extracellular water, it was assumed that no preexisting fluid deficits existed preoperatively, despite no fluid intake. Operative losses were replaced at surgery. Postoperative fluids were calculated from maintenance requirements and an anticipated small loss from the gastrostomy tube drainage. Electrolyte replacement in excess of that present in standard maintenance solution was not necessary. This quantity of fluid was given daily until gastrostomy feedings were started.

Case 2.   *Preoperative preparation of an infant with pyloric stenosis; upper gastrointestinal losses.*

A 6-week-old infant, weighing 3.2 kg at birth, with a 2-week history of progressive vomiting was found to have pyloric stenosis. On admission, his weight was 3 kg with clinical signs of marked dehydration and chronic starvation. The serum electrolyte levels were Na 135, K 2.2, Cl 84, and total CO_2 of 36 mEq/L. A number 21 scalp vein needle was inserted, and fluids and electrolytes were given according to the following calculations to replace losses on the day before surgery:

MAINTENANCE REQUIREMENTS (75 ml/kg)		225 ml
DEFICIT	(½ × 10% B.W.)	150 ml
		375 ml
REPLACEMENT FLUID 5% D in ½ normal saline		375 ml
4 mEq KCL/100 ml		

Following this infusion over a 24-hour period, preoperatively he voided 5 times, signs of dehydration disappeared, and pyloromyotomy was performed. The serum electrolyte concentrations immediately prior to surgery were Na 138, K 3.0, Cl 95, and total CO_2 of 28 mEq/L. Since only half the calculated deficit was replaced preoperatively, the remainder was given during the next 24 hours. The replacement solution of ½ normal saline with 4 mEq K Cl/100 ml provided the necessary Na, Cl, K, and water to reverse the hypochloremic hypokalemic acidosis. Fifteen mEq of K, more than twice the amount required for maintenance, were administered.

Case 3. *Management of infant with ileal atresia; large volume loss of intestinal fluid.*

A 4-day-old infant with a birth weight of 3.6 kg had abdominal distention and bilious vomiting which started in the second day of life. He was transferred for surgery at age 4 days with a diagnosis of low intestinal obstruction. His weight on admission was 3 kg and he was markedly dehydrated. The serum Na was 130, Cl 105, K 2.8, and total CO_2 20 mEq/L. The hematocrit was 65 percent and the base deficit was calculated at 8 mEq/L. Preoperatively a nasogastric tube was placed on suction and a cutdown made in the saphenous vein. Fluid needs calculated for the first 24 hours were:

MAINTENANCE REQUIREMENTS (75 ml/kg)		225 ml
DEFICIT	($\frac{1}{2} \times$ 10% B.W.)	150 ml
		375 ml
REPLACEMENT FLUID 5% D in $\frac{1}{2}$ normal saline		375 ml
	4 mEq KCL/100 ml	15 mEq
	10 mEq Na HCO_3 (.8 mEq/ml)	12 ml
HOURLY INFUSION RATE		15 ml

Six hours after the start of intravenous fluid replacement after a volume of 90 ml had been given, his clinical status improved and hematocrit fell to 60 percent. At this point, surgery was started. During and following the surgical procedure, the previous rate of fluid replacement was maintained, and an additional 60 ml of Ringer's lactate (10 ml/kg/hr) was added during the two-hour operation. The calculated fluid requirement for the day following surgery was:

MAINTENANCE REQUIREMENT (75 ml/kg)		225 ml
DEFICIT	($\frac{1}{2} \times$ 10% B.W.)	150 ml
GASTROSTOMY LOSS (Anticipated)		100 ml
		475 ml
REPLACEMENT FLUID 5% D in $\frac{1}{2}$ normal saline		475 ml
	4 mEq KCL/100 ml	19 mEq
HOURLY INFUSION RATE		20 ml

In the initial 24 hours of therapy, the volume infused included the maintenance fluids, half the estimated deficit, and intraoperative requirements. A solution of 5 percent dextrose in $\frac{1}{2}$ normal saline was chosen to provide for the large electrolyte loss from intestinal fluids. The mild acidosis (base deficit of 8 mEq/L) was corrected by adding 12 ml of $NaCHO_3$ (10 mEq). This amount was obtained by multiplying the base deficit by the extracellular fluid volume (40 percent body weight) estimated to be 1.2 liter in this infant. In the second 24-hour period, the remainder of the calculated deficit was added to the maintenance volume and the anticipated gastrostomy loss. Appropriate quantities of Ringer's lactate solution, instead of saline and $NaHCO_3$, could have been used to replace intestinal fluid losses.

Case 4.   *Management of older child with ulcerative colitis and per-nicious diarrhea; large-volume electrolyte-poor water loss.*
A 14-year-old, chronically ill child with known ulcerative colitis currently treated with steroids was admitted with severe diarrhea and abdominal pain. He was severely dehydrated and weighed 40 kg. The hematocrit was 43 percent and serum electrolytes were Na 150, Cl 110, K 3.5, and total CO_2 20 mEq/L. The first day, fluid program was:

MAINTENANCE REQUIREMENT			1500 ml
DEFICIT	($\frac{1}{2} \times$ 10% B.W.)		2000 ml
PERSISTENT DIARRHEA (Anticipated)			1000 ml
			4500 ml
REPLACEMENT FLUID 5% Dextrose in $\frac{1}{4}$ normal saline			4500 ml
	3 mEq KCL/100 ml		135 mEq

Maintenance fluid requirements are 1500 cc per day for older children over 20 kg. A dilute replacement fluid, 5% dextrose in $\frac{1}{4}$ normal saline, was selected because of the relatively large volumes of water lost in the diarrheal stools. Large quantities of potassium were needed because of the low serum potassium, the high potassium content of the stool, and excessive urinary loss of potassium resulting from steroid therapy.

LONG-TERM PARENTERAL NUTRITION (HYPERALIMENTATION)

Insufficient caloric intake over a long period contributes appreciably to mortality in infants and children with lesions of the gastrointestinal tract. Not uncommonly, patients with persistent intestinal obstruction, bowel fistulas, short-bowel syndrome, and chronic nonspecific diarrhea die solely from inanition and its complications before curative treatment can be completed.

Dudrick and co-workers first demonstrated that the intravenous infusion of a fat-free, amino acid, glucose solution could support normal growth and development. Filler and co-workers reported the successful long-term use of this solution in 14 critically ill infants, and to date 134 infants and children have been treated at the Children's Hospital Medical Center in Boston. This experience and reports from other institutions confirm the contention that satisfactory total intravenous nutrition is possible even in the very small infant.

The success of the method depends on the infusion of glucose for calories and a protein hydrolysate as a source of nitrogen. Special equipment is required to administer this hypertonic solution at a uniform rate into the vena cava. Because of problems not ordinarily seen with routine intravenous therapy, intelligent use of this life-sustaining system requires the careful selection of patients for therapy, constant surveillance for the development of complications, and persistent attention to the minute details of procedures which minimize the dangers.

Indications

Total intravenous nutrition is reserved for those infants and children whose lives are threatened because feeding by way of the gastrointestinal tract is impossible, inadequate, or hazardous. The goal of treatment depends on the patient's underlying condition. In some instances, such as in those infants with chronic nonspecific diarrhea, placing the gastrointestinal tract at rest for a prolonged period is curative. In others, the restoration and maintenance of adequate nutrition will permit corrective surgery.

The common conditions for which this treatment has been used include chronic intestinal obstruction due to adhesions or peritoneal sepsis, complicated omphalocele and gastroschisis, bowel fistulae, inadequate intestinal length, chronic nonremitting severe diarrhea, extensive body burns, and enteritis arising during tumor therapy (Table 9–4). Although total intravenous nutrition is used to replete the malnourished child, it may be started prophylactically in clinical situations in which prolonged starvation is expected.

Table 9–4
Indications for Long-term IV Nutrition in 134 Children

Diagnosis	No. of Pts
Chronic intestinal obstruction	23
Intraperitoneal sepsis and bowel fistulae	6
Omphalocele and gastroschisis	16
Complicated esophageal abnormalities	15
Chronic diarrhea	24
Enteritis during tumor therapy	13
Prematurity (less than 1000 gm)	3
Miscellaneous	34

As confidence and experience with the method have grown, new indications have developed. For example, with certain modifications we have employed this method of total intravenous nutrition in very small premature infants (weighing less than 1 kg) who constantly regurgitate feedings placed in the stomach either by gavage or by gastrostomy despite an apparently normal gastrointestinal tract. Dudrick has successfully treated the uremia and hyperkalemia of acute renal failure with intravenous infusions of purified amino acids and glucose, thus completely eliminating the need for dialysis.

The decision to begin a program of total intravenous nutrition requires mature clinical judgment. Such a decision can be made readily in the case of an infant with complicated omphalocele or in the case of one in whom a large portion of the midgut has been resected because of volvulus. In other cases, the decision may be more difficult. For example, in treating a child with chronic diarrhea and malnutrition, one must be certain that customary therapy has failed before beginning total intravenous therapy. Although anorexia, vomiting, and diarrhea commonly accompany irradiation and chemotherapy, only the occasional patient becomes so markedly debilitated that such treatment is required.

One must cautiously weigh the need for improved nutrition to save life and reduce morbidity against the possibility of serious complications. Intravenous alimentation should not be employed in those children in whom nutrients can be safely delivered and absorbed from the gastrointestinal tract by careful oral feedings, gavage, or gastrostomy.

Methods

The fat-free infusate which is prepared in the hospital pharmacy by mixing 50 percent glucose and a 5 percent casein or fibrin hydrolysate contains 20 percent glucose, 3.5 percent protein (as amino acids and polypeptides), and 0.8 calories per milliliter. Vitamins and minerals are then added and final concentrations are noted in Table 9–5. The sodium, potassium, and chloride concentrations in the infusate are further adjusted to the needs of the individual patient at the bedside. In general, 30 mEq NaCl and 20 mEq KCl are added to each liter to raise the concentration of sodium to 45 mEq/L, potassium to 35 mEq/L, and chloride to 61 mEq/L. These quantities supply maintenance electrolytes without overloading the normal infant kidney or cardiovascular system. An infusion of 135 ml/kg/day provides approximately 110 calories kg/day, the amount necessary to meet the normal infant's need for tissue repair and growth. In the older child whose basic caloric requirements are somewhat less, 135 ml/kg/day may still be administered safely. Purified amino-acid solutions are also commercially available. We have employed a solution containing 4.2 percent purified amino-acids (Fre-Amine) and 25 percent glucose in 15 children. With the more concentrated solutions, lesser volumes are needed to supply the same number of calories. In addition, the electrolyte content of the stock solution is different for each amino-acid preparation, a factor which must be considered before final electrolyte adjustment at the bedside. Plasma (10 cc/kg) is given twice weekly to provide trace elements and essential fatty acids which are not present in the mixture. In general, plasma infusions are not necessary during the first two weeks of therapy. Iron requirements are met either by weekly intramuscular injections of iron dextran or by blood transfusions. Daily requirements of all vitamins are supplied in the mixture.

Table 9–5
Contents of Infusate

Constituent	Content/Liter
Protein hydrolysate (Hyprotigen)*	30.0 gm
Dextrose (hydrous)	196.6 gm
Sodium†	15.0 mEq
Potassium†	16.0 mEq
Calcium	27.0 mEq
Phosphorous	19.0 mEq
Magnesium	7.6 mEq
Chloride†	10.8 mEq
Folic Acid	0.5 mg
Multivitamin infusion‡	5.0 ml
Vitamin K_1	0.2 mg
Vitamin B_{12}	6.6 mcg

* Casein Hydrolysate, McGaw Laboratories.
† Further adjusted at bedside.
‡ U. S. Vitamin & Pharmaceutical Corp. Each liter provides 4.8 gm nitrogen and 800 calories.

This hypertonic infusate must be delivered through a central venous catheter to avoid peripheral venous inflammation and thrombosis. For this purpose, a silicone rubber catheter is passed through the internal or external jugular vein to the superior vena cava. This procedure is best carried out in an operating room or cardiac catheterization laboratory where adequate exposure, proper instruments, and strict aseptic conditions are available. To minimize bloodstream contamination, the venous catheter is tunneled from the vein entry point to a skin exit site which is placed two to four inches away. In the infant, it is brought out on the scalp, whereas in the older child, the exit site may be the neck or upper extremity. Central venous intubation by percutaneous subclavian vein puncture has also been used by others. The silicone rubber venous line may be left in place until the completion of therapy, unless it becomes accidentally dislodged or septic complications develop. We have had a single catheter in place for as long as 90 days.

The central venous catheter can be inserted under local or general anesthesia. The head is turned to the side and the scalp carefully shaved. A transverse incision, 1 to 2 cm long, is made over the sterno-cleidomastoid muscle at the junction of the middle and lower third of the neck. The external or internal jugular vein is prepared for can-nulation. The external jugular vein is ordinarily preferred and can usu-ally be successfully cannulated even in the premature infant. However, if neither external jugular vein is available because of previous use or small calibre or if entrance of the catheter from the external jugular vein into the vena cava is not possible, the internal jugular vein can be used for cannulation. A long hollow needle (number 15) with an obturator in place is passed beneath the skin of the neck from the in-cision to the scalp (Figure 9–3). If the internal jugular vein is being used,

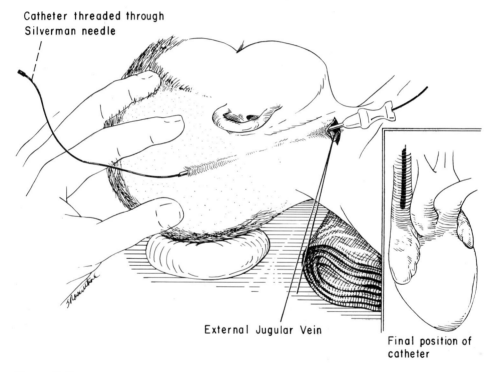

Catheter threaded through
Silverman needle

External Jugular Vein

Final position of
catheter

Figure 9–3
The method of tunneling indwelling silicone rubber catheter from its entrance into a jugular vein to a site on the scalp (see text).

the needle also pierces the belly of the sternocleidomastoid muscle. After the obturator is removed, the silicone rubber catheter (for an infant, the internal diameter is 0.025 inch and the outside diameter is 0.047 inch) is passed through the needle. When the needle is with-drawn, the catheter resides in its subcutaneous tract. Prior to cannula-tion, the vein is ligated distally and an incision made between this point and a proximal controlling ligature. If the internal jugular vein has been selected, ligature of the vein can sometimes be avoided by passing the cannula into the vein through an incision made in the center of a purse-string suture. The jugular vein is then cannulated and the tubing advanced to the region of the right atrium (approximately 5 cm in an infant). Occasionally, manipulation of the neck is necessary to obtain entry into the superior vena cava from the external jugular vein. The exact location of the catheter is confirmed radiographically by taking a single x-ray with the catheter filled with radio-opaque contrast material.

The silicone rubber catheter slides easily and is soft and compressible. Therefore, the ligature which holds it in the lumen of the vein must be tied so that it neither occludes the lumen of the tube nor allows it to slip out of the vessel. To fix the tube properly, we use a circular sleeve of silicone rubber to which dacron wings have been bonded (manufactured by Medical Devices, Inc.). After venous cannulation, the sleeve of silicone rubber is opened, and, at its entrance into the jugular vein, the venous catheter is placed within the lumen of the sleeve. The venous catheter is glued to the sleeve with silicone cement. The dacron wings are sutured with nonabsorbable sutures to the surrounding tissues. To remove the central venous line, the sleeve and its dacron attachments must be cut by opening the neck wound under local anesthesia.

Antibiotics are administered only when indicated by the child's primary illness, but not specifically to prevent sepsis which might occur from the presence of a central venous line.

An antibacterial ointment and sterile dressing are applied to the skin exit site, and, to avoid accidental displacement, a coil of catheter is included in the dressing. Every three days, the dressing is removed aseptically, the skin cleansed with an antiseptic, and a sterile dressing and antibacterial ointment reapplied. Povidone-iodine (Betadine) ointment is now used routinely because of its effectiveness against both bacteria and fungi. Before the infusion is started, a Millipore filter (0.22μ) is placed in line to remove particulate matter and/or microorganisms which may have contaminated the solution. A calibrated burette is placed in the circuit to accurately monitor the volume delivered. An injection tubing ("T" connector, manufactured by Abbott Laboratories) may also be added to the circuit so that intravenous drugs can be administered aseptically above the filter.

The infusate must be delivered at a slow uniform rate to insure proper utilization of the glucose and amino acids. In the small infant, this is most readily accomplished by the use of a constant infusion pump (Sigmamotor pump, TM 20-2, manufactured by Sigmamotor, Inc.) which functions by compressing a section of disposable tubing. The particular pump we employ avoids frequent uncoupling of the tubing. In some centers, infusion to the older patients has been accomplished by gravity drip. The entire system, locally referred to as the "lifeline," is shown in Figure 9–4.

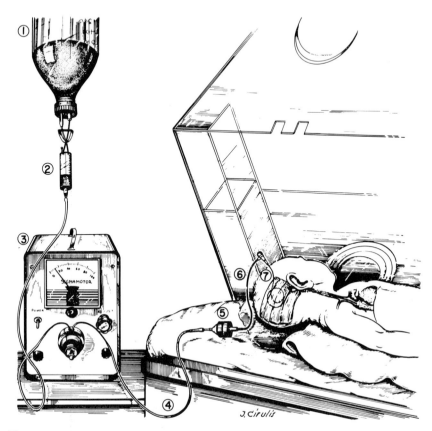

Figure 9–4
System for long-term intravenous alimentation ("lifeline"). (1) Amino acid-glucose infusate. (2) Calibrated burette. (3) Constant infusion pump. (4) Disposable tubing with a compressible section which adapts to pump head. (5) Millipore filter. (6) "T" connector. (7) Silicone rubber intravenous catheter.

Metabolic Observations and Responses

Early in our experience, patients receiving all nutrients by vein were admitted to the Metabolic Unit of the Clinical Research Center at the Children's Hospital Medical Center so that careful extensive observations could be obtained. As a result of this experience, a simplified protocol of care has evolved so that patients can now be adequately cared for on general medical and surgical divisions.

Clinical measurements which have been found essential to evaluate the child's metabolic response include daily body weight, accurate volume of urine, and other body fluid losses. The important laboratory tests include qualitative urinary sugar analysis, blood sugar concentrations, and serum electrolyte content and osmolarity. The urine sugar content is monitored at each voiding. In the stable patient, the other tests are obtained every three days for the first two weeks, and thereafter only as indicated. These determinations will indicate the child's nutritional progress and readily detect the occurrence of an osmotic diuresis or abnormal fluid retention.

Weight change during the period of intravenous feeding will vary with the patient's overall clinical status. Weight gains comparable to those of normal infants may be expected in those children who are not malnourished at the time intravenous feedings are instituted or in whom sepsis is not a part of the clinical picture. In the patient with infection or another clinical problem which increases metabolic requirements, a flatter growth curve may be observed. A significant weight gain in the first two weeks of therapy is not usually seen in those infants and children who are severely depleted at the start of treatment. Typical weight curves are shown in Figure 9–5.

Despite the variations in weight curves, positive nitrogen balance has been noted in all patients studied in detail. On the intravenous diet providing 0.65 gm N/kg/day (equivalent to 4.05 gm protein/kg/day), persistent positive balance of nitrogen of 100 to 300 mg/kg/day has been observed (Figure 9–5). Fecal loss of nitrogen is usually negligible since stools are infrequent and scanty during periods of intravenous feeding. Urinary amino-acid losses have been found to be negligible and not sufficient to produce an osmotic diuresis except in infants weighing under 1 kg and in those children with severe renal disease.

In most patients, the large quantity of intravenous glucose (27 mg/kg/day) is well tolerated without the addition of exogenous insulin. Blood sugar levels remain in the normal range, but urinary sugar content usually varies between 0 and 3+ by the Clinitest method. Quantitative glucose excretion studies have shown that this represents less than one percent of the total glucose infused. Urinary sugar levels are generally highest during the first day or two of treatment. Qualitative urine sugars consistently above 3+ may cause an osmotic diuresis and often signal the likelihood of bloodstream infection especially in the patient who has been treated for many days without glycosuria. A temporary decrease in hourly infusion rate or use of a more dilute solution usually corrects the problem if it is not due to sepsis.

Water balance is maintained even in infants weighing under 2.5 kg and in those following surgery despite the infusion of this hypertonic solution (1600 mOsm/L) at the rate of 135 ml/kg/day. Urinary solute excretion on this intravenous diet is usually greater than that observed during oral feeding, but this increased load does not exceed the concentrating capability of the normal infant kidney.

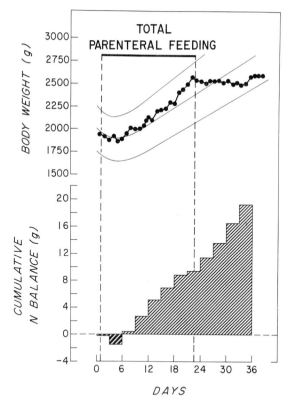

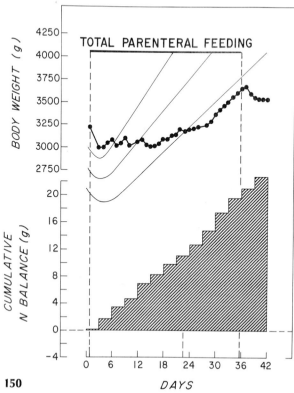

Figure 9–5

Weight response of two neonates to total parenteral feeding during multistaged repair of an omphalocele, with daily weights charted adjacent to expected weight curves for normal infants (cumulative nitrogen balance is indicated). (Top) A 1.9-kg premature infant with antenatal rupture of an omphalocele. A central venous catheter was inserted, and first-stage repair with gastrostomy was performed on the first day of life. Total parenteral feedings were continued for 19 days during three subsequent operative procedures. Daily weight increases paralleled those of a normal infant. When oral feedings were started, weight gain diminished, although positive nitrogen balance persisted. (Bottom) A 2.9-kg infant with antenatal rupture of an omphalocele, received all nutrients by vein for 34 days while a five-stage repair was completed. During the first three weeks of parenteral nutrition, less than expected weight gain was observed. During this time, localized infection at the wound edges was evident. When this subsided, greater daily weight gain was noted. Although weight gain differed from (A), nitrogen balance was similar. (Reprinted with permission of *New Eng J Med* 281:589–594, 1969.)

Complications

Although most patients tolerate this infusate, an occasional patient will develop hyperglycemia, glycosuria, and an osmotic diuresis. This inappropriate response in the absence of sepsis has been seen in children with severe renal disease, central nervous system abnormalities, and in the smallest premature infants. In the premature infant, the osmotic diuresis can usually be controlled by temporarily decreasing the content of glucose and amino acids in the mixture. In others, insulin administration may be tried, but often therapy must be discontinued.

The presence of a catheter in the superior vena cava for prolonged periods adds the hazard of venous thrombosis and pulmonary embolus. The use of nonreactive silicone rubber tubes minimizes this danger.

Accidental withdrawal of the venous line is a common problem. This complication ordinarily causes swelling near the venotomy site and may be confirmed by x-ray visualization of the catheter tip. If the tip is not in the superior vena cava, the catheter should be completely removed and a new line inserted at another site. Accidental withdrawal occurs more frequently when a soft silicone rubber catheter, which is difficult to secure, is used. Perforation of the vena cava has been reported with central catheters, but we have not encountered this problem.

The most serious complication of this method is sepsis. Long-term indwelling venous cannulae are a well-documented source of bloodstream infection. Organisms may enter the bloodstream along the catheter tract or with a contaminated intravenous solution. The catheter, a foreign body in the bloodstream, may act as a focus for bacterial growth even if organisms enter from a distant septic site. Sepsis should be suspected when fever or glycosuria without any apparent cause occurs. To minimize the risk of sepsis, the following measures and precautions should be taken. Catheters should be placed under aseptic conditions in an operating room. Silicone rubber catheters, rather than polyethylene or polyvinyl catheters, should be used because they cause less tissue reaction and are less likely to produce a thrombus which will support the growth of microorganisms along the wall of the intubated vein. The skin exit site for the catheter should be placed in an area which can be aseptically and meticulously cleansed. Routine dressing changes at the skin exit site should be performed every three days, and, after adequately prepping the skin, an antimicrobial ointment should be applied to the catheter where it exits from the skin. Povidone-iodine (Betadine), which is available as a solution and an ointment, is now used routinely to clean the skin and to cover the skin exit site because it is both bactericidal and fungicidal. Use of the central venous catheter for blood sampling (except for blood culture) or central venous pressure measurements should be avoided. Nutrient solutions should be prepared aseptically in the hospital pharmacy preferably in a laminar flow hood and not on the open ward. Intravenous bottles and tubing should be changed daily. A bacterial filter is placed in-line to remove any organisms which may have contaminated the solution. Since the high sugar content of these infusates support the growth of yeast, the external surface of the intravenous tubing should be washed with Betadine solution twice a day to remove any traces of nutrient solution which may have inadvertently dripped from the bottle onto the tubing. Betadine ointment should also be applied to all joints in the circuit to prevent entry of microorganisms at these points. Antibiotics need not be employed unless warranted by the child's primary illness. The intravenous infusion should be cared for only by a team of specially trained individuals who are alert to all the hazards.

In spite of our taking these precautions with our 134 patients, 21 instances of septicemia occurred between the 8th and 9th day of treatment. Fever and/or unexplained glycosuria are usually the first clues to bloodstream infection. Blood culture obtained through the central venous line is diagnostic. In our series, Candida albicans grew from the blood in 10 patients, staph aureus in four, strep fecalis in three, diphtheroids in two, E. coli in one, and enterobacter in one. Infants with proven bloodstream infection were treated by removal of the central venous line. In addition, appropriate antibiotics were given to those with bacterial sepsis. Of these 21 children with septicemia, only two deaths could be attributed directly to catheter sepsis. However, sepsis contributed to death in two others because nutrition could not be maintained after the catheter was withdrawn. Recovery from septicemia was generally rapid, indicating that early detection and treatment of this complication can prevent serious sequelae.

In our series of 134 infants and children, 102 are alive. Four infants died of malnutrition, two because they were unable to tolerate the infusate, and two because sepsis required withdrawal of the intravenous catheter. Two infants died because of a complication of the method. Other causes of death included surgical complications, tumor metastases, extensive burns, and immune deficiency disease.

The risk of sepsis becomes acceptable when one treats only those children whose lives are seriously threatened because the gastrointestinal tract cannot be utilized to prevent starvation.

BIBLIOGRAPHY

Short-Term Intravenous Therapy
1. Edelman, C.M., Jr., Barnett, H.L., and Troupkou, V.: Renal concentrating mechanism in newborn infants. *J Clin Invest* 39:1062, 1960.
2. Holliday, M.A., and Segar, W.E.: The maintenance need for water in parenteral fluid therapy. *Pediatrics* 19:823, 1957.
3. Knutrud, O.: *The Water and Electrolyte Metabolism in the Newborn Child After Major Surgery.* Oslo: Universitetsforlaget, 1965.

4. Kinney, J.M., Egdahl, R.H., Zuidema, G.D.: *Manual of Preoperative and Post-operative Care,* ed 2, Philadelphia: W.B. Saunders, 1971.

5. Metcoff, I.: Regulation of the Body Fluids. In Cook, R.E., ed: *Biologic Basis of Pediatric Practice.* New York: McGraw-Hill, 1968.

Intravenous Nutrition

6. Dudrick, S.J., et al: Long-term total parenteral nutrition with growth, development, and positive nitrogen balance. *Surgery* 64:134–142, 1968.

7. Dudrick, S.J., and Steiger, J.M.: Renal failure in surgical patients treatment with intravenous essential amino acids and hypertonic glucose. *Surgery* 68:180, 1970.

8. Filler, R.M., et al: Long-term parenteral nutrition in infants. *New Eng J Med* 281:589–594, 1969.

Catheter Sepsis

9. Fuchs, P.C.: Indwelling intravenous polyethylene catheters: Factors influencing the risk of microbial colonization and sepsis. *J Amer Med Assoc* 216:1447, 1971.

10. Moran, J.M., Atwood, R.P., and Rowe, M.I.: A clinical and bacteriologic study of infections associated with venous cutdowns. *New Eng J Med* 272:554, 1965.

11. Smits, J., and Freedman, L.R.: Prolonged venous catheterization as a cause of sepsis. *New Eng J Med* 276:1229, 1967.

10

Blood and
Its Components in
Transfusion Therapy

Harry J. Sacks, M.D.

Over seven million units of blood are used every year. Despite the relatively precise nosology that has evolved relative to indications for its use, a large body of obsolete traditional beliefs clouds this therapeutic arm of medical practice, and results in overuse of whole blood and inappropriate attention to blood component therapy. The concept that appropriate blood components exist for a given clinical need and that whole blood should not be used as a form of shotgun therapy for all needs will be developed in this chapter.

THE SHORT SUPPLY

Shortage of blood is a constant problem, periodically aggravated by negative donor response during the summer, vacation time, and bad weather. Fifteen to 30 percent of all stored blood across the country becomes outdated and unusable, an additional drain on the available supply.

Potential solutions are available, some requiring the physician's participation, some requiring innovation and discovery, and some financial support. Advances in blood storage may extend shelf life at 4°C up to as much as 35–40 days, or at −80°C, indefinitely. Difficulty in procurement must be eliminated and an artificial fluid with hemoglobin's attributes developed.

The physician's role must include active solicitation of donors from among his patients and their families and from among his circle of social acquaintances for only when the physician is deeply committed to this task will donors begin to appear in numbers appropriate to supply the community's blood-component needs. He must also become thoroughly familiar with the available blood components, their advantages and disadvantages, and with their physiological indications in order to use each available component to fullest advantage, and thus indirectly to expand the available total supply of blood and its components.

BLOOD COMPONENTS [1]

Blood consists of a cellular phase (containing red cells, white cells, and platelets) and a fluid phase (containing plasma proteins, biochemicals, coagulants, antibodies, and so on).

Procedures are now available to separate the various components of each phase, and experience and experimentation have shown the areas of greatest usefulness for each.

Blood is most commonly collected in acid citrate dextrose (ACD) preservative and, in many areas, in citrate phosphate dextrose (CPD). The former's shelf life is 21 days and the latter's 28–40 days.

A second method of separating blood into its components is by plasmapheresis. In this process, a patient is bled into a preservative solution. The collected bag or bottle is then centrifuged lightly to sediment the red cells, and the supernatant platelet-rich plasma is removed. The sedimented red cells are reinfused into the donor. The plasma is separated into platelets and platelet-poor plasma. The platelet-poor plasma can be frozen or lyophilized; it can be converted to cryoprecipitate, and the supernatant plasma then used as an albumin-containing component; it can be sent to a manufacturer who will separate the gamma globulin and albumin components, who will concentrate the Factor VIII content or the Factors II, VII, IX, and X content.

Finally, the recent development of a separatory centrifuge makes possible the automatic separation of blood into plasma, red cells, platelets, and leukocytes.

Red Blood Cells

Preparations

Stored red cell units are prepared in two ways: by centrifugation of whole blood followed by removal of the supernatant plasma resulting in a component called *packed red cells* (PRC); and by permitting sedimentation of the red cells at 4°C for 18–24 hours followed by removal of the supernatant plasma (*sedimented red cells* or SRC).

The hematocrit of PRC is about 70 volumes percent while that of SRC is about 60 volumes percent. ACD, PRC, or SRC can be stored for 21 days and CPD preparations for 28 days, if the container is not entered during the processing, e.g. if a dual plastic bag system is used.

Washed red cells (WRC) are prepared by washing PRC or SRC with salinous fluids in order to remove leukocytes, platelets, plasma, chemicals, proteins, and complement or other hemolytic components. Washing is relatively effective in removing the former two and probably 99 percent plus effective for the latter ones. Its effect on removal of Au antigen is at present unknown, but one would surmise that washing should remove that amount of Au antigen which is in the plasma, and possibly wash off at least *some* of the Au antigen on the surface of the red cells.

Frozen red cells (FRC) are prepared in several ways, the most common of which is by freezing of fresh PRC in glycerol and reconstituting them by thawing and washing the FRC in large amounts of salinous fluids.

"Fresh" PRC has several connotations as to age of the preparations. For the purpose of this discussion, "fresh" will refer to ACD blood that has been processed into PRC (and other components) within 6–12 hours (and up to 5 days for CDP blood) of its collection. Such PRC will contain significant amounts of 2,3 diphosphoglycerate (2,3 DPG) while red cells older than 12 hours have lost substantial amounts of 2,3 DPG and so cannot be expected to immediately afford proper oxygen release in the tissues (2,3). The latter may well be a significant issue following exchange transfusion, especially in the newborn with hyaline membrane disease and in older children and adults where pulmonary oxygen diffusion problems exist. The solution to this problem is thought by some to relate to additives such as adenine or fresh blood no older than that referred to above. From a positive point of view, the 2,3 DPG content of transfused red cells is known to return to normal levels within 24–36 hours.

Indications

In general, increasing the oxygen-carrying capacity of the blood by transfusion is required only when the anoxemia syndrome is present. Under such a circumstance, red cells are needed. Whole blood should be used only when both red cells and plasma are required. The situations in which red cells are useful are:

1. Acute anemias
    a. Hemolytic anemia unassociated with autoimmune antibodies. (Transfusion is best avoided in autoimmune hemolytic anemia in favor of steroid and/or other therapies unless imminent or probable circulatory collapse forces the use of red cells as a calculated risk.)

   b. Medical, surgical, or traumatic blood loss where blood
       volume has been replaced with a predominance of albu-
       min and salinous fluids. In many such patients, if the
       anoxemia can be safely managed with bed rest and, if
       necessary, with oxygen therapy, red cell transfusions can
       be properly deferred in favor of iron therapy.
   c. Where underlying heart disease contributes to the hy-
       poxia. In this circumstance, care against overloading of
       the circulation is mandatory because red cells are also
       volemic substances, although considerably less so than
       the plasma proteins of a unit of whole blood. Those red
       cell units which are given should be infused slowly. Fi-
       nally, fast-acting diuretics can also be of value when con-
       gestive heart failure exists, is a possibility, or develops
       after the transfusion.
2. Any chronic anemia in which fatiguability, weakness, and las-
   situde are not due to the underlying illness. Many chronic
   illnesses are associated with such symptoms although unrelated to or minimally due to hypoxia. Transfusion is *not* indicated in this instance. On the other hand, where it can be
   shown that hypoxia is a significant factor in the disability,
   serial transfusions titrated to the point of reversing the hypoxic symptoms are in order. Examples of such situations
   are:
   a. The aplastic crisis in chronic hemolytic anemia. This crisis
       is generally limited in duration and often can be managed
       symptomatically. In some patients, the crisis is due to folic
       acid deficiency and the anemia responds dramatically to
       folic acid therapy. When hemoglobin levels fall to 5 gm
       percent or less, red cell transfusion should be undertaken
       as a calculated risk toward the avoidance or reversal of
       circulatory failure.
   b. Hypoplastic anemias.
   c. Chronic uremia, leukoses, malignancy, and other debili-
       tating diseases.
   d. When the chronic anemia is specifically due to deficiency
       of iron, or vitamin B_{12}, or folic acid, transfusion should be
       deferred in favor of the specific therapy, if circulatory col-
       lapse is not imminent. If major surgery is necessary, trans-
       fusion to the level of 10 gm percent is appropriate.

Advantages
1. The oxygen-carrying effect of a unit of whole blood is provided in approximately one-half that volume of red cells. This
   is especially useful when there is need to improve the oxygen
   capacity of the blood in patients with congestive heart failure,

with normovolemia, and in infants and children whose normal blood volume is small. In short, the danger of circulatory overload is lessened because a lesser volume can be used for the same net effect in augmenting oxygen-carrying capacity.

2. The sodium, potassium, and ammonia content is reduced by that amount which is in the removed supernatant plasma.

3. Increased use will expand the community's blood supply by permitting use of the supernatant plasma (and its components) and platelets for other patients.

4. Frozen red cells
   a. Stockpiled FRC should eventually do away with the recurrent blood shortages which result over holiday periods, during the summer, and during bad weather. Likewise, outdating of 4°C stored blood will be minimized or become a thing of the past.
   b. Because hepatitis has rarely been reported after transfusion of frozen cells, this is the safest red cell preparation.
   c. The possibility of white cell antibodies [Human Leukocyte Antigen (HL-A)] being formed following the transfusion of leukocytes is virtually prevented, presumably as a result of removal of the leukocytes during preparation for freezing, by destruction of the leukocyte during freezing and thawing, and by further removal by abundant washing during reconstitution from the frozen glycerolized state.
   d. Rare bloods can be stockpiled.

5. Pyrogenic, allergic, biochemical, and isoantibody complications of donor blood are minimized by PRC and SRC and avoided with WRC and FRC.

Disadvantages
   1. All red cell preparations must be typed and crossmatched to prevent incompatible transfusion.
   2. All red cell preparations must be properly stored to avoid unexpected freezing and overheating.
   3. Accidental addition of water produces pretransfusion lysis.
   4. Contamination, as with whole blood, is a serious but extremely rare possibility.
   5. Serum hepatitis may follow use of any of the preparations of red cells except FRC.
   6. Virtually any infectious agent can be transmitted, e.g. plasmodia, leishmania, and viruses including hepatitis A and B, cytomogalic inclusion disease, and so on.
   7. Isosensitization may set the stage for hemolytic disease of the newborn in a later pregnancy, and for the risk of a hemolytic reaction at a later date in either male or female.
   8. Red cells have a limited storage life.

9. All red cell preparations require special facilities and special handling.
10. It is expensive.

Whole Blood

Whole blood is prepared by collection into ACD or CPD and stored at 4°C.

Indications
1. Whenever both red cells and plasma proteins are needed.
2. Whenever needed red cells are not available.
3. Whenever needed platelet packs are unavailable, fresh whole blood may be used to the limit of volemic tolerance.
4. Whenever needed coagulants are unavailable, fresh whole blood may be used to the limit of volemic tolerance for all coagulant deficiencies. Likewise, stored blood may be used for coagulation deficiencies other than Factor V and Factor VIII for which fresh blood is best.

Advantages
1. It is the "complete" replacement for blood loss.
2. It can be used for any component deficiency if component products are not available.
3. One unit can be "exploded" into several components thus expanding available blood supplies.

Disadvantages
1. All disadvantages that apply to red cells apply to whole blood.
2. Doses of components are limited to the volume of whole blood which can be transfused, in contrast to component concentrates which permit large doses by virtue of the small volume of plasma that contains them.
3. Massive transfusions introduce hazards related to:
    a. The biochemical contents of the supernatant plasma, e.g. sodium, K, citrate, NH_3, and organic and inorganic acids.
    b. Depletion of platelets and coagulants.
    c. Depression of temperature of body tissues by cold blood.

Leukocytes

White cell concentrates are prepared by differential centrifugation. They have been effective in some cases of serious sepsis. Unfortunately, they are only available, and in limited amounts, at some research centers.

Platelets

Preparations

Platelets are generally available as a part of fresh whole blood, platelet-rich plasma, and as packed platelet concentrate P.C. The latter are prepared by slow (7 g) centrifugation of whole blood to sediment the red cells; after separation from the red cells, the platelet-rich plasma is centrifuged at 13 g's to sediment the platelets into a button. Following this, all but 25 ml of plasma is removed.

The preparation always contains some red cells and leukocytes and so offers the hazard of immunologic complications to either or both. Because typing for HL-A antigen is not generally available, this risk cannot be minimized. Rh_o typing will, however, minimize this most common cause of red cell isosensitization and consequently rh individuals should receive platelets from rh donors insofar as it is possible. ABO specificity is also best observed to afford improved viability of future transfused platelet and to avoid increase of existing anti-A or anti-B titers.

P.C. is best used as soon after preparation as possible. Storage at 4°C augments the expected in vitro degradation of platelets in comparison to storage at 22°C. Clinical and experimental studies have shown that packs stored at 22°C for 24 hours are as effective as packs which have been stored up to 6 hours at 4°C, and considerably more so than packs at 4°C storage for 24 hours.[4] There is evidence that even 48 hours storage at 22°C is considerably more effective than is storage at 4°C for 24 hours. Although the U.S. Department of Biological Sciences has issued regulations which limit the maximum age for use to 24 hours for packs which are distributed across interstate lines, there is an advantage to using up to 48-hour-old platelets if the clinical situation demands their use and none other are available. When whole blood is used for its platelet content, a reasonable platelet effect can be expected only when blood less than six hours old is used because of the 4°C exposure necessary for whole blood storage.

Indications [5]

In general, fresh whole blood or platelet-rich packed red cells or plasma are not the primary modality of treatment for thrombocytopenia, unless red cells and plasma are also needed. Even when massive thrombocytopenic hemorrhage requires the use of whole blood, platelet packs will still be required because the number of platelets in a given unit of blood is inadequate to provide sufficient platelet effect in such a situation. Obviously, if packs are not available, platelet-rich packed cells or plasma, or whole blood should be used to the limit of volemic tolerance.

1. In aplastic anemia associated with thrombocytopenic bleeding.

2. As supportive therapy for the thrombocytopenia produced by chemotherapeutic agents in the treatment of malignancy.
3. In bleeding states associated with thrombocytopenia which follows massive or exchange blood transfusions.
4. As supportive therapy immediately before and after surgery in thrombocytopenic patients to achieve platelet levels of 50–70,000/mm^3.
5. Platelet transfusions are not primarily indicated in the treatment of idiopathic thrombocytopenic purpura (ITP).

Dosage [6]

Each platelet pack contains 1×10^{11} platelets for the purpose of this determination. The dose is ascertained by the following formulas and relates to up to 6-hour-old refrigerated packs, and up to 24-hour-old 22°C stored packs:

(1) $\dfrac{C - B}{A} \times E = F$ $\qquad$ (2) $\dfrac{D - B}{G} \times E = H$

(3) $\dfrac{C - B}{H} \times E = I$ $\qquad$ (4) $\dfrac{(C - B)}{D - B} \times G \times E = I$

Where:

A = 15,000/mm^3 = expected rise in platelets (per m^2 of body surface) one hour after transfusion
B = pretransfusion platelet count per mm^3
C = posttransfusion platelet count per mm^3
D = one hour posttransfusion platelet count per mm^3
E = number of square meters (m^2) of body surface
F = number of platelet units to be infused
G = number of platelet units actually infused
H = actual increase in platelets per mm^3 per unit transfused
I = actual number of units needed for next infusion to attain an increase of 15,000 platelets per mm^3

Formlua (1) is the primary one. It relates to a rise of 15,000 platelets/mm^3 for each unit of platelets per m^2 of body surface one hour after transfusion. Inasmuch as thrombocytopenic bleeding seldom occurs below 40–50,000/mm^3 of platelets, and clinical experience indicates that bleeding is aborted and prevented when platelet transfusions yield levels between 20,000 and 40,000, it is advisable to aim for 40,000 when platelets are readily available, and even for 20,000 or less when they are in short supply. As a rule of thumb 2 packs of platelets given to a 30-kg child will raise the platelet count by 20,000/mm^3, a level that will generally stop thrombocytopenic bleeding.

Formula (2) is of sequential value in determining the actual increment (H) per transfused pack to provide and estimate for actual future needs. Formula (3) permits calculation of the actual needs based upon the value of H. Formula (4) combines (2) and (3) and can be used in their stead.

Less than optimal rise in platelets may be due to any one of the following.[7]

1. Miscalculation.
2. Less than 1×10^{11} platelets per pack are present in those used.
3. Less survival than expected of platelets due to:
   a. Platelet damage in vitro
   b. Platelet antibodies in patient as is the case in ITP and after previous platelet transfusions
   c. Greater utilization in the vascular bed than expected
   d. Fever and/or sepsis
   e. Splenic sequestration (especially with splenomegaly)
   f. Active bleeding
   g. Massive transfusion therapy

Advantages
1. Large doses of platelets can be readily given to any patient in relatively small volumes of fluid.
2. Hemolytic reaction is not a problem to be reckoned with.

Disadvantages
1. The most serious complication is an immediate one, namely the presence of significant bacterial contamination. To date, the use of the closed plastic bag systems for collection and preparation under rigidly controlled and specified directions has avoided this problem.
2. Hepatitis A or B transmission remains a serious risk for two reasons:
   a. Because multiple units are necessary for an effect, exposure is proportionately increased.
   b. Because the need is frequently urgent, packs are often used before hepatitis screening can be performed.
3. Other infectious agents may be transmitted.
4. Isosensitization to irregular red cell antigens is possible.
5. HL-A sensitization is possible.
6. Storage life is short.
7. Platelet packs are in short supply.

Universal Donor [25]

The universal donor concept relates to compatibility in the ABO blood group system of donor Group O red cells with the plasma of any other recipient of ABO group. The corollary universal recipient concept is that the plasma of a Group AB recipient will be compatible with the red cells of any other donor ABO group.

These principles hold absolutely if only red cells are transfused (the supernatant plasma having been completely removed), but only generally hold when whole blood or SRC or PRC are given because transfused along with the red cells is all the plasma (whole blood) or a variable portion of the plasma (SRC or PRC) in the unit.

Thus the ABO antibody content of the donor plasma becomes the determining factor and is reflected in the minor crossmatch's compatibility or noncompatibility. This circumstance has led to the use of low titer Group O blood. This refers to Group O whole blood (or SRC or PRC) which is free of anti-A and anti-B as measured by tests for hemolytic activity of these antibodies. The same is true of the antibody content of Group A or Group B blood when it is to be transfused into a Group AB patient.

Notwithstanding the low hemolytic titer of universal donor blood the introduction into the recipient of antibodies via the donor plasma may produce destruction of recipient's cells. In infants and small children because of their small blood and body fluid volume such antibodies from a unit of whole blood, SRC or PRC may result in a sufficiently high concentration to compromise survival of the recipient's own red cells.[26] Obviously then the best preparation of universal donor blood is WRC.

Another shortcoming of the universal donor transfusion is that the different ABO types of donor and recipient red cells that are present in the blood may cause some difficulty in later ABO typing and crossmatching. However, knowledge of this circumstance will obviate this problem.

Finally, the use of ABO specific plasmas is essential and especially so in the infant and small child, if the above problem is to be avoided.

Compatibility Testing

In the modern sense this refers to the provision of compatible blood by following three testing steps:

1. Providing type specific red cells. This is routine for the ABO and RH_o positive and RH_o negative. However, when irregular antibodies are known to be present, donor red cells which avoid these antibodies are sought after, e.g. an rh' patient with rh" antibodies is provided with rh' donor red cells.
2. Antibody detection by precrossmatch screening of donor and recipient plasmas against a panel of selected reagent red cells known to contain 99 percent of red cell antigens associated with hemolytic reactions. Reagent cells, because of their high

sensitivity, are more sensitive than is the crossmatch in detecting incompatibility. They will also detect antibodies not possible of detection by the crossmatch, because any given donor may *not* contain the corresponding antigen. Thus, although such crossmatched blood is compatible and safe for transfusion, the next crossmatch may be found to be incompatible at a time when the need is urgent, or the second crossmatch may miss an incompatible situation. Thus advance knowledge of the presence of an antibody makes blood transfusion safer.

3. Antibody detection by the crossmatch. The crossmatch acts as a recheck on the accuracy of some aspects of ABO typing, the antibody screening (if the recipient plasma has an antibody corresponding to the antigen in the donor's red cells, and vice versa for the minor crossmatch). It is, however, the sole determiner of low-incidence antigen-antibody systems, such as Lu^{a+}, because these systems are most often not present in the screening panel of red cells simply because such low incidence red cells suitable for the panel are difficult to obtain.

The blood bank which performs appropriate antibody-screening procedures can make available virtually safe uncrossmatched blood in an emergency be it ABO and Rh_o type specific; or Group O, Rh_o negative universal donor blood when the blood group is not known. Of course, a rapid emergency type crossmatch is always set up when such blood is released so that incompatibility can be seen if the emergency procedure is able to detect it. At the same time, a standard crossmatch is also set up as a backup for the rapid procedure.

Plasma

Plasma is the source of components for (1) passive immunization (general gamma globulin, specific gamma globulin as for prevention of Rh_o sensitization, an experimental gamma globulin from patients who have recovered from hepatitis, and various immune sera); (2) blood volume replacement (albumin); and (3) for replacement of coagulant deficiencies.

This text goes beyond the scope of item (1) above. In regard to item (2), plasma per se is no longer used as a primary agent for hypovolemia, having been supplanted by intravenous fluids and albumin, because of plasma's icterogenicity. However, fresh plasma may be used as a volemic agent if albumin is unavailable.

Plasma is useful for all coagulant deficiencies. Fresh plasma ("fresh" is defined as less than six to twelve hours in age after phlebotomy) provides the highest content of the labile Factors V and VIII.

Factor VIII Preparations

Fresh plasma is prepared in limited amounts as a byproduct of PRC and/or platelet pack preparations, and specifically for use as a co-agulant, and especially for Factor VIII (F-VIII) deficiencies. This component is then generally frozen or lyophilized and reconstituted just before use.

F-VIII is concentrated in the precipitate of the thawed frozen plasma. This cryoprecipitate contains the average equivalent of the F-VIII content in one unit of whole blood, e.g. about 125 units. The material is stored in one of two ways: as fresh frozen plasma. When the need for the cryoprecipitate occurs, the unit is thawed and the supernatant plasma is removed, leaving behind the precipitate containing the F-VIII in approximately 25–30 ml of plasma as a diluent. In this way, the fresh frozen plasma may be thawed and used as such when there is need for both the volemic effect of plasma protein and for its F-VIII content or the precipitate alone may be used when renewal doses are required. The second mode of storage is to prepare the cryoprecipitate at the time of separation of the blood into PRC, platelets, and plasma. The cryoprecipitate is then stored as such at minus 20°C, while the plasma, if not used for its volemic effect, is sent for separation into albumin and gamma globulin. Just before use, 10 ml of normal saline is added to each cryoprecipitate bag. All bags to be used are pooled and then the pool is ready for administration. Alternatively, each unit can be infused in rapid sequence, followed by a rinse of each bag with a small amount of normal saline.

The other principal preparation is the commercial concentrate, which contains 300–900 units of F-VIII and which can be stored at refrigerator or room temperature. This material is prepared from large pools of fresh plasma.

Indications.   Contrary to empiric impressions, F-VIII is normal to elevated in most patients given massive transfusions and so cryoprecipitate is seldom indicated in this situation.[8] By all odds, the principal use relates to F-VIII hemophilia.[9] In general, multiple single units of cryoprecipitate are preferred to the commercial concentrate, because of lesser cost and lesser icterogenicity.

Dosage.   To stop bleeding, a loading dose is necessary to bring the F-VIII level to about 50 percent of normal, and this is based upon an assumed average 125 units of F-VIII per bag of cryoprecipitate, and an assumption of a 40 vol% hematocrit. Dr. Pool uses a rule-of-thumb dosage of one bag of cryoprecipitate for each 6 kg of body weight for the priming dose. If maintenance therapy is needed, one half of priming dose is recommended every twelve hours or two-thirds the initial dose if infusions are to be given every 24 hours.[10]

For elective surgery, a level of 25 percent of F-VIII activity should be attained and maintained for 7–10 days before and for 7–10 days after surgery.[10]

In infants, the dosage is preferably doubled, because of the uncertainty of the exact F-VIII unitage in any given bag of cryoprecipitate (occasional bags have very low unitage), a situation that is overcome by "averaging" in larger children and adults because of the need for more than one bag of cryoprecipitate.

Advantages
1. The F-VIII content of a whole unit of blood is present in 25–30 ml, thus avoiding the hypervolemic effects of whole blood or plasma when large amounts of the Factor are needed.
2. It is relatively low in cost.
3. Its icterogenicity per unit is the same as for an equivalent number of units of whole blood.
4. Its use permits the expansion of the community's blood component supplies as its red cell, platelet, albumin, and gamma globulin content can be utilized for specific needs of other patients.

Disadvantages
1. It requires storage at $-20°C$.
2. It must be used promptly upon reconstitution.
3. It is not readily available in rural and remote areas (the lyophilized preparation is invaluable under such conditions because it can be transported along with the patient as a part of baggage).
4. It is icterogenic—although no more so than whole blood or plasma, because each unit is derived from a single unit of blood.

In contrast to cryoprecipitate, the commercial concentrate while containing 3–6 times as much F-VIII in the same volume of solution has several serious disadvantages.

1. It is 5–15 times as costly per dose.
2. It is highly icterogenic—presumably because the hepatitis virus is concentrated along with the F-VIII precipitate of every infected unit of plasma that goes into the large pools. As a consequence these preparations should only be used if single unit cryoprecipitate is unavailable or if effective blood levels cannot rapidly be attained by cryoprecipitate units.

Von Willebrand's Factor
Von Willebrand's disease is associated with a defect in platelet adhesiveness and a deficiency in F-VIII.[10] The former commonly results in a prolonged bleeding time and the latter occasionally in hemophilic

bleeding. The F-VIII deficiency is related to the absence of a precursor substance present in fresh plasma. Plasma or cryoprecipitate regularly correct this deficiency. While plasma contains the platelet adhesiveness factor, only in occasional patients is such a deficiency corrected by cryoprecipitate.[10]

Treatment is undertaken when the underlying F-VIII disorder results in bleeding, usually following surgery, or trauma. Prophylactic treatment for elective surgery is also a consideration when F-VIII levels are below 20–30 percent of normal. In both instances it is directed at the F-VIII deficiency in the manner described earlier. Tests for capillary integrity such as the Ivy Bleeding Time tend to remain abnormal even though effective hemostasis ensues after treatment (or is assured following prophylactic F-VIII therapy.[10]

Because of its negative effect on platelet adhesiveness, aspirin or any of its derivatives must not be given to the patient. It is, in fact, also possible that aspirin therapy given to a patient with a mild Von Willebrand's disorder that ordinarily might be unassociated with bleeding or with minimal bleeding could lead to severe hemorrhage following trauma, surgery, or even spontaneously.

Factors II, VII, IV, and X Concentrate [12,13]

This is a commercial product having high icterogenicity because it is prepared from pools of plasma. It is also expensive compared to fresh plasma. It contains only about twice the content of II, VII, and X, and about three times the average amount of IX found in a single unit of plasma or whole blood.

Because of its high icterogenicity, its use should be deferred in favor of whole blood (when red cells and plasma are needed) or fresh frozen plasma. It should also be noted, that except for F-IX hemophilia and dicumarol toxicity, that the most common cause of deficiency of these factors relates to liver disease in which F-V also is invariably a most important deficiency. F-V replacement can only be achieved by use of fresh whole blood and/or plasma. At the same time, this therapy will supply enough of the other factors. In hemophilia B (F-IX) treatment with single-unit plasma should be attempted before use of the concentrate is resorted to.

Except for F-V,[14] stored blood or plasma may be used for the stable Factors II, VII, IX, and X.[15,16] From a practical point of view, if plasma is needed, the most commonly available single-unit preparation is the fresh-frozen one, which of course is as effective as stored plasma.

Fibrinogen

Fibrinogen is rarely needed by infants and children, except in the very rare case of congenital afibrinogenemia, when bleeding occurs or surgery is contemplated. As a rule, in disseminated intravascular coagulation (DIC), the acquired fibrinogen deficiency is best treated by heparin therapy directed at the DIC.

Volemic Agents

Plasma Substitutes

Plasma substitutes, in reality, are substitutes for the albumin content of plasma and enjoy their usage because of volemic effects.

Dextran has a place in the modern treatment of plasma volume replacement only if albumin and salinous fluids are unavailable, because of the known incidence, albeit low, of pyrogenic, allergic, and rarely anaphylactic reactions and thrombocytopenia when administered a second time.

Electrolyte solutions [17,18,19,20,21] have assumed an increasingly greater role as a supplement to albumin and blood in volemic replacement of blood and plasma loss. In the infant and small child, blood lost should be replaced with blood for reasons given under "Indications" below. On the other hand, plasma lost, as in burns, should be replaced primarily by albumin. In both situations, tissue fluid and electrolyte replacement is also invariably necessary and so should be included in the therapeutic plan.

Of interest is the finding that hemodilution for extracorporeal circulation [22] is perfectly compatible with survival. In fact, experimental evidence suggests that tissue perfusion is less than optimal under conditions of stress when the hematocrit is high and when lost blood is replaced only with blood.[18,23,24] From this experimental and clinical experience, it would appear advisable, after blood loss, to initiate treatment of the hypovolemia with Ringer's lactate and albumin solution and to complement this with enough whole blood and/or red cell units to keep the hematocrit in the neighborhood of 30 vol%.

Albumin Solutions

Albumin is prepared in a variety of ways from plasma separated from blood or from plasma extracted from placentas. It is available in five percent and 25 percent concentrations.

Indications. Its prime value is for replacement of blood volume after blood or plasma loss, sepsis, or trauma. Its use in the hypoalbuminemic states due to such conditions as the nephrotic syndrome, cirrhosis, and malnutrition is now seldom entertained. In the infant and small child, blood lost should be replaced with whole blood because the amount of albumin which can be given is small before severe anemia sets in. For larger children, the use of albumin and salinous fluids in lieu of blood may be useful (see below).

Advantages
1. It is the perfect blood-volume expander.
2. The 25 percent solution is particularly useful when one wishes to quickly replenish circulatory volume through its oncotic

action on the extravascular fluids. Depleted tissue fluid can be replaced subsequently. This action may be especially valuable in the newborn who has actually lost a large volume of its blood.

3. Hepatitis transmission is not recorded.
4. Other infectious disease transmission has not been recorded.
5. Pyrogenic and allergic reactions are extremely rare.
6. Red blood cell incompatibility is obviated.
7. Patients on low salt restriction will get the minimal salt dosage (20 mEq/L) with the 25 percent solution.
8. There are no chemical problems.

Disadvantages
1. Overload, especially when using the 25 percent solution is a hazard.
2. Acute extravascular dehydration has been observed when the 25 percent solution is used, since it will expand the blood volume by approximately 3½ times the volume of albumin solution given, by attracting extracellular fluids into the circulation. The hazard is particularly great in dehydrated patients, especially infants and young children. The problem is obviated by the use of the five percent solution and concomitant attention to hydration.
3. It is costly. The questionable practice of marking up its pharmaceutical wares by 100 percent has led hospitals to charge $90 to $100 for 25 gm of albumin (equivalent to 500 ml of five percent albumin).
4. Occasionally pyrogenic reactions have been observed by the writer and by others. This usually occurs in a series and is often related to a given batch. While no explanation is immediately available, considered thought relates the problem to variations in the quality of the plasticizers used in the manufacture of the tubing that is supplied with the albumin.
5. It will produce hemodilution. This is of relatively small hazard if anoxemia does not result. In any event, PRC can be used later to supplement oxygen-carrying ability.
6. While not in itself a disadvantage, albumin derived from placental source contains great alkaline phosphatase activity (of placental isoenzyme type) and will result in mild to prominent elevations of serum levels of the phosphatase after infusion.

HAZARDS

The constant admonition of the blood banker to examine the indications for any given transfusion is only due in small part to the need to conserve our available supply. It is overwhelmingly directed to the reality that hemotherapy is a two-edged sword, with serious hazards lying in opposition to its usefulness.

It is for this reason that the use of blood must be reduced to its barest minimum. The hazards may be listed as immediate and delayed.

Immediate	*Delayed*
Pyrogenic	Immunization
Allergic	Red cell
Sepsis	Delayed hemolysis
Circulatory overload	Isosensitization
Chemistry toxicity	Platelet
Cold arrythmia	Anti A or B platelet antibodies
Anti-cell	Anti HL-A platelet antibodies
anti-red cell (hemolysis)	Leukocytes
antineutrophile	Anti HL-A leukocyte antibodies
antiplatelet	Graft vs host reaction
Acquired platelet deficiency	Siderosis
Acquired coagulant deficiency	Transmission of disease
Air embolism	Virus
	Hepatitis
	Epstein-Barr
	Cytomegalic Inclusion Disease
	Other
	Protozoan
	Malaria
	Leishmaniasis
	Trypanosomiasis
	Syphilis
	Infectious carrier state is produced (i.e. Au antigenemia)

Immediate

Pyrogenic reactions are so classified after a search for specific causes of fever is unrevealing. While it is entirely possible that any of the "immediate" complications could be present in a forme fruste that is unrecognizable, the reaction is for the moment treated as a nonspecific one, while reservations remain in the mind of the observer. At the same time, a posttransfusion blood sample, the pretransfusion and donor samples, and the donor blood in the bottle, are retyped, rescreened for antibodies and recrossmatched to ensure the absence of a red cell antibody-antigen reaction. The donor bottle (or bag) contents are cultured at 30°C and at 37°C in anaerobic and aerobic media. The posttransfusion serum specimen is examined grossly for hemolysis. Urine, if available, is examined grossly for hemoglobinuria. Treatment with antipyretics generally suffices.

Allergic reactions relate to transmission of an antiallergen or of an allergen to the patient. Hives, fever, itching, and discomfort are the usual obvious symptoms. The sudden onset of stridor always is a sign of laryngeal and/or glottic involvement. Treatment is with antihistamines and, if severe, adrenalin may be most valuable. Steroids should be given if there is inadequate response to the former drugs.

Transmission of grossly infected blood is a fortunate rarity when the blood is collected in an approved manner.

Circulatory overload remains an often overlooked disorder. It most commonly occurs when whole blood and/or red cells and/or fluids are given too zealously. It is seen most commonly in patients with severe chronic anemia, whose blood volumes are normal or increased and whose cardiac status is already compromised as a consequence of the anemia and/or intrinsic cardiac disease. A recent report attests to the frequency of this complication by reporting four of 27 deaths of 6199 consecutively monitored patients receiving some drug therapy, as due to this complication.[27] How many escape death by prompt treatment or by eventual resolution cannot even be surmised. Treatment is by prompt phlebotomy and/or use of a fast-acting diuretic *other than a volemic one such as mannitol.* Furosemide and ethacrynic acid are two that are quite effective. However, their potential toxicity is something to be reckoned with.

Chemical toxicity chiefly relates to citrate, potassium, ammonia ion, and acid metabolites. These can be virtually avoided by resorting to red cell packs whenever anoxemia is to be combatted. If volume is also needed, electrolyte and albumin solutions should also be used in required amounts.

Cold blood may induce arrythmia if given as an exchange transfusion or as part of massive transfusion. Prevention is easily effected through the use of electrical coil warmers now generally available.

Another possible complication is the activation of a cold hemolytic reaction on the exceedingly rare occasion when a high-titer cold antibody exists in the patient and the patient is under hypothermia. Knowledge of the presence of such an antibody will permit use of blood lacking the antigen in question.

Antineutrophilic leukocyte antibodies are the leukoagglutinins commonly referred to. They can cause mild to severe pyrogenic reactions. Treatment consists of antipyretic and symptomatic care. If very severe, and occurring in a severely ill patient, a single large dose of steroid can be given. Prevention is effected by using buffy-coat poor red cells and if this is unsuccessful, washed or frozen red cells will obviate the problem.

Antiplatelet antibodies specifically to platelet antigens may uncommonly induce a febrile reaction.

Anti-red cell antibodies are the most feared, and properly so, because about 50 percent of hemolytic reactions are serious or fatal. The problem most often relates to a clerical error such as (1) blood sample for crossmatch is obtained from the wrong patient, (2) errors of transcription and labeling in the laboratory, and (3) properly labeled blood is transfused to the incorrect patient.

Symptoms consist of chest, loin, back or abdominal pain, dyspnea, fever, discomfort, and in short, almost any other symptom to appear suddenly. Objective signs are dyspnea, hypotension, unexpected hypertension, bradycardia, or tachypnea and tachycardia.

Treatment consists of immediate discontinuance of the transfusion, but keeping the iv open.[28] Then the procedure as outlined above under pyrogenic reaction is carried out.

If the symptoms are classical, 20 percent mannitol should be injected in three to four minutes in an amount appropriate for the weight of the person. This is followed by an alkalinizing agent and a large dose of steroid. Urine flow should ensue promptly. Forced diuresis with appropriate electrolyte solutions should continue the diuresis. If urine suppression occurs and is not responsive to one or two doses of mannitol, a presumption of renal insufficiency is in order.

The treatment of shock, if present, is with electrolyte solutions and albumin. Blood is not used until the cause of hemolysis is ascertained.

Platelet deficiency regularly occurs after massive transfusion. Because it rarely falls below 50,000–100,000/mm^3 and does not cause bleeding when in this range, replacement is unnecessary. Return to normal ensues in four to ten days. Where bleeding occurs and levels lower than 50,000/mm^3 are present, replacement therapy would seem to be a judicious move.

Coagulant deficiency is a most unlikely result of massive transfusion [8] unless disseminated intravascular coagulation (DIC) is also present. However, multiple borderline deficiencies of coagulants associated with platelets in the 50,000–75,000/mm^3 range may be responsible for bleeding. In such a situation, the use of fresh blood complemented by fresh frozen plasma will generally turn the tide. If available, platelet-rich plasma can be used in lieu of the fresh frozen plasma. In general, this problem can be avoided if a unit of fresh frozen plasma is used for every three to five units of whole blood that is given. If anoxemia ensues, PRC can be given. Likewise, if severe thrombocytopenia results, platelet packs may be given. If DIC is present, heparin therapy must be started with replacement of Factor VIII, Factor V, platelets, and fibrinogen as complementary therapy.

Air embolism is a serious complication, most often occurring when blood in glass bottles is infused rapidly under pressure. While plastic bags are safer in this regard, air embolism has been observed as a result of entry of air into the bag at the time the entry port is opened just prior to insertion of the filter tubing's nozzle.[29] The complication can be obviated by careful observation of the emptying blood bottle and by clamping the tubing with a hemostat kept readily available for this purpose as soon as a last few milliliters of blood are left in the bottle or bag. When air embolism occurs, treatment consists of

placing the patient on his right side and providing supportive symptomatic therapy.

Delayed Reactions

Hemolytic reactions occasionally occur seven to 15 days after transfusion in a recipient having a low titer or absence of previously present
antibodies. While generally mild or even asymptomatic, occasionally a
full-blown reaction takes place. In the latter, treatment is as with the
acute hemolysis. The former is by far the most common and requires
no treatment.

Immunization commonly results following transfusion. For Rh_o
(D), it is known that immunization approximates 80 percent when an
rh person receives Rh_o blood. The serious problem associated with such
immunization is the future risk of hemolytic disease in the newborn of
an rh girl given Rh_o blood, and the risk of hemolytic transfusion should
Rh_o blood be given again to a sensitized person of either sex. Similar
risks apply to other red cell antigen systems.

Immunization to lymphocytes produces antibodies to the HL-A
antigen system and as such would present a hurdle if future isologous
transplantation is attempted in the sensitized person.

Antibodies to neutrophiles may be formed to provide leukoagglu-
tinin problems at a later date.

Siderosis occurs only in the patient who is repeatedly transfused
for chronic non-blood loss anemia.

By all odds, hepatitis is the most serious delayed reaction, because
it is at present impossible, other than by history and the HAA test, to
ascertain the presence of most of the infectious agents. In the areas of
the world where the protozoan diseases and HAA positivity are endemic and/or epidemic, it may be extremely difficult to collect non-
infective donors. Similarly, during virus epidemics in this country, we
undoubtedly transfuse the blood of some donors who carry the epidemic virus. Be that as it may, the threat is serum hepatitis, for which
incidences of 15 percent, 14.9 percent, and 12 percent[30] are an indication of the serious nature of this complication.

Some progress has been made in recent years in uncovering the
hepatitis-associated antigen (HAA) or as it is also called, the Australia
(Au) antigen.[31] The HAA antigen is a 200–300 angstrom particle, largely
protein, and is stable after freezing for transmission and immunologic
action. It is stable immunologically after heating to 60°C, but is no
longer transmissible, as witness the lack of icterogenicity of albumin
solutions, which are subjected to this temperature. The agent's icterogenicity is transmissible through all other transfusable blood components. Transfusion of blood containing HAA carries up to a 74-percent
risk of producing hepatitis, transmitting the antigen or inducing anti-
HAA antibodies in the recipient.[32,33,34]

Methodology for HAA detection in donor blood is rapidly changing. At present, some 0.1 percent of community type donors and about four percent of skid row–type donors have been found to contain the antigen by the available procedures. Improved sensitivity is expected in the near future. Notwithstanding this, the test detects only about 25 percent of the cases of icteric hepatitis that follow transfusion. It follows that most cases are not related to HAA and as such are due to another agent, or that HAA is only one of a variety of forms the agent of hepatitis takes, or HAA is present in too low a titer for detection. Suffice it to say that HAA screening is universally done, and donors positive for HAA are excluded from giving blood.

Its impact on our understanding of the relationship of endemic or epidemic hepatitis to the serum variety is great. We now recognize that HAA is transmitted either parenterally or nonparenterally, and that epidemics of HAA hepatitis have occurred and continue to occur.[35,36] Further, about one to two percent of patients with hepatitis become carriers and some of these go on to chronic liver disease.

Prevention

The observation that in some patients antibody titer can be elicited after Au injection and the titer boosted by a second injection has led to the exploration of passive immunization in Au contacts or recipients.

Ordinary gamma globulin, according to a recent cooperative study, has no effect.[38] More recently, several reports suggest protection with HAA immune serum globulin.[39,40,41]

CONCLUSION

1.   Blood is composed of several components, each of which have specific indications.
2.   Whole blood should be used only when there is need for the effects of both red cells and plasma or when one of its components is needed, but is unavailable as such.
3.   Red cells should be used as the primary mode of therapy in chronic anemia and in the hemodiluted normovolemic state of post-hemorrhagic anemia.
4.   Blood loss should be primarily treated with large amounts of Ringer's lactate and albumin and complemented with enough whole blood and/or red cell unit to keep the hematocrit around 30 volumes percent.
5.   Coagulant effect can be obtained from fresh frozen plasma for any deficiency.
6.   Cryoprecipitate is the preferred material for treatment of hemorrhage due to Factor VIII deficiency.

7. In general, commercial concentrates made from large pools of plasma should be avoided because of their high hepatitis risk.
8. Blood and its components have a very decided hazard.
9. Resolution of the chronic blood shortage will be greatly assisted by the involvement of physicians in donor procurement.

REFERENCES

1. Blood component therapy. American Association of Blood Banks, 1969.
2. Brewer, G.J., and Eaton, J.W.: Erythrocyte metabolism: Interaction with oxygen transport. American Assoc. for the Advancement of Sciences 717:1205–1211, 1971.
3. Oski, F.A., and Gottlieb, A.J.: The inter-relationships between red blood cell metabolites, hemoglobin, and the oxygen equilibrium curve. Progr Hemat 7:33–68, 1971.
4. Murphy, S., and Gardner, F.H.: Platelet preservation. Effect of storage temperature on platelet viability. Deleterious effect of refrigerated storage. New Eng J Med 280:1094–1098, 1969.
5. Hirsh, J., and Dobry, J.C.G.: Platelet function in health and disease. Prog Hemat 7:185–234, 1971.
6. Levin, R.H.: Response to transfusion of platelets pooled from multiple donors and the effects of various techniques of concentrating platelets. Transfusion 5:54–63, 1965.
7. Freireich, E.J.: Response to repeated platelet transfusions from the same donor. Ann Intern Med 59:277–287, 1963.
8. Schmidt, P.J., and Gridon, A.J.: Blood and blood components in the prevention and control of bleeding. JAMA 202:967–969, 1967.
9. Pool, J.G.: Cryoprecipitated Factor VIII concentrate, Thrombosis, et Diathesis Haemorrhagica. 35:35–40, 1969.
10. Dallman, P.R., and Pool, J.G.: Treatment of hemophilia with Factor VIII concentrate. New Eng J Med 278:199–202, 1968.
11. Perkins, H.A.: Correction of the hemostatic defects in Von Willebrand's disease. Blood 30:375, 1967.
12. Breen, F.A., Jr., and Tullis, J.L.: Prothrombin concentration in treatment of Christmas Disease and allied disorders. JAMA 208:1848–1852, 1969.
13. Kasper, C.K.: Surgical operation in hemophilia B, use of Factor IX concentrate. Calif Med 113:4–8, 1970.
14. Roberts, H.R., and Penick, G.D.: Hemostasis in Factor V deficiency. Amer J Med Sci 248:194, 1964.
15. Spector, I., Corn, M., and Ticktin, H.E.: Plasma transfusions in liver disease. New Eng J Med 275:1032–1037, 1966.
16. Strauss, H.S.: Surgery in patients with congenital Factor VII deficiency. Blood 25:325–334, 1965.
17. Trudnowski, R.J.: Hydration with Ringer's lactate solution: Its effectiveness in maintaining stable circulation during and after surgery. JAMA 195:545–548, 1966.
18. McCleland, R.N., et al: Balanced salt solution in the treatment of hemorrhagic shock: Studies in dogs. JAMA 199:830–834, 1967.
19. Rigor, B., Bosomworth, P., and Rush, B.F., Jr.: Replacement of operative blood loss of more than 1 liter with Hartmann's solution. JAMA 203:399–402, 1968.
20. Bridenbaugh, P.D., et al: Limitations of lactated Ringer's solution in massive fluid replacement. JAMA 206:2313–2315, 1968.

21. Lowery, B.D.: Electrolyte solutions on resuscitation in human hemorrhagic shock. *Surg Gynec Obstet* 133:273–283, 1971.

22. Moffitt, E.A., et al: Myocardial metabolisms in open heart surgery using whole blood in the pump oxygenator. *Mayo Clin Proc* 46:333–338, 1971.

23. Takaori, M., and Safar, P.: Treatment of massive hemorrhage with colloid crystalloid solutions. *JAMA* 199:297–302, 1967.

24. Marty, A.T., et al: Rheologic effects of hypothermia on blood with high hematocrit values. *J Thorac Cardiovasc Surg* 61:735–738, 1971.

25. Standards for blood banks and transfusion services. American Association of Blood Banks, 1970.

26. Wood, M., Price, W.R., Childer, D.: Hidden danger of pooled plasma. *Amer J Surg* 114:629–635, 1967.

27. Shapiro, S., et al: Fetal drug reactions among medical inpatients. *JAMA* 216:467–472, 1971.

28. Sacks, H.J.: Hemolytic reaction to transfusion of incompatible blood, *Current Pediatric Therapy*. Philadelphia: W.B. Saunders, 1971, pp 260–261.

29. Yeakel, A.C.: Lethal air embolism from plastic blood storage containers. *JAMA* 204:267–269, 1968.

30. Gruber, U.F.: *Blood Replacement*. New York. Springer Verlag, 1969, pp 22–26.

31. Blumberg, B.S., et al: Australian antigen and hepatitis, a comprehensive review. CRC Critical Reviews in *Clinical Laboratory Science*, p 473, September 1971.

32. Gocke, D.J., Greenberg, H.B., and Kavey, N.B.: Correlation of Australia antigen with post-transfusion hepatitis. *JAMA* 212:877–979, 1970.

33. Widman, F.K.: The Australia antigen: Where do we stand?, Part I. *Postgrad Med* 50:167–169, 1971.

34. ———: The Australian antigen: Where do we stand?, Part II. *Postgrad Med* 51:257–260, 1972.

35. Kelan, A.E., et al: Hepatitis-associated antigen in sporadic cases of acute viral hepatitis. *Canad Med Ass J* 106:32–35, 1972.

36. Krugman, S., and Giles, J.P.: Viral hepatitis: New light on old disease. *JAMA* 212:1019–1029, 1970.

37. Kern, F., Jr., et al: The elusive hepatitis virus. *Audiodigest: Internal Medicine* 18, September 15, 1971.

38. Grady, G., and Bennett, A.J.E.: Prevention of post-transfusion hepatitis by gamma globulin. *JAMA* 214:140–142, 1970.

39. Prince, A.M.: Antibody against serum hepatitis antigen prevalence and potential use as immune serum globulin in prevention of serum hepatitis infections. *New Eng J Med* 285:933–937, 1971.

40. Krugman, S., Giles, J.P., and Hammond, J.: Viral hepatitis, Type B (MS-2 strain): Prevention with specific hepatitis B immune serum globulin. *JAMA* 218:1665–1670, 1971.

41. Katz, R., Rodriguez, J., and Ward, R.: Post-transfusion hepatitis: Effect of modified gamma globulin added to blood in vitro. *New Eng J Med* 285:925–932, 1971.

11

Physiologic Monitoring

Marc I. Rowe, M.D.

This chapter deals with the management of the seriously ill pediatric surgical patient with emphasis placed almost exclusively on the newborn and the infant. The baby, because of his unique physiologic adjustments and pathologic processes, presents complex management problems and, because of his small size, difficult technical obstacles. Principles and techniques discussed will be those with which we have had personal experience either in the nursery or in our clinical or newborn animal research laboratories. The views are personal and at times controversial.

THE PHILOSOPHY OF INTENSIVE CARE

At mortality conferences, the death of an infant is often described as follows: "He was doing well postoperatively when he suddenly became unresponsive and, in spite of vigorous efforts, died." Many of the physicians present will sadly shake their heads and agree that babies are fragile and can deteriorate with alarming speed. It is our contention that the infant surgical patient is a hardy organism who has already coped with the difficult and complex adjustments of birth and who gives ample warning when he is in trouble. The problem is that the warnings are not those we expect if we use the adult patient as our guide. One of the prime goals of intensive care is to search out and identify subtle signs of trouble before deterioration has progressed to the point where therapy is unsuccessful. Elaborate physical facilities and electronic monitoring equipment simply aid us in this task. Monitoring devices offer to the attending personnel a method of extending their physical faculties so that slight changes may be rapidly recognized and measured. No matter how sophisticated this equipment has become, the basic monitor still remains the highly skilled nurse. The computer system has not replaced the sound clinical judgment of a trained surgeon who is well versed in basic physiology.

MONITORING EQUIPMENT

Many physicians find it difficult to properly evaluate the impressive, costly, and, at times, seemingly magic hardware that is offered at scientific exhibits, in brochures, journals, and by manufacturers' representatives for monitoring and treating the sick infant. The doctor must first decide whether he needs equipment for patient care or clinical research. Then he must determine the actual function of the instrument considered for purchase. Some equipment gives significant data that are easy to interpret and useful in almost all situations. Other devices may be of value for research purposes or only in special clinical situations. If the budget is low and the prime mission of the staff is care, not research, a minimum of elaborate, specialized equipment should be purchased.

There are three factors that must be considered before monitoring devices are purchased: simplicity of operation, reliability, and service. Equipment becomes less valuable for patient care if its operation is so complex that only highly skilled and trained technicians can obtain accurate results. Such a device often becomes useless at night, on weekends, or on holidays when trained personnel are not available. Equipment should be relatively simple to operate so that a number of people can be trained in its use and the manufacturer must provide simple and accurate operating instructions. A surprisingly high percentage of costly monitoring equipment arrives from the manufacturer nonoperational. Often, a long and frustrating delay takes place while a vigorous communication is carried on between the manufacturer and the physician, adjustments are made, and improperly functioning elements are replaced. It is essential that the doctor investigate the reliability of the firm before he purchases its product. This can best be done by contacting other hospitals and laboratories who use the same equipment and questioning their personnel about the dependability of the manufacturer. Service is often a geographic problem. If the company that sells the equipment is a great distance from the intensive care unit and there are no local skilled service representatives available, malfunction of the equipment can lead to long delays and costly repair and transportation bills. The potential purchaser must explore the service record of the company and the availability of skilled repairmen.

ELECTRICAL SAFETY

With the advent of electronic monitoring devices, a new hazard faces the neonatal surgical patient—electrocution. An idea of the amount of electrical power required during the course of intensive care can be gathered from recent design recommendation for maximal care areas of newborn intensive care units. It was recommended that at least eight electrical outlets be available for each newborn patient. Documented cases of electrocution have occurred in adult intensive care units, but as yet there have been no known cases of infant death due to electrocution. The amount of current necessary to produce ventricular fibrillation in a newborn is unknown. In the normal adult it is about 10 ma. The sick patient can develop cardiac arrest from exposure to 1 ma and the "electrically susceptible" patient, suffering from cardiac arrhythmias, 10 μa.[1] Available information suggests that infants and children are more vulnerable to electric shock than adults. Electrical safety involves several phases: the design of the monitoring equipment, the local grounding system of the patient and his environment, the isolation from the building and electrical power systems, and the knowledge of the attending personnel. The following recommendations will reduce electrical hazards in a newborn intensive care unit:

1. All attending staff should have basic training in the safe use of electricity.
2. A common ground should be installed for all electrical outlets.
3. Adaptors, extension cords, and junction boxes should not be used.
4. Electrical apparatus should be checked for current leak.
5. No electrical equipment with a leak of 10 μa or more should be used in a nursery.
6. Monthly electrical checks of the nursery should be done for grounding and current leakage.

VASCULAR CANNULATION

The future of monitoring rests with the development of noninvasive methods of measuring bodily functions. Unfortunately, many important monitoring and therapeutic arrangements presently require a connection with the vascular system. This necessitates cannulation of arteries and veins. The placement of a foreign body into the vascular system can result in serious complications—sepsis, thrombosis, perforation, and embolization. Before a vascular cannula is placed, the physician should be sure that the condition of the patient warrants the risks. Vascular catheterization will be discussed in detail since there are many difficulties associated with the insertion and maintenance of a relatively large cannula in the small blood vessel of the sick infant.

The Intravascular Catheter

The ideal vascular catheter should be nonreactive, thin walled, and rigid enough not to dampen pulse waves. It should be slippery to allow easy passage through the vessel, radiopaque so that the position of the catheter can be checked by x-ray, and made of a material that will retard the clotting of blood within its lumen. I do not believe that the perfect catheter has yet been developed.

Silastic cannulae cause little endothelial reaction and blood within their lumen does not clot rapidly. They are soft and difficult to pass into small blood vessels. Because of their soft walls, they dampen pulse waves and are of little use for pressure monitoring. Silastic catheters distend when blood is pumped under pressure and should not be used during operations when blood loss is expected. They are excellent for long-term intravenous nutrition. (See Chapter 9.)

Teflon catheters have a slippery external surface. Their walls are rigid and they transmit pulse waves accurately. Catheters made of this material can be constructed with thin walls so that the inside diameter is relatively large, allowing a larger lumen size for the overall size of the catheter. Unfortunately, because of their rigid walls, teflon cannulae tend to kink and, more important, can perforate the infant's blood vessels.

Polyvinyl chloride catheters are usually made by the manufacturer with a radiopaque filler for x-ray localization. They are easy to pass and transmit pulse waves accurately, but are more reactive than teflon or silastic catheters. Although teflon cannulae have thinner walls and are more slippery, there is less danger of vascular perforation with the polyvinyl catheters. We prefer the polyvinyl catheters for arterial and venous pressure monitoring and for short-term intravenous therapy.

Surgical Technique

It is possible to insert plastic cannulae percutaneously into the vein of even a small infant using one of the specially designed kits commercially available (see pages 128–129). The advantages of the percutaneous method over a formal cutdown are speed and the avoidance of a surgical procedure. However, since the catheter must usually be placed in a peripheral vein, it is not suitable for measuring central venous pressure and delivering hypertonic fluids. The percutaneous route is often impossible to use in small patients profoundly dehydrated or in shock. Percutaneous catheters usually cannot be placed in peripheral arteries of small infants. In the seriously ill baby who requires venous and arterial cannulation, we prefer placement of the cannula by a formal cutdown procedure.

Because the blood vessels of the baby are fragile and tiny, there are technical difficulties associated with performing a venous or arterial cutdown. However, if the proper equipment is available and a precise technique is developed, cannulation can usually be accomplished without difficulty (see Figure 9–1 on page 129). One of the most critical and frequently neglected aids to the rapid and safe placement of an intravascular catheter is proper lighting. It is unusual to perform a cutdown in a well-lighted operating room. More often, catheterization is done as an emergency in the nursery or emergency room. We keep available a powerful fibre-optic headlight that plugs into the standard hospital electrical outlet. This lamp directs a circle of cold, bright light at the blood vessel and simplifies a difficult procedure immeasurably.

In many hospitals, the instruments necessary to perform a cutdown on an infant are not available. The surgeon must insist that small, well-maintained instruments be made up as a kit and placed in the pediatric facilities. The instruments that determine the success or failure of the cutdown are scissors. These are usually in poor repair and dull from repeated autoclaving and misuse. The points are often blunt and bent. We use microvascular scissors that have sharp, fine, curved points. This instrument is separately packaged and gas sterilized. Microvascular scissors serve two functions: to make a clean, controlled incision into the blood vessel and to act as a vascular dilator (Figure 11–1). After the vessel is isolated, a transverse incision is made at a right angle to the long axis of the blood vessel with the tips of the scissors. The scissors are then closed and the points inserted through the in-

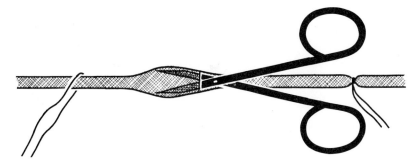

Figure 11–1
Microvascular scissors' blades spread within the vessel lumen dilating vessel lumen, relieving spasm and opening the vascular incision.

cision into the vessel lumen. The blades are spread and the scissors withdrawn with open blades. The catheter is then quickly inserted into the blood vessel and passed to the desired distance. We believe that dilatation of the blood vessel before catheter insertion is the most important maneuvre in the performance of a venous or arterial cut-down. If the scissors points cannot be passed into the lumen, it will be impossible to pass the catheter. The dilatation relieves vascular spasm, opens the incision, and pushes aside the strands of adventitia that hang into the vessel lumen and inhibit catheterization. This simple maneuver has made it possible for us to successfully perform over 2000 vascular cannulations in newborn puppies weighing as little as 180 gm.

The Saphenous Vein

The saphenous vein at the ankle is a reliable route for the routine administration of intravenous fluids. We do not use this vessel when central venous pressure is to be measured, irritating hypertonic fluids are to be administered, or large-volume blood replacement will be needed.

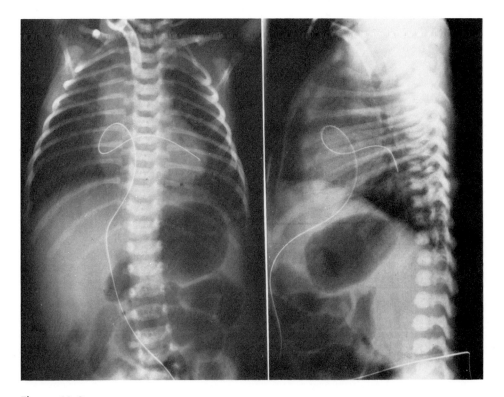

Figure 11–2
Umbilical vein catheter passed upward through inferior vena cava into right atrium across the foramen ovale into the left atrium.

The Umbilical Vein

The umbilical vein can serve as an emergency site for catheter placement when a large vein is needed in a newborn. Except in critical emergencies this vessel should be avoided because of the high complication rate associated with catheter placement. Sepsis is a serious risk, and thrombosis can lead to portal vein obstruction, portal hypertension, and bleeding esophageal varices. Bowel necrosis has been reported as a complication of umbilical vein cannulation. Umbilical vein catheters are frequently misdirected. We have seen the tip passed into the superior mesenteric vein, the right portal vein, the coronary sinus, and into various chambers of the heart (Figure 11–2). If it is used, an x-ray check of its position must always be done.

The Brachial Vein System

The antebrachial vein located in the medial aspect of the antecubital fossa is usually of sufficient size for easy cannulation. Catheters can be passed into the brachial vein and with manipulation of the arm and shoulder upward into the subclavian vein and the superior vena cava. The cephalic vein is also found in the antecubital fossa. Passage of a catheter through this vessel into the central veins is difficult because of the sharp angle where the cephalic vein joins the subclavian vein at the deltopectoral groove.

Jugular Veins

Both external jugular veins are large and superficial, but passage of a catheter through them into the superior vena cava is difficult at times. The final position of the catheter tip must be checked by x-ray. The internal jugular vein gives direct access to the superior vena cava, but is not used until both external juglar veins have been utilized (see Figure 9–3 on page 131 and Figure 9–4 on pages 145–146).

The Umbilical Artery

The umbilical arteries are easily cannulated during the first two or three days of life. Once the catheter is in place, arterial blood pressure, pH, and blood gases can be monitored from the abdominal and ascending aorta. Sepsis presents a problem because of the frequent bacterial colonization of the umbilical stump. In one study positive bacterial cultures were obtained from 56 percent of the umbilical catheters.[2]

Umbilical artery catheterization has resulted in thrombosis of major aortic branches, particularly the renal and mesenteric, with organ necrosis and death. With uncontrolled advancement, the tip can be passed into the ascending aorta through the ductus arteriosus and into

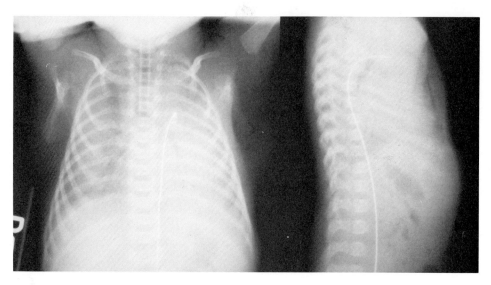

Figure 11–3
Umbilical artery catheter advanced to the ductus arteriosus and into the pulmonary artery. Confusing pO_2 measurements were obtained from this infant managed on a mechanical respirator.

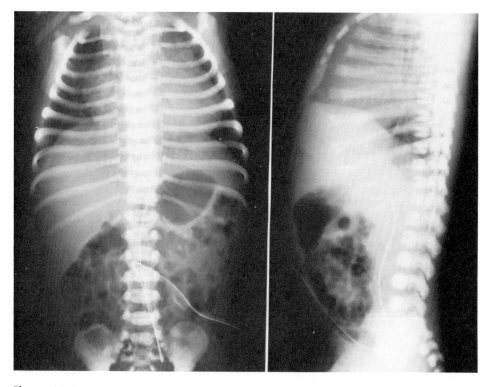

Figure 11–4
Post mortem examination of this newborn revealed that the umbilical catheter tip was wedged into the celiac artery with thrombosis of this vessel.

the pulmonary artery, causing dangerously confusing oxygen tension (pO_2) readings (Figure 11–3). Serious obstruction of blood flow can be produced if the catheter is inadvertently passed into the blood supply of an organ (Figure 11–4).

In spite of these hazards, with proper precautions, the umbilical arteries are useful routes for arterial cannulization. No anesthesia is necessary, the cord is transected, and the ends of the arteries identified. The umbilical vein is a single, large, thin-walled vessel with its end lying open in the superior aspect of the cord. The arteries lie on either side of the inferior aspect of the cut surface of the cord. The vessels on cross section are white, their lumens are collapsed, and their walls thicker than the vein. The tissue adherent to one of the arteries is grasped with a forceps and the lumen dilated with fine forceps or the microvascular scissors. A number 3 or 5 French umbilical catheter is then inserted into the vessel lumen and passed downward. We prefer soft thermosensitive catheters with rounded ends made from polyvinyl chloride that have a radiopaque strip for x-ray localization. As the catheter is advanced, it reaches the iliac artery and then passes upward into the abdominal aorta. The safest position for the catheter tip is at the level of the diaphragm approximately (T 12) or just above the aortic bifurcation (L 2 or 3) (Figure 11–5). The position of the catheter must

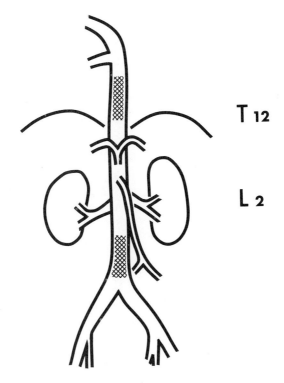

Figure 11–5
The two safe areas for placement of the umbilical artery catheter tip—just above the diaphragm and at the level of the bifurcation of the aorta.

always be checked by x-ray to avoid incorrect placement (Figure 11–4). Immediately after insertion of the catheter, the physician should observe the color of the infant's lower extremities and palpate the femoral pulsations. Occasionally, the catheter can induce vascular spasm or pass downward into the femoral vessels. If the femoral pulses cannot be felt, the cannula should immediately be withdrawn.

The Radial Artery

This artery is usually sufficiently large and superficial that it can be easily cannulated even in the small infant. It gives access to the blood above the ductus arteriosus, which is helpful if a right to left shunt develops. However, use of this vessel carries serious risk, and we only use it when no other artery is available. If peripheral circulation is poor and the color of the hand is dusky we will not cannulate the radial artery. To insure adequate circulation to the hand we always ascertain that the ulnar artery is functional. If pulsations cannot be felt, a Doppler ultrasonic probe is helpful in determining if there is blood flow in the ulnar artery. No attempt should be made to cannulate the radial artery if there is any question about the integrity of the ulnar artery. Care must be taken not to pass the catheter into the brachial artery or higher into the arterial tree, since the catheter may then occlude the blood flow into the arm. Irritating solutions containing sugar should not be used for irrigation since they cause endothelial reaction and may lead to thrombosis. The radial artery should never be used as a route for fluid infusion. Rapid flow of fluid against the arterial stream can inhibit blood flow to the hand and lead to gangrene.

Temporal Artery

We prefer to use the temporal artery rather than the radial artery for cannulation when the umbilical artery is no longer available or there is a right-to-left shunt across the ductus arteriosus. The temporal artery is expendable. Thrombosis has not led to complications. Its position can accurately be determined in most cases by palpation, and it is easily found by making a short transverse incision just anterior to the helical ring of the ear, above the tragus. Unfortunately, it is a small vessel, making cannulation a difficult chore if the infant weighs less than 6 lbs. We have successfully catheterized the temporal artery in infants weighing as little as 2 lbs, but feel that this would be impossible unless proper lighting and instruments are available. The fibre-optic headlight and the microvascular scissors are absolutely essential. Temporal artery cannulae lie above the ductus arteriosus and give an accurate index of oxygen tension of the blood perfusing the eyes and brain, even if a right-to-left shunt across the ductus develops in an hypoxic infant.

Management of Intravascular Catheters

The presence of a foreign body that communicates with the external surface of the body and lies within the lumen of a blood vessel frequently leads to sepsis. The risk of infection increases with the time the catheter remains in place. As soon as a vascular cannula is no longer needed, it should be removed. The incidence of infection can be reduced if meticulous sterile technique is maintained during the actual performance of the cutdown. When possible, the catheter should emerge from a site distant from the cutdown incisions. Daily application of an antibacterial ointment to the catheter and exit wound appears to reduce the incidence of sepsis. Betadine preparation has been used as a defence against fungal infections. Redness, swelling, or drainage about the catheter suggests infection and prompts removal of the catheter. When infection is suspected, blood culture should be drawn and the tip of the catheter cultured. Once an intravascular line has been established, its continuity should be broken as infrequently as possible.

Blockage of an intravascular catheter by blood clot is a common problem. If a constant flow of fluid is delivered through the catheter, the danger of obstruction is reduced. In some institutions, infusions are run through umbilical artery catheters to prevent blockage. Although this can be done with apparent safety, we avoid this route of fluid administration. Fluid should never be infused into a peripheral artery of an infant. To prevent catheter obstruction, arterial cannulae are usually filled with a heparinized saline solution and flushed intermittently. If flushing is not done with care, fluid overload, hypernatremia, and systemic heparinization can develop in a baby. By using dilute heparin-saline solution, the amount of heparin and sodium chloride the patient receives is reduced. To minimize the volume of fluid delivered during catheter irrigation, a tuberculin syringe or a flushing setup employing a pressurized bag (Figure 11–6) can be used. A common error when attaching arterial lines to blood pressure transducers is to employ long, plastic connecting tubes that can hold more than 10 ml of fluid. If vigorous flushing is then done proximal to the tube, the entire dead space will be injected into the baby's circulation. Transducers should be attached as close as possible or directly to the catheter.

Significant blood loss is a constant danger when frequent blood gas and pH determinations are made. A small infant maintained on a respirator can have as many as 15 samples drawn from an arterial line by an enthusiastic house officer. In a 5-lb baby, this may represent a loss of almost nine percent of the total blood volume in 24 hours. We attempt to limit the number of samples drawn, replace blood loss with plasma or plasma substitute, and insist that our technicians do determinations on 0.5 ml of blood.

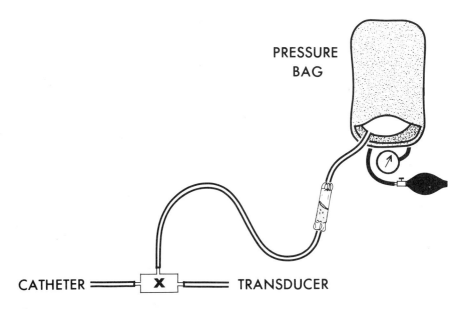

Figure 11–6
Pressure flushing system. Inflatable bag and three-way stopcock allow small volumes of irrigating solution to be injected through the catheter.

PHYSIOLOGIC MONITORING

Pulse Rate

The heart rate can be accurately and continuously measured electronically. The ventricular (QRS) complex of the electrocardiogram (ECG) can be displayed on an oscilloscope or permanently recorded. By introducing a meter into the system, it is possible to digitally display the rate in beats per minute and broadcast each beat as an audible tone. An alarm included in the system will signal a fall or rise in rate. The weakest link in the heart rate monitoring system is the junction between the electrode and the patient. Improper fixation of the electrodes causes artifacts, patient discomfiture, and requires frequent replacement. Large electrodes may cover a premature infant's entire chest. Needle electrodes give good contact, but necessitate a break in the skin. We prefer the disposable silver–silver chloride electrodes that are small and remain in place over several days.

Keep in mind when monitoring the pulse rate of the newborn patient that a rapid rate, usually around 120 beats per minute, is normal. An increase in pulse rate is often due to hyperthermia, produced by overheating of the infant's incubator. Unlike the adult, who responds to difficulties with tachycardia, life-threatening challenges such as hypoxia, blood loss, and sepsis result in bradycardia in the newborn. Slowing of the pulse rate is an ominous sign often followed by seizures or cardiac arrest.

Arterial Blood Pressure

The measurement of arterial blood pressure is still an important cornerstone in assessing the circulation, although flow measurements may prove to be of greater value in the future. In both the adult and the newborn baby, a fall in pressure suggests blood volume reduction or inadequate cardiac output. Significant hypotension is often found in infants suffering from hyaline membrane disease, asphyxia neonatorum, and sepsis. Kitterman, Phibbs, and Tooley found that the aortic blood pressure of the newborn infant correlates closely with birth weight.[3] The lower limits of normal during the first 12 hours of life were 30 mm Hg at 1001–2000 gm, 35 mm Hg at 3000 gm, and 43 mm Hg at 4000 gm. A rough estimate of the cardiac output can be determined from the pulse pressure and the pulse wave contour.

Arterial blood-pressure monitoring of the infant has been neglected because of past technical difficulties. The pneumatic cuff and stethoscope serve well for intermittent measurements of large infants and children, but are difficult to use and unreliable in the small baby. Blood pressure can be accurately measured and continuously displayed through an arterial catheter attached to a strain-gauge transducer and recording device. The major objection to direct measurement of blood pressure is the necessity for intravascular cannulation. In seriously ill infants, the risks are justified and the arterial line can also serve as a blood-sampling site for blood gas and pH determinations.

The recent introduction of the Doppler ultrasonic shiftsensor for measuring blood pressure in infants has proven simple, safe, and relatively inexpensive. Blood pressure can be measured from either the leg or the arm. The method utilizes an ultrasonic transducer that senses arterial wall motion. Both systolic and diastolic pressure can be measured. Several studies have shown excellent correlation between arterial blood pressure measured by the Doppler and by intraarterial lines and strain gauges.[4,5] The proper placement and fixation of the probe over the baby's artery, usually the radial, popliteal, or brachial is important.

Central Venous Pressure

Central venous pressure monitoring has been used in the adult to prevent circulatory overload during rapid intravenous replacement therapy, as a method of determining the adequacy of blood-volume replacement, and as a means of differentiating the various forms of shock.

The following general principles must be kept in mind when this technique is used to monitor the infant.

Baseline

The zero point for measuring central venous pressure should be at the level of the right atrium. A convenient reference point is the midaxillary line. For consistent readings, as the baby's position is shifted, the manometer or transducer's zero point must be realigned with the reference point of the patient. This can be done with the aid of a carpenter's or line, level (Figure 11–7) or by holding the manometer near the chest at the zero point during the measurement.

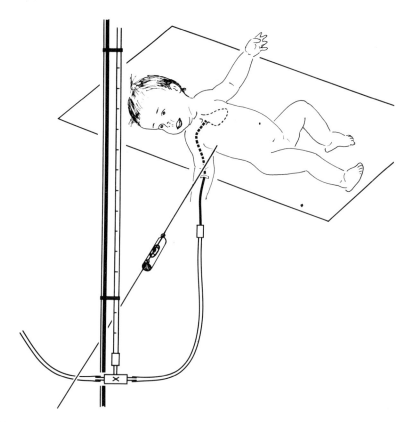

Figure 11–7
Line level used to find the zero reference on the infant's chest when measuring central venous pressure. Mid-axillary line is a convenient point.

Intraabdominal Pressure

Abdominal distention from intestinal obstruction or intraperitoneal fluid or tight abdominal closure can produce a rapid rise in intraabdominal pressure and cause inferior vena cava compression. Figure 11–8 illustrates the pressure differential between the superior vena cava

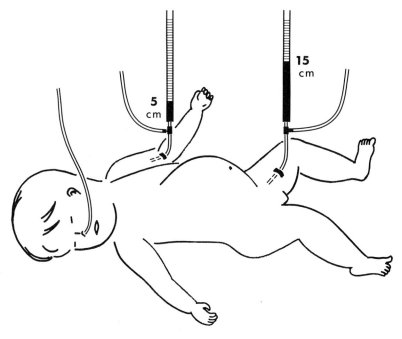

Figure 11–8
This newborn infant had peritonitis and marked abdominal distention. In spite of hypovolemia, venous pressure measured in the inferior vena cava was 15 cm of water. Simultaneous measurement in the superior vena cava was 5 cm of water.

and the inferior vena cava with marked abdominal distention. This newborn infant had an ileal perforation and peritonitis. The abdomen was markedly distended. Venous pressure measured in the inferior vena cava was 15 cm of water, a high figure that suggests an adequate blood volume. A simultaneous measurement in the superior vena cava was 5 cm of water, suggesting inadequate blood volume. Intraabdominal pressure is frequently high in the newborn surgical patient, and a more valid reading can be obtained from the superior vena cava.

The Respiratory Effect

Central venous pressure fluctuates with respiratory effort. This effect can be clearly seen when venous pressure is measured by a transducer and continuously recorded. Grunting, forceful respirations produce gross fluctuations in the atrial pulse waves. With inspiration there is a fall, and with expiration a rise, and a sine wave pattern is produced. This effect is usually not appreciated when central venous pressure is measured by a water manometer because only gross changes are noted.

The infant responds to many serious insults, pneumonia, hyaline membrane disease, and peritonitis with respiratory distress. Figure 11–9 demonstrates the effect of respiratory distress on venous pressure. This infant responded to a massive hemorrhage with grunting respirations. Central venous pressure was measured by a manometer as 12

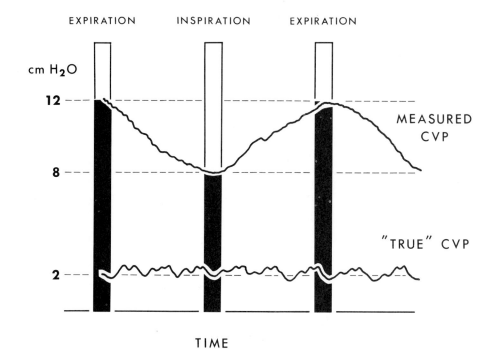

Figure 11–9
Continuous central venous pressure measurements of an infant with massive hemorrhage and grunting respirations. The initial pressure was 12 cm of water. With inspiration, venous pressure fell, but with expiration it again rose. Because of the frequent expiratory efforts, venous pressure never fell to "true" atrial level.

cm of water, a high figure in the face of hemorrhage. With inspiration, his venous pressure began to fall towards atrial pressure, but a grunting expiration occurred and venous pressure rose. Because of the frequent expiratory efforts, venous pressure never fell to "true" atrial level. When blood was rapidly infused, respiratory distress ceased, and central venous pressure paradoxically fell. A "high central venous" pressure can also be produced by positive pressure breathing during endotracheal anesthesia or during artificial ventilation by a mechanical respirator.

The Volley Technique

Central venous pressure monitoring is most helpful when the measurements are made serially and the changes with therapy observed. A method we use to resuscitate the profoundly hypovolemic infant, the volley technique, is illustrated in Figure 11–10. This baby was suffering from peritonitis as the result of a colon perforation that occurred 1½ days before admission. The infant was greatly distended, nonresponsive, and appeared markedly hypovolemic. Central venous pressure,

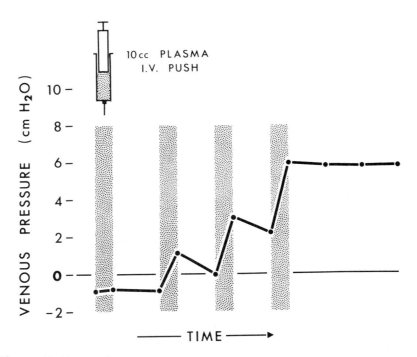

Figure 11–10

The volley technique. A markedly hypovolemic infant suffering from peritonitis due to a colon perforation. Central venous pressure initially was less than zero. A rapid injection of 10 ml of plasma did not alter the measurement. A second injection caused a slight temporary rise. A third 10 ml infusion produced a moderate rise in pressure while a final injection resulted in a stable reading of 6 cm of water. When a plateau is reached without further injections, this suggests correction of the hypovolemic state.

measured from the superior vena cava, was less than 1 cm of water. There was no respiratory distress. A rapid injection of 10 ml of plasma was given and central venous pressure measured again. There was no change. Repeated injections were given until the level of venous pressure rose and remained elevated at 6 cm of water for a period of over 15 minutes. When this plateau was reached, injections were discontinued. A total of 40 ml of plasma was given in 50 minutes to this 5-lb infant with improvement in his general condition and no signs of circulatory overload.

Muscle pH Monitoring

Filler and his associates have recently introduced the continuous measurement of muscle pH by an implanted electrode as a means of monitoring the critically ill pediatric patient.[6] Muscle pH falls before arterial pH or blood pressure with hypoperfusion and can thus serve as an early warning sign of conditions leading to poor peripheral perfusion. This method has the advantage of avoiding vascular cannulation, not requiring blood sampling, and giving minute-to-minute information. The equipment is relatively inexpensive, and the technique of placing the probe is not difficult.

Cardiac Output

Cardiac output appears to be a more direct index to the circulatory status of the patient than vascular pressure measurements, since flow rather than pressure is monitored. Unfortunately, the majority of techniques for measuring cardiac output are complex, often require multiple vascular cannulations and the removal of large volumes of blood, only indirectly measure the output of the heart, and give no insight into the distribution of blood flow.

The dye indicator dilution technique has several drawbacks when used to serially measure cardiac output in the infant. The technique requires at least two cannulations, an artery and a central vein, involves the withdrawal of a relatively large volume of blood for calibration, and may require heparinization. When blood is withdrawn through the cuvette densitometer during the performance of a dye curve, a large volume of blood is rapidly lost unless a continuous circuit system is employed.[7] The method is subject to errors during low flow states and when vascular shunts are present. Calculation of the cardiac output from the dye curve requires replotting of the curve to correct for recirculation and time-consuming calculations. Computers are available for rapid calculation, but are expensive and some are not accurate. Several have to be modified because they are not designed to measure the small output of the infant. The dye indicator dilution technique has the advantage of visually demonstrating right-to-left shunts. The indicator dilution method can be utilized without blood withdrawal if a thermal dilution probe or fibre-optic densitometer is used. A "solid" catheter must be placed in the artery with these techniques, necessitating a second arterial catheterization if blood samples need to be drawn for pH and blood gas measurements.

Use of the Fick Principle for determining cardiac output requires the measurement of oxygen consumption and arterial and venous oxygen concentrations. For consistent results, venous samples must be drawn from the pulmonary artery to ensure a true mixed venous blood. Oxygen consumption must be measured during a relatively steady state and usually requires a tight-fitting mask or endotracheal intubation.

Weintraub, Cuderman, Hunt, Stauffer, Roback, and Leonard studied the arterial pulse contour as a means of measuring cardiac output in infants.[8] This method requires only one arterial cannula, and the output can be measured continuously without blood loss. The catheter is available for obtaining blood samples for pH and blood gas determinations. Certain theoretic assumptions must be made with this method and an elaborate computer setup was utilized. The distentability characteristics of the aortic wall must be known, and these vary from patient to patient depending on size, age, and maturity. Shunts are not identified. A cardiac output measured by the pulse curve system is not an absolute number. An output must first be determined by another system such as the dye indicator dilution method and the information entered into the computer. To avoid the separate measurements of cardiac output, Weintraub et al have compared their first pulse contour measurement with subsequent readings and determined a "cardiac trend."

Although cardiac output determinations would be helpful clinically, it is our feeling that until techniques are simplified this measurement is not essential for successful management of the newborn surgical patient. The great value of cardiac output determinations presently lies in the information that can be collected on the hemodynamic changes of the newborn surgical patient as he responds to various life-threatening challenges.

Monitoring Arterial pO_2

One of the most valuable guides to safe management of the seriously ill newborn is serial measurements of arterial oxygen tension (pO_2). It is the most helpful means of detecting hypoxia. Clinical signs such as lethargy, tachypnea, hypotonia, and seizures are nonspecific. Even cyanosis in the newborn cannot be depended upon as a sign of hypoxia.[8] Oxygen tension measurements are mandatory when high oxygen concentrations are administered or the baby is being maintained on a mechanical ventilator.

Oxygen tension has been measured from "arterialized" capillary, venous, and arterial blood. Blood pH and carbon dioxide tension (pCO_2) vary only slightly when measured from any of these sites. This is not true of pO_2. Venous pO_2 is lower than arterial pO_2 and varies considerably depending on the vein sampled. Consistent venous samples can only be obtained from true mixed venous blood obtained from the pulmonary artery. To place a catheter accurately in the pulmonary artery usually requires fluoroscopy. Balloon catheters as small as number 3 French catheters have recently been developed to enable the physician to "float" the catheter into the pulmonary artery at the bedside. The position must be confirmed by x-ray.

Properly sampled arterialized capillary blood pO_2 correlates well with arterial blood samples in the older infant and child with good peripheral circulation. In the normal newborn baby and the sick infant with reduced peripheral circulation, the pO_2 is usually much lower and inconsistent when compared with arterial samples.[9,10] We feel that the most reliable source of sampling for determining the pO_2 is the artery.

The relationship of the catheter tip to the ductus arteriosus is of importance when monitoring arterial oxygen tension in the newborn. With hypoxia and acidosis, the transitional circulation of the newborn responds by pulmonary arteriolar vasconstriction and dilation of the ductus arteriosus. A right-to-left shunt can develop across the ductus and a large volume of blood can enter the descending aorta without passing through the lungs.[11,12] Arterial oxygen tension as a result can be 20–80 mm Hg higher in the aortic arch above the ductus arteriosus than in the abdominal aorta. Figure 11–11 illustrates the simultaneous arterial pO_2 measurements from temporal and umbilical artery catheters. The pO_2 in the temporal artery is 50 mm Hg higher than in the abdominal aorta. Presumably, temporal artery blood is more representative of blood perfusing the heart, brains, and eyes. Figure 11–12 demonstrates a group of experiments illustrating the pO_2 differential above and below the ductus arteriosus following hemorrhage in the newborn puppy.

Many neonatal surgical conditions result in hypoxia. The marked abdominal distention that accompanies bowel obstruction and peritonitis inhibits diaphragmatic movement and leads to hypoventilation. A similar situation is produced when closure of an omphalocele or gastroschisis is done under great tension. The newborn with a diaphragmatic hernia often has an extremely low pO_2 as the result of hypoplasia of the ipsilateral lung, compression of the contralateral lung, and shunting from right to left across the ductus arteriosus. It is well documented that the newborn has an increased tolerance to hypoxia. The physician aware of this and impressed by the stable appearance of the baby in spite of a low arterial pO_2 often ignores the hypoxic state. However, the infant with decreased arterial pO_2 may respond ineffectually to trauma. This may account for the sudden deterioration of a surgical patient with a low arterial pO_2 who appears to be tolerating hypoxia well, but suddenly becomes unresponsive or suffers a cardiac arrest during the course of a minor hemorrhage, difficult operative procedure, or the induction of anesthesia. We attempted to objectify this concept by a series of experiments in the newborn pig. Two groups of piglets were studied. One group breathed room air, the other 10 percent oxygen. After four hours, both groups appeared healthy and had similar hemodynamic and metabolic findings. The 10 percent oxygen group had a lower pO_2 and pCO_2. Both groups were then subjected to a modest challenge—a hemorrhage of 25 percent of their total blood volume. None of the animals breathing room air died and suffered only temporary cardiovascular and hemodynamic alterations. Over 50 percent of the hypoxic animals died. The average time of death was 17 minutes following hemorrhage.

We believe that every effort should be made to rapidly correct

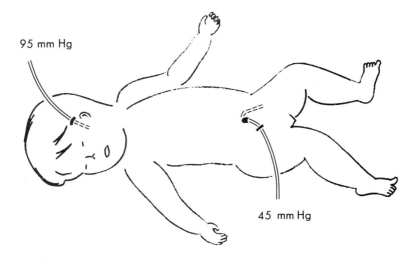

Figure 11–11
Simultaneous measurements of arterial blood oxygen tension from the umbilical
artery and temporal artery in a hypoxic newborn with a diaphragmatic hernia. The
pO₂ differential from measurements above and below the ductus arteriosus suggests
that a right-to-left shunt is present.

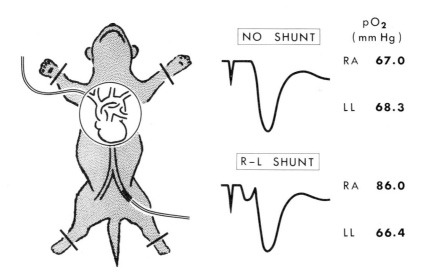

Figure 11–12
A group of ten puppies less than 48 hours old had dye indicator dilution measurements of cardiac output performed and simultaneous measurements of arterial blood
pO₂ made above and below the ductus arteriosus. Preliminary measurements showed
that the pO₂ values were essentially the same and there was not a right-to-left shunt.
The animals then were subjected to a hemorrhage of 35 percent of their total blood
volume. A right-to-left shunt was seen on the dye curve and there was an average
pO₂ difference of 20 mm Hg between the pO₂ measured above and below the ductus
arteriosus.

hypoxia in the pediatric surgical patient in spite of the patient's seeming tolerance for this state. When hypoxia is suspected or may develop, an arterial line should be placed and serial pO_2 measurements done. A pO_2 below 60 mm Hg in a newborn infant should be considered abnormal and attempts made to improve oxygenation. A value below 50 mm Hg suggests hypoxia. The airway should be cleared and the concentration of inspired oxygen increased. Obstruction should be relieved utilizing an oral or nasotracheal tube or, when necessary, a tracheostomy should be performed. Abdominal distention can sometimes be lessened by nasogastric suction or by aspiration of free air or fluid from the peritoneal cavity. Other mechanical causes for hypoxia such as pneumothorax or atelectasis should be searched for and corrected. If these general measures and the administration of 100 percent oxygen do not increase arterial pO_2 to above 40 mm Hg, mechanical ventilation is necessary.

Careful monitoring of arterial oxygen tension is particularly important in the premature infant receiving inspired oxygen concentrations over 40 percent. High oxygen concentrations in the immature baby can lead to retrolental fibroplasia and permanent blindness.[13] The level of arterial oxygen tension and the duration of exposure necessary to produce retrolental fibroplasia is not known. Cases of permanent blindness have developed after exposure to arterial pO_2 levels of 150 mm Hg.[14] We attempt to keep the pO_2 level below 100 mm Hg in all newborn infants receiving concentrations of oxygen above 40 percent.

Recently, an automated system of pH and blood gas determination was described by Veasy and his associates.[15] Small samples of blood are automatically withdrawn from an arterial line, measurements made, and the results continuously displayed. The cost of this elaborate system has been estimated at $20,000.

There are a number of methods currently available that measure tissue oxygen by electrodes. These techniques avoid vascular cannulation and blood loss from sampling. At present, the technical difficulties related to maintaining constant reliable readings has made this an impractical clinical tool, but a valuable research instrument. Further refinement of tissue electrodes in the future will be an important advance in clinical monitoring.

Arterial Blood pH

A falling arterial blood pH signals developing acidosis and to many is an indication for buffering with sodium bicarbonate or Tham. In the newborn surgical patient, acidosis is a secondary manifestation of a serious underlying disease process. The prime goal of treatment should be directed towards correcting the condition that led to the acidosis.

Accurate therapy will result in a rising pH and correction of the acidosis without buffering.

Buffering can produce serious side effects. Tham may cause an osmotic diuresis or hypoglycemia and, when infused into a patient with respiratory acidosis, respiratory arrest.[16] Sodium bicarbonate infusions will further increase the CO_2 concentration if acidosis is the result of respiratory insufficiency. The standard ampule of sodium bicarbonate contains 880 mEq/L of sodium and has an osmolality of 1640 mOsm/L. Sudden infusions of this high sodium, hyperosmolar solution into a critically ill neonate may be dangerous.[17]

When acidosis results from respiratory insufficiency with CO_2 retention, relief of airway obstruction, increased oxygenation, and correcting mechanical difficulties such as pneumothorax or herniated viscus will increase pO_2, reduce pCO_2, and pH will rise without the addition of buffers. Metabolic acidosis often can be corrected by improving tissue perfusion by blood-volume replacement, treating infection, increasing oxygenation, and reducing metabolic work. The metabolic activity of the sick newborn can be lowered towards normal by placing him in a thermally neutral environment and reducing respiratory effort. A rising pH will suggest therapy has been adequate, and a low or falling pH suggests inadequate treatment.

It is still not clear to what extent the acidotic state itself is dangerous to the organism and if correction of the blood picture by buffering improves prognosis. We believe that buffering may become necessary during the course of resuscitation of the critically ill infant, but that indescriminate buffering may not produce significant physiologic benefits, is not without risk, and may obscure important clinical signs. The major therapeutic effort should be directed at the etiology of the acidotic state.

Monitoring of Fluid and Electrolyte Balance in the Infant

It is impossible to generalize about the newborn surgical patient's fluid and electrolyte needs. The infant's internal environment is rapidly changing due to extrauterine adaptation and pathologic processes. There is a marked variability in blood volume, renal function, and metabolic activity between individual babies. We are at a further disadvantage because our knowledge of newborn physiology is incomplete. A multiplicity of systems for fluid and electrolyte management have developed over the years in an attempt to deal with these problems. We believe that these systems are, at best, rough estimates of fluid and electrolyte requirements of the newborn surgical patient. We must "read the baby" and base our management on what the infant needs rather than following rules of thumb, formulas, or physiologic principles. There are several methods that help us to "read the baby," give us a clearer picture of his water and electrolyte needs, and help us gauge the effectiveness of our treatment.

Body Weight

To take frequent and accurate measurements of body weight is a simple method of monitoring the fluid balance of the infant. Fluctuations in weight over a 24-hour period are primarily related to a loss or gain of fluid. One can estimate roughly that 1 ml of fluid is equal to 1 gm of body weight. It is possible, by weighing the baby every 4 hours, to estimate the fluid deficit or gain of a postoperative infant receiving intravenous fluids who is losing large and immeasurable quantities of fluid. A loss of 50 gm of body weight over the four-hour period suggests that fluid volume replacement is inadequate while a gain in weight suggests that fluid replacement was overestimated.

The scales must be checked for accuracy every few days with standard weights. To avoid the variability associated with the weight of dressings, diapers, and gowns, we avoid dressings in the postoperative period, and nurse the infant naked. If nasogastric tubes or other devices are inserted, they are weighed first and the added weight accounted for. For the usual clinical situation, standard nursery scales are satisfactory as monitoring devices.

Serum Osmolality

Serial measurements of serum osmolality is a rapid, simple, and inexpensive method that the physician may use himself to monitor the fluid and electrolyte balance of the infant. Osmolality is a measure of the concentration or number of solute particles in a kilogram of solvent, not their size, weight, shape, or charge. For this reason, albumin, a heavy but not numerous particle, contributes only slightly to serum osmolality, while sodium ion, a minute but numerous particle, is the major determinant of serum osmolality. Osmolality is measured clinically by determining the freezing point of a serum sample and correlating freezing point with concentration. It is possible to train a house officer in 15 minutes to operate the osmometer. Only 0.2 ml of serum is necessary. Capillary and venous blood samples give identical readings. For infants, the normal serum osmolality is 270–280 mOsm/L.[18] Serum osmolality can be calculated if the serum sodium, blood urea nitrogen, and sugar concentrations are known by using the Na(1.86) + blood urea nitrogen/2.8 + glucose/18 + 5.[19] When monitoring serial serum osmolality in a newborn surgical patient, it is important to initially determine serum electrolytes, blood urea nitrogen and sugar, and calculate osmolality. This gives a clear picture of what solutes in the serum account for the osmolality reading. During the course of monitoring, an unexpected rise in osmolality necessitates remeasuring of serum sodium, blood urea nitrogen, and blood sugar. Osmolality can then be calculated and compared with the measured osmolality. With this information, it is possible to determine if the elevation resulted from an increase in serum sodium, a rise in blood sugar, or blood urea nitrogen. It will also indicate whether another osmolar substance, either produced by the patient or added to his bloodstream, is increasing osmolality.

Figure 11–13 illustrates the serial changes in serum osmolality in

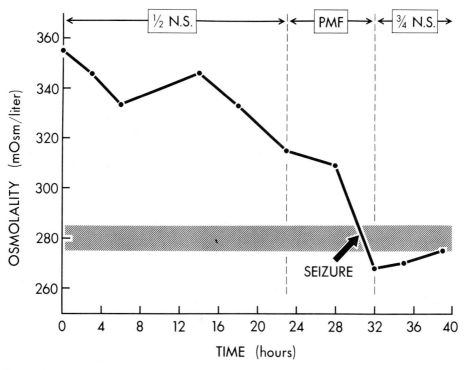

Figure 11–13

An infant with severe diarrhea from enterocolitis. Hypertonic dehydration was marked. The initial serum osmolality was 359 mOsm/L. Gradual reduction of the osmolality and volume replacement was accomplished without event by infusion of 5% dextrose and 0.45 normal saline over an 18 hour period. A more dilute solution was then inadvertently administered and osmolality fell from 318 to 280 mOsm/L in 4½ hours and grand mal seizures developed.

an infant suffering from Hirschsprung's disease and enterocolitis. Serum osmolality was initially high, 359 mOsm/L. The hyperosmolality was gradually reduced over an 18-hour period to avoid brain damage. Serial osmolality measurements were of great help in regulating the speed of correction. However, due to a physician error, a sudden infusion of a hypotonic solution was given before normal osmolality had been reached. Osmolality fell from 318 to 280 in 4½ hours and grand mal seizures developed. The fall in tonicity was recognized, corrective steps were taken, and permanent brain damage was averted.

Urine Osmolality

In general, when dehydration is present, a small amount of concentrated urine is produced, whereas, with overhydration, large quantities of dilute urine is excreted. The measurement of urine osmolality by the freezing-point determination is a simple and rapid method of evaluating the renal excretion of solute and water and serves as a guide to the state of hydration of the surgical patient. Serial changes in urine osmolality reflect the effectiveness of fluid therapy.

We have studied the urine osmolality of over 100 normal newborn babies. There is a good deal of variability from day to day and between individual infants, but, in general, urine osmolality remains slightly below serum osmolality. The average well-hydrated infant in the first three days of life has a urine osmolality of 268 mOsm/L. The lowest urine osmolality we have noted, 62 mOsm/L, was in a markedly overhydrated newborn surgical patient. The highest osmolality, 500 mOsm/L, was recorded in a 2-day-old baby with severe dehydration. The adult kidney can produce urine with an osmolality as high as 1400 mOsm/L. The important fact to keep in mind is that while a urine osmolality of 400 in an adult would be considered normal, the same value in a 2-day-old infant suggests marked dehydration and maximum concentration of the urine.

Urine Output

A urinary catheter to measure hourly urine output will almost certainly be used on an adult suffering from peritonitis or a major burn. The physician accepts this as a good guide to the adequacy of fluid intake and renal perfusion. However, the accurate measurement of urine output is often neglected in the baby. Infants, like adults, will produce significant volumes of urine when well hydrated and scant urine when underhydrated, but one must keep in mind what is a large or small volume of urine in a baby. We roughly estimate that a newborn surgical patient receiving intravenous fluids should produce approximately 500–600 ml of urine per square meter of body surface per 24 hours. This figure is somewhat arbitrary, and our main concern is the change in output as a result of fluid therapy. We routinely place a small Foley catheter or feeding tube into the bladder and measure hourly urine output of severely hypovolemic infants. When urine flow is scanty, we increase the rate of fluid administration until urine output rises. Too great a urine output suggests that the volume of fluid administered should be decreased. We do not consider the hourly urine output as an isolated measurement, but interpret its significance in relation to serum osmolality measurements, changes in body weight, and serial measurements or urine osmolality.

Plasma Oncotic Pressure Monitoring

Serum and urine osmolality determinations and the measurement of urine output are valuable guides to fluid and electrolye management. However, they give only one view of a multidimensional picture. Plasma proteins have an important effect on fluid balance. The distribution of fluid between blood and tissue is regulated primarily by the interaction of capillary hydrostatic pressure and plasma colloid oncotic pressure according to the thesis of Starling. It is important not to confuse serum osmolality with plasma oncotic or osmotic pressure. Serum osmolality is a measure of the number of solute particles in a kilogram of serum. Plasma oncotic pressure is a measure of the pressure, usually recorded in centimeters of water, generated by the plasma proteins separated from non–protein-containing fluid by a semipermiable membrane.

A fall in plasma oncotic pressure would presumably lead to an increased movement of fluid and electrolytes across the capillary membrane into the tissues. In conditions such as neonatal peritonitis, widespread capillary injury results in the loss of protein, water, and electrolytes into the surrounding tissue and peritoneal cavity. As protein is lost from the vascular space, colloid oncotic pressure falls. Protein-free infusions of electrolyte solutions may result in further reduction in plasma protein by dilution and a portion of the infused fluid may be lost into the tissues and peritoneal cavity. Theoretically, increasing the serum oncotic pressure by infusion of colloid may prevent this loss of fluid across the capillary membrane and increase reabsorption of fluid into the circulation. Before colloid therapy can be placed on more than an empiric basis, much more needs to be learned about the normal colloid oncotic pressure of the newborn and infant, the changes that take place during various diseased states, and the response of oncotic pressure to colloid infusions.

Measurements of the total protein and albumin would appear to be an accurate method of estimating colloid oncotic pressure. From a practical point of view, these determinations usually require a well-set-up clinical laboratory, and the results are not immediately available to the physician. A drawback to the utilization of total protein measurements to estimate oncotic pressure is the fact that proteins do not behave as ideal solutes and the relationship of plasma proteins to osmotic properties is nonlinear.[20] There is a disproportionate rise in protein osmotic pressure as protein concentration increases. All the factors that contribute to this discrepancy are not known, but in the past, the nonlinear relationship is produced by the Donnan effect and chloride binding on the albumin molecule.

The measurements of total serum solids by a refractometer is a simple technique requiring only a drop of plasma.[19,21] This instrument is relatively inexpensive and a determination can be performed in seconds at the bedside. There is a close correlation between total serum solids and total protein. However, the relationship of total solids to colloid oncotic pressure, like the relationship of proteins to oncotic pressure, is not linear.

Colloid oncotic pressure can be measured by recording the changes in the pressure that occur when a colloid and colloid-free solution are separated by a membrane that is not permeable to protein. This method, in the past, was cumbersome and inaccurate because of the deterioration that took place in the biologic membranes that were then available and because it was necessary to utilize manometers to measure pressure. With the new synthetic membranes and sensitive transducers, there is now available a device that can rapidly and accurately measure serum oncotic pressure on samples as small as 0.1 ml. This instrument was first described by Hansen[22] and was modified and refined by Zweifach and Intaglietta.[23] Baum, Eisenberg, Franklin, Meschia, and Battaglia were the first to study colloid oncotic pressure in the newborn with this apparatus.[24] They found that the pressure increased with gestational age and tended to be low for infants that were small for date. We have found that newborn infants suffering from such conditions as peritonitis and gastroschisis have extremely low oncotic pressure values while patients suffering from simple obstructive phenomena such as duodenal and jejunal atresia have normal pressures. The colloid osmometer is a valuable research instrument and may, in the future, be a helpful clinical tool for gauging intravenous colloid therapy.

REFERENCES

1. Kilpatrick, D.G.: The electrical environment. *Med Clin N Amer* 55:1095–1105, 1971.
2. Krauss, A.N., Albert, R.F., and Kannan, M.M.: Contamination of umbilical catheters in the newborn infant. *J Pediat* 77:965–969, 1970.
3. Kitterman, J.A., Phibbs, R.H., and Tooley, W.H.: Aortic blood pressure in normal newborn infants during the first 12 hours of life. *Pediatrics* 44:959–968, 1969.
4. McLaughlin, G.W., et al: Indirect measurement of blood pressure in infants utilizing doppler ultrasound. *J. Pediat* 79:300–303, 1971.
5. Hochberg, H.M., and Saltzman, M.B.: Accuracy of an ultrasound blood pressure instrument in neonates, infants and children. *Curr Ther Res* 13:482–488, 1971.
6. Filler, R.M., and Das, J.B.: Muscle surface pH: A new parameter in monitoring of the critically ill child. *Pediatrics* 47:880–885, 1971.
7. Arcilla, R., and Rowe, M.I.: Modified dye dilution technique for cardiac output studies in tiny subjects. *Amer Heart J* 77:804, 1969.

8. Weintraub, W.H., et al: Computer monitoring of cardiodynamics in the newborn. *J Pediat Surg* 6:251–255, 1971.

9. Mountain, K.R., and Campbell, D.G.: Reliability of oxygen tension measurements on centralized capillary blood in the newborn. *Arch Dis Child* 45:134–138, 1970.

10. Koch, G., and Wendel, H.: Comparison of pH, carbon dioxide tension, standard bicarbonate and oxygen tension in capillary blood and in arterial blood during the neonatal period. *Acta Paediat Scand* 56:10–16, 1967.

11. Chu, J., et al: Neonatal pulmonary ischemia: I. Clinical and physiological studies. *Pediatrics* 40 (suppl):709–766, 1968.

12. Dawes, G.S.: "Changes in the circulation after birth," *Foetal and Neonatal Physiology*. Chicago: Year Book Medical Publishers, 1969, pp 160–176.

13. De Leon, A.S., Elliott, J.H., and Jones, D.B.: The resurgence of retrolental fibroplasia. *Pediat Clin N Amer* 17:309–322, 1970.

14. Silverman, W.A.: What is the present status of retrolental fibroplasia, in problems of neonatal intensive care units? 59th Ross Conference of Pediatric Research, Library No. 53:22189, 1969.

15. Veasy, L.G., et al: A system for computerized automated blood gas analysis. *Pediatrics* 48:5–17, 1971.

16. Strauss, J.: Tris: A pediatric evaluation. *Pediatrics* 41:667–689, 1968.

17. Finberg, L.: Dangers to infants caused by changes in osmolar concentration. *Pediatrics* 40:1031–1034, 1967.

18. Rowe, M.I.: The role of serial serum osmolality measurements in the management of the neonatal surgical patient. *Surg Gynec Obstet* 133:93–96, 1971.

19. Mansberger, A.R., et al. Refractometry and osmometry in clinical surgery. *Ann Surg* 169:672, 1969.

20. Landis, E.M., and Pappenheimer, J.R.: Circulation II. In Hamilton, W.F., ed: *Handbook of Physiology*. Washington, D.C.: American Physiological Society, 1963, p 974.

21. Talbert, J.L., and Haller, J.A.: Recent advances in the postoperative management of infants. *J Surg Res* 6:502–509, 1966.

22. Hansen, A.T.: Self-recording electronic osmometer for quick, direct measurement of colloid osmotic pressure in small samples. *Acta Physiol Scand* 24:602, 1968.

23. Intaglietta, M., and Zweifach, B.W.: Measurement of blood plasma osmotic pressure: I. Technical aspects; II. Comparative study of different species. Microvascular Research 3:72–88, 1971.

24. Baum, J.D., et al: Studies of colloid osmotic pressure in the fetus and newborn infant. *Biol Neonat* 18:311–320, 1971.

12

Postoperative Respiratory Care in Infants and Children

Eric W. Fonkalsrud, M.D.
Leonard M. Linde, M.D.

PHYSIOLOGIC BACKGROUND

A rational approach to the management of respiratory problems in infants and children is properly based on knowledge of respiratory and circulatory physiology. Because of the frequency of cardiopulmonary difficulties related to the transition from fetus to neonate, a brief discussion of this subject is warranted here.

Central nervous system respiratory receptors are functional by the fifth or sixth month of gestation, but cellular changes in the lung and vascularization are not adequate to permit survival until about the 28th week of gestation. Although the *volume* of blood in the fetal lung has recently been shown to be similar to that of the neonate, dynamic lung flow represents only a small fraction of the total cardiac output in the fetus. High pulmonary vascular resistance is explained by increased pressure on blood vessels by fluid-filled alveoli, mechanical effects of vascular tortuosity, and, primarily, by pulmonary vascular constriction maintained by chemical and blood-gas effects. The ability of the lungs to resist collapse is enhanced, starting at approximately 28 weeks of gestation, with the appearance of surfactant which lines the alveoli.

At birth, with the onset of respiration and cessation of blood flow through the placenta, the lungs become air-filled, pulmonary vascular resistance falls, and pulmonary blood flow becomes equal to the entire cardiac output. Initiation and maintenance of these profound and rapid changes require adequate central nervous system development, integrity of respiratory muscles and thoracic movement, and adequate maturation of lung air passages and blood vessels. In the normal infant, these changes result in an increase in left atrial pressure above right atrial pressure and functionally close the foramen ovale, while increased oxygen tension closes the ductus arteriosus. For initial air expansion of the lungs, large surface forces must be overcome, requiring pressures of up to 50 cm of water. Spontaneous alveolar rupture is not uncommon, but this complication is much more likely with artificial respiration, partly related to difficulties in controlling pressure and partly due to the lung disease which necessitated it.

Alveolar ventilation and control of blood-gas and acid-base levels are functions of medullary and peripheral chemoreceptors. In the newborn, a low pCO_2 is maintained, possibly to compensate for metabolic acidosis. Periodic breathing is common in premature infants, but also is seen in full-term babies. Apneic spells, seen in prematures, are more common in infants with lower birth weights and may indicate serious underlying central nervous system disease. However, the possibility of a maturational integrational delay is suggested by complete recovery without sequelae in many.

The main control of ventilation is probably related to a localized fall in pH associated with an increased pCO_2, with the response to hypoxia held in reserve under normal conditions. Prolonged and severe hypercarbia and hypoxia, on the contrary, are respiratory depressants and require prompt treatment to reverse their effects.

The *vital capacity* is made up of three components: (1) the *tidal volume* is the amount of air that moves with normal ventilation, (2) which can be increased involuntarily by a maximal voluntary inspiration (*inspiratory reserve*), and (3) maximal voluntary expiration (*expiratory reserve*). The expiratory reserve and the air remaining in the lung after maximal voluntary expiration (*residual volume*) together make up the *functional residual capacity*. The stretchability, or *compliance,* of the lung is measured as volume change per unit of pressure required to change it. Whereas the pressure to expand the lung in the infant is closely related to lung compliance, in older children, as in adults, an equal amount of ventilatory pressure is required to overcome the effect of the more resistive rib cage and abdominal wall and contents.

Adequate respiration involves *ventilation* or movement and distribution of gas from the outside into position for exchange. *Diffusion* is concerned with the passage of O_2 and CO_2 across the alveolar capillary membranes. *Circulation* or pulmonary capillary blood flow must be adequate in total volume and in even distribution to ventilated alveoli.

Ventilation defects are seen in emphysema, cystic fibrosis, and in cases of congenital or acquired airway obstructions. Diffusion defects are rare in children and usually are involved with problems in oxygenation rather than with CO_2 diffusion, such as in pulmonary fibrosis. Pulmonary circulatory problems are seen in congenital cardiac disease, particularly in patients with increased pulmonary blood flow who develop pulmonary hypertension. Frequent pneumonia in these children may be related to pulmonary vasoconstriction and increased resistance, but is often due to vascular engorgement and airway compression.

Although ventilation and perfusion normally exist in balance, there are many exceptions. Hydrostatic forces produce a greater decrease in blood flow than in ventilation to the lung apices in normal children in the erect position, but this difference in vascular filling is less than in adults and is abolished in the supine position and with left-to-right shunts. In some cyanotic children with decreased pulmonary blood flow, ventilation remains close to normal so that ventilation/perfusion ratios are abnormally increased.

The pulmonary vessels normally are thin-walled and distensible and offer minimal resistance to flow. Cardiac output can triple, causing distension of perfused vessels or opening of previously closed vessels, such as in the apex, so that little increase in vascular pressure results. These mechanical geometric changes in the lung vessels are the main determinants of pulmonary vascular resistance changes, but many factors may affect the pulmonary vessels, usually causing vasoconstriction, as occurs with hypoxia, hypercarbia, and acidosis, as well as with several chemical agents. Positive pressure breathing must be used judiciously to prevent decreased systemic venous return and secondary increase in pulmonary vascular resistance.

RESPIRATION THERAPY

Respiratory complications are among the most common and serious causes of postoperative morbidity and mortality in infants and children, although many diagnostic and therapeutic techniques developed during the past decade have reduced their frequency and severity.

One of the major reasons for the current decrease in respiratory complications in pediatric patients is the use of inhalation therapy, an inclusive term that refers to the theory and practice of treatment by changes in the composition, volume, or pressure of inspired gases. These techniques are used to achieve bronchial drainage, to provide ventilation, to oxygenate the blood, and to correct hypoxia due to any cause. The therapeutic results are accomplished by increasing the fractional concentration of oxygen (oxygen therapy), increasing the water vapor content of inspired gas (humidification), adding airborne particles with beneficial properties (aerosol therapy), removing bronchial secretions, and assisting respiration (intermittent or continuous positive pressure breathing). Thus, it is important that any physician caring for infants and children be familiar with the indications and techniques for these procedures.

OXYGEN THERAPY

Oxygen therapy is recommended when arterial oxygen concentration is significantly reduced and can be elevated by increasing alveolar oxygen concentrations. Cyanosis, although not detectable until a considerable drop in the partial pressure of oxygen in arterial blood has occurred, still remains the best single criterion for the use of supplemental oxygen. The basic treatment of hypoxia is determined by the causative mechanism, e.g. pneumonia or hypoventilation. The volume deficit of oxygen in the alveoli usually is not very great, and a small increase in the volume of inspired oxygen is generally effective. Repeated arterial oxygen and CO_2 saturation and pH determinations obtained from umbilical or superficial temporal arterial cannulation in the infant, or by radial artery cannulation in the child, should be used to monitor the volume of oxygen administered. Oxygen alone will not relieve dyspnea, and, depending on its cause, more rational therapy might be the use of a bronchodilator, such as epinephrine, aerosol therapy with 10 percent propylene glycol, or a mucolytic agent.

The rationale for use of oxygen therapy is based upon the fact that most of the circulating oxygen is carried as oxyhemoglobin.[1] In the patient with a normal hemoglobin level, oxyhemoglobin carries about 19.4 volume percent of oxygen (19.4 ml O_2 measured at standard temperature and pressure, per 100 ml of blood). At the same time, approximately 0.3 volume percent of oxygen is dissolved in the plasma. This small amount is seldom considered when the oxygen capacity of the blood is discussed, but it becomes important in pathologic situations. Since hemoglobin cannot be saturated beyond 100 percent, any additional oxygen must be carried in solution. If the normal oxygen partial pressure of 100 mm Hg in the alveolus is increased to 600 mm Hg, the dissolved oxygen in the plasma may be increased from 0.3 volume percent to 1.8 volumes percent. This 1.5 volumes percent increase plus 0.6 volume percent, representing the completion of hemoglobin saturation, means that 2.1 ml oxygen has been added to every 100 ml of blood, giving the blood 21.8 ml instead of the normal 19.7. Since the oxygen difference between arterial and venous blood is normally less than 5 volume percent, the amount added by oxygen therapy is equal to almost half of the oxygen normally removed from a given volume of blood by the tissues. It is possible, therefore, to obtain a higher level of oxygen in the tissues even before the circulation is improved.

When oxygen therapy is indicated, it may be administered by placing the child in an oxygen mist tent, Isolette, or head tent, or by using a face mask, endotracheal tube, or occasionally a nasopharyngeal catheter. The method of choice depends on the size of the child, the degree of oxygen desaturation, the percentage of oxygen desired in the inspired air, and the ventilatory status of the patient. In most cases, an inspired oxygen concentration of 40–60 volume percent is satisfactory. A well-sealed oxygen tent or face mask seldom yields more than a 40 percent oxygen concentration to the patient. A nasal catheter generally yields an oxygen concentration of only 30–35 percent, whereas an endotracheal tube or airtight face mask may yield over 70 percent. Face masks have been very effective in some centers in providing prolonged respiratory support in infants while eliminating the complications of prolonged intubation.[2] A nasogastric tube should be employed routinely when a face mask is used with assisted respiration. Oxygen therapy should be discontinued when its use is no longer indicated, as determined by repeated monitoring of arterial oxygen saturation or partial pressure. Although oxygen must be regarded as being of great therapeutic utility, toxicity will result if an overdose is given. The syndrome of "oxygen toxicity," which has been described with increasing frequency during the past few years, is characterized by heavy and beefy lungs with two merging phases microscopically: an early exudative phase with congestion, edema, and hyaline membranes, and a later proliferative phase with interstitial edema and early fibrosis.[3,4] This bronchopulmonary dysplasia has been seen in infants who received more than 150 hours of continuous high concentrations of oxygen or more than 800 hours of total supplemental oxygen.[5] The American Academy of Pediatrics has indicated that there is a causal relationship between a higher-than-normal oxygen tension in arterial blood (100 mm Hg) and retrolental fibroplasia, and that the arterial blood oxygen tension should not be permitted to exceed 80 mm Hg.[6]

HUMIDIFICATION

Since oxygen is dry, regardless of its source, some provision must be made for humidification, especially in infants. Water mist serves to liquefy the thick secretions of the tracheobronchial tree and also tends to decrease mucosal edema. The loss of body water, that might occur otherwise, may be minimized by inhalation of fully humidified gas at body temperature. The temperature within the mist tent or Isolette should be monitored frequently to provide an optimal environment of 23°–25°C.[7] Cold mist is used only temporarily when the body temperature must be lowered, since persistent exposure induces shivering and vasoconstriction and increases oxygen consumption.

Although mist is generally considered a benign form of treatment, this is not always true in the younger patient. In the infant, concentrations of water vapor greater than 60 percent in the inspired air are rarely indicated and may result in water condensation, which predisposes to infection or aspiration of a water bolus. A problem unique to the small infant is the hazard of water intoxication from moisture absorbed in the process of nebulization. Use of an ultrasonic nebulizer may result in a net gain of 200–400 ml of body water per 24 hours in the normally respiring infant.[8] The risk of such a water load in a newborn infant with a cardiac or other serious malformation is obvious.

AEROSOL THERAPY

Aerosol therapy consists of the deposition within the airway of particles suspended in inspired air or gases and has been used effectively in children with bronchiectasis, atelectasis, pneumonia, cystic fibrosis, and bronchitis, as well as before and after bronchoscopy, bronchography, tracheostomy, and thoracic surgery. Although usually consisting of droplets of water, aerosols may contain sodium chloride, stabilizing agents which inhibit evaporation of particles after they have been generated (propylene glycol, glycerine), or medications (bronchodilators, vasoconstrictors, mucolytics, steroids, antibiotics). The particle size usually varies from 1 to 20 microns in diameter, based upon the density and method of humidification. Particles measuring larger than 3 microns usually are deposited in the main bronchi or in the trachea or above. Only particles smaller than one micron pass into the alveoli.

The effectiveness of aerosol therapy is dependent upon the ability of the nebulized material to be distributed within the lung. There is a direct relationship between the effective use of aerosol therapy and bronchial drainage. Unventilated areas of the lung, as occur in atelectasis, receive no aerosolized particles. Aerosols for clinical use are produced by nebulizers which generate visible mists when attached to a source of gas or oxygen. Nebulizers may be constructed to filter out large particles and thus produce a mist with particles of desired size.

Intermittent use of a hand nebulizer (with a capacity of less than 10 ml) and a face mask is adequate to deliver aerosolized mist to most children without severe respiratory distress. Five to 10 minutes of mist inhalation every four hours is followed by extensive postural drainage and nasopharyngeal suctioning. For the patient who requires intensive and continuous mist therapy, the ultrasonic nebulizer delivering mist into a tent, Isolette, or head bubble is desirable. Heated or tepid aerosols slightly warmer than body temperature are fully saturated, thus minimizing water loss from the respiratory tract, and may be used for short periods.

When aerosol therapy is used for more than a few hours, preparations should be made to clean the entire nebulizer and mechanical respirator with acetic acid (0.25 percent) or activated gluteraldehyde at least every 24 hours to prevent contamination of the equipment with the "water bugs," pseudomonas and aerobacter, in particular. (See Chapter 14.)

In 1962, the first extensive clinical trials of a new mucolytic agent, acetylcysteine, were reported.[9] This potent drug, which also liquefies pus, has been used extensively in the treatment of cystic fibrosis. It has not been generally appreciated that acetylcysteine is destroyed by high concentrations of oxygen and that it has an antagonistic effect on certain antibiotics when they are administered in aerosol form.[10] Untoward effects may accompany its use, including buccal irritation, stomatitis, nausea, and rhinorrhea. The most important side effect is a potent bronchoconstrictive activity in certain patients, especially those with asthma, in whom its use is contraindicated.[11] Despite these limitations, the drug has proved to be quite effective in liquefying thick bronchial secretions. Tergemist, a combination of a detergent and mucolytic, has also proved to be a highly effective aerosol with minimal irritative effects on the bronchial epithelium. Use of mucolytic agents must be accompanied by aggressive bronchial drainage techniques and cough stimulation to remove the profuse secretions.

Adrenocortical steroids have been used extensively as aerosols in children with asthma in an attempt to minimize the side effects and still maintain the antiinflammatory and bronchodilatory effects of the drugs. These preparations rarely have been used as aerosols in the treatment of infants, although they have been used systemically in the treatment of gastric aspiration or tracheitis.

A variety of enzymes have been used in aerosol form in an attempt to liquefy tenacious, thick secretions in children. There are few studies proving the efficacy of aerosolized enzymes, however, and these agents are associated with a number of potential hazards, including allergic reactions, bronchial constriction, and tracheobronchial irritation.

The most common bronchodilators administered by means of aerosol are epinephrine and isoproterenol. A high local concentration of the drugs may be achieved with minimal systemic effects, although caution is necessary to avoid overdosage.

Although detergents or wetting agents often are used in mist therapy, most are irritating to the respiratory mucosa and have not been shown to be more effective than water mist alone.

REMOVAL OF SECRETIONS

Removal of secretions from the middle and lower respiratory tract of infants and young children who seldom cough and deep breathe voluntarily during the postoperative periods has posed a serious problem in the pediatric surgical patient. Although nasotracheal suction at frequent intervals has long been recommended during the early postoperative period, the value of this procedure has been questioned in view of the difficulty of passing such tubes accurately on repeated occasions without direct trauma to the larynx and vocal cords, which may in turn compound the respiratory distress. Caution should be exercised when tracheal or nasopharyngeal suctioning are used since cardiac arrhythmias may be induced due to vagal stimulation.[12] Such arrhythmias may be less common if 100 percent oxygen is administered for five minutes prior to suctioning.[13] The primary benefit from endotracheal suction is stimulation of the cough reflex, which may be accomplished by nasopharyngeal suction or aerosol therapy. When the trachea of a small infant is partially obstructed by a large mucous plug, direct laryngoscopy and endotracheal suction are recommended. Sterile catheters should be used each time the trachea is suctioned, whether through a tracheostomy or endotracheal tube or by direct laryngoscopy, in order to minimize the risk of secondary bacterial infection with virulent pathogens.

Perhaps one of the most effective and safe methods of mobilizing bronchial secretions which are not removed by normal ciliary activity and cough is postural drainage. After the area of poor ventilation is localized by auscultation or chest roentgenograms, postural drainage directed to that area four to six times daily may effectively loosen the secretions so that they may be coughed up with stimulation of the cough reflex. With proper positioning of the patient and effective cupping or clapping of the chest by the nurse, even the most tenacious secretions are frequently mobilized. The techniques of postural drainage are well summarized in several reviews of cystic fibrosis.[14]

Bronchoscopy is as important an adjunct in removing bronchial secretions in the pediatric patient as it is in the adult, although it is much less commonly used. General anesthesia or heavy sedation is usually required in young children. Traumatic manipulation of a bronchoscope may be more harmful than helpful, and laryngeal trauma during bronchoscopy may require subsequent tracheostomy, especially in small infants. A desperately ill child, with multiple sites of distal bronchial obstruction, usually does not benefit from bronchoscopy and may be further exhausted by the operative manipulations. Direct laryngoscopy with endotracheal suction has been effective and less difficult than bronchoscopy in infants.

Percutaneous transtracheal catheterization and tracheobronchial lavage, using a small-bore plastic catheter inserted into the lower cervical trachea through a needle, has been effective in stimulation of coughing and in insertion of mucolytic agents, especially in children with chronic pulmonary disease such as cystic fibrosis. This procedure is not usually recommended for children under 6 years of age because of the small size of the trachea and the likelihood of dislodgment of the catheter.

ASSISTED RESPIRATION

The method of respiratory support recommended for the infant or small child who requires assisted ventilation has been the subject of considerable controversy during the past few years. Tracheostomy has been avoided in most infants because of the great difficulty encountered during decannulation, which has frequently made it necessary to leave the tracheostomy tube in place until the child is 1 year of age or older. Removal of the tracheostomy tube in young infants has frequently been followed by tracheal collapse and airway obstruction. The recommendation by Aberdeen [15] that infant tracheostomy be performed by using a single vertical slit through two or three tracheal rings, instead of removing a segment of cartilage, has resulted during the past five years in much easier decannulation and more frequent survival of infants. Removal of a window of tracheal cartilage in infants appears (in contrast to adults) to decrease the tracheal support to a significant degree.

Whenever possible, tracheostomy in an infant should be preceded by endotracheal intubation to assure good ventilation. The tracheostomy should be performed in an operating room or treatment room where adequate instruments, lighting, suction equipment, and personnel are available. Although the most commonly used tube is still the silver cannula with removable inner liner, Silastic catheters appear to be more satisfactory since they are less irritating to the trachea, may be trimmed to a proper length, and do not require an inner cannula because secretions are much less likely to adhere to the inner wall.[16] A number 0 or 00 tracheostomy tube is generally recommended for infants under 6 months of age. It is rarely possible to use a cuffed tube in children under 3 years of age because of the small size of the tracheal lumen.[17] Auscultation and a chest roentgenogram should follow tracheostomy to assure good ventilation in both lungs, proper placement of the tube in the trachea without passage into either mainstem bronchus, and prevention or detection of pneumothorax.

Prolonged endotracheal intubation for infants with respiratory distress has gained in popularity as compared to tracheostomy, because of the relative ease with which the tube may be inserted and ventilating assistance administered. Because of the difficulty of fixing the *oral* endotracheal tube to the face to prevent movement or dislodgment of the tube from the trachea, *nasotracheal* intubation has received greater acceptance.[19] The use of Silastic, Portilex, and other soft plastic tubes has decreased the number of complications compared to those seen when hard rubber tubes were employed. Although nasotracheal tubes may be safely left in place for periods of two weeks or more, providing optimal care is given, frequent complications include hoarseness, laryngeal edema, subglottic cicatrical narrowing, and pressure necrosis of the ala nasi.[19] Our policy has been to use nasotracheal intubation initially in all infants and young children with postoperative respiratory distress. If prolonged intubation is anticipated (more than two to five days), tracheostomy is usually employed, even in infants.

Recent reports indicate that continuous positive pressure respiration using pressures from 4–10 mm Hg has been of great benefit to both infants and adults who require respiratory support.[20,21] The continuous pressure may be applied through an endotracheal tube or by placing the patient's head into a chamber with a loosely fitting collar about the neck.[21] A nonrebreathing system is used with a pop-off valve to prevent development of excessive pressure. Arterial oxygen tension should be monitored frequently and the oxygen concentration in the environment decreased if the pO_2 increases above 70 mm Hg. This system has significantly increased the survival of infants with respiratory distress syndrome and offers great promise in postoperative patients.

Mechanical ventilators may be required to treat a variety of conditions which could result in postoperative respiratory failure and hypoventilation in infants and children. Respiratory assistance for several hours or even days is advisable in many infants who undergo operations for congenital heart disease, certain other major anomalies, or major trauma. Two basic types of mechanical ventilators are available: a pressure-controlled ventilator that develops a predetermined maximum airway pressure while providing the tidal volume, and a volume-controlled respirator that discharges a set volume of gas during inspiration. With appropriate adjustment of the controlling mechanisms, however, similar airflow and pressure patterns and inspiratory volumes can be produced in a given patient with either type of ventilator, as long as full adjustment capabilities are available. A thorough understanding of the details of operation of any ventilator is of far greater importance than the simple selection of a machine. Although most ventilators in common use function satisfactorily when operated properly, none is totally foolproof, reliable, and capable.[22,23] Although many advantages and disadvantages have been cited for each, the pressure respirator appears to be more satisfactory in infants in whom a cuffed endotracheal tube cannot be used, provided pulmonary compliance remains approximately the same, since the air leak around the tube may result in highly variable tidal volumes.

Respirators augment or replace the patient's own respiratory effort and may function as an assister or as a controller. When functioning as an assister, as in most patients who are not comatose, the respirator inflates the patient's lungs in response to an inspiratory effort or sudden small reduction in airway pressure initiated by the patient. When set as a controller, the respirator will cycle automatically, but an assister-controller can be triggered on the next phase at an earlier time by the patient-generated signals.

When respirators are employed, constant medical nursing supervision is necessary. Initial respiratory pressures may be set at 20–25 cm of water, but may be increased to 35 cm under certain conditions.

Higher pressures may be followed by alveolar rupture and pneumo-thorax, decreased cardiac output, and hypotension, particularly in in-fants. Patients ventilated at a steady rate for long periods of time tend to develop small areas of atelectasis and progressive pulmonary in-sufficiency unless periodic hyperventilation for two to three breaths at a high pressure is used. If the ventilator does not have provision for automatic "sighing," this should be done manually at frequent inter-vals. Care must be taken to avoid prolonged hyperventilation, which may result in an arterial pH above 7.55 and hypokalemia. This is best prevented by frequent determinations of the blood arterial pH and serum electrolytes. In most situations, minimal oxygen concentrations should be used after initial resuscitation.[24] When increased oxygen is required for a prolonged period, oxygen concentrations should be maintained below 50 percent and 300 mm Hg partial pressure in the inspired air, especially in neonates.

In most instances, it is necessary to wean the patient from the respirator by gradually increasing the intervals of time without venti-latory support or by switching to an assister if controlled ventilation has been used. The sensitivity setting of the respirator may be de-creased gradually to stimulate more patient effort to trigger the respi-rator. The oxygen concentration of the inspired gas should be reduced gradually to that of room air when weaning is undertaken. The infant must be observed very closely during periods without respiratory sup-port and kept in a high mist environment with 40–50 percent oxygen supplied to the endotracheal tube.

SUMMARY

Respiratory therapy techniques have served as a valuable adjunct in alleviating difficulties in respiration in infants and children receiving surgical care. By judicious use of oxygen therapy, humidification, aero-sol therapy, removal of bronchial secretions, and assisted respirations by physicians, nurses, and allied personnel familiar with the techniques and equipment available, a significant reduction in postoperative mor-bidity and mortality may be achieved in pediatric patients.

REFERENCES

1. Waring, W.W.: Diagnostic and therapeutic procedures. In Kendig, E.L., ed: *Dis-orders of the Respiratory Tract in Children*. Philadelphia: W.B. Saunders, 1967, p 101.
2. Oliver, T.: personal communication.
3. Nash, G., Blennerhassett, J.B., and Pontoppidan, H.: Pulmonary lesions in patients receiving oxygen therapy and artificial ventilation. *New Engl J Med* 276:368–373, 1967.

4. Northway, W.H., Rosan, R.C., and Porter, D.Y.: Pulmonary disease following respirator therapy of hyaline membrane disease: Bronchopulmonary dysplasia. *New Engl J Med* 276:357–367, 1967.

5. Northway, W.H., and Rosan, R.C.: Oxygen therapy hazards in neonates. *Hosp Pract* 4:59–61, 66–67, 1969.

6. Committee on Fetus and Newborn, American Academy of Pediatrics: Oxygen therapy in the newborn infant. *Pediatrics* 47:1086–1087, 1971.

7. Avery, M.E., Galina, M., and Nachman, R.: Mist therapy. *Pediatrics* 39:160–165, 1967.

8. Herzog, P., Norlander, O.P., and Engstrom, C.G.: Ultrasonic generation of aerosol for the humidification of inspired gas during volume-controlled ventilation. *Acta anaesth Scand* 8:79–95, 1964.

9. Webb, W.R.: Clinical evaluation of a new mucolytic agent: Acetylcysteine. *J. Thorac Cardiov Surg* 44:330–343, 1962.

10. Harris, R.L., and Riley, H.D., Jr.: Reactions to aerosol medication in infants and children. *JAMA* 201:953–955, 1967.

11. *New Drugs 1967*. Chicago: American Medical Association, 1967.

12. Cordero, L., Jr., and Hon, E.H.: Neonatal bradycardia following nasopharyngeal stimulation. *J Pediat* 78:441–447, 1971.

13. Shim, C., et al: Cardiac arrhythmias resulting from tracheal suctioning. *Ann Intern Med* 71:1149–1153, 1969.

14. Guide to diagnosis and management of cystic fibrosis. New York National Cystic Fibrosis Research Foundation, 1963.

15. Aberdeen, E.: Mechanical pulmonary ventilation in infants: Tracheostomy and tracheostomy care in infants. *Proc Roy Soc Med* 58:900, 1965.

16. Haller, J.A., and Talbert, J.L.: Clinical evaluation of a new Silastic tracheostomy tube for respiratory support of infants and young children. *Ann Surg* 171:915–922, 1970.

17. Hollinger, P.N., Brown, W.T., and Maurizi, D.G.: Tracheostomy in the newborn. *Amer J Surg* 109:771–779, 1965.

18. Smith, R.M.: Diagnosis and treatment: Nasotracheal intubation as a substitute for tracheostomy. *Pediatrics* 38:652–654, 1966.

19. Hatcher, C.R., Jr., et al: Prolonged endotracheal intubation. *Surg Gynec Obstet* 127:759–762, 1968.

20. Ashbaugh, D.G., Petty, T.L., and Bigelow, D.B.: Continuous positive pressure breathing (CPPB) in adult respiratory distress syndrome. *J Thorac Cardiovasc Surg* 57:31–41, 1969.

21. Gregory, G.A., et al: Treatment of the idiopathic respiratory-distress syndrome with continuous positive airway pressure. *New Engl J Med* 284:1333–1340, 1971.

22. Anderson, M.N.: Ventilatory support. *Surgery* 66:1112–1119, 1969.

23. Peters, R.M., and Hutchin, P.: Adequacy of available respirators to their tasks. *Ann Thorac Surg* 3:414, 1967.

24. Bryant, L.R.: Mechanical respirators, their use and application in lung trauma. *JAMA* 199:149–154, 1967.

13

Resuscitation Following Cardiopulmonary Arrest

Arnold G. Coran, M.D.

Although the majority of cases of cardiopulmonary arrest occur in adults, this catastrophic event also occurs often in infants and children. The general principles of management are the same regardless of the patient's age—only the finer details of management differ. It is very important that each physician who may be confronted by a patient who has suffered a cardiac arrest, have all the steps that must be taken to resuscitate the patient clearly outlined in his mind. In this way, the ultimate objective of treatment, i.e. the return of the patient to his prearrest state, with spontaneous respiration and circulation, can be achieved most effectively.

PATHOPHYSIOLOGY

Whatever the etiology of the cardiac arrest, the sequence of physiological events that follows is the same. Ineffective cardiac action leads to diminished oxygenation of tissues, including the myocardium. The resulting hypoxemia leads to the accumulation of acid metabolites such as lactic acid. The hypoxic and acidotic myocardium becomes more irritable and more and more difficult to resuscitate. As the process continues, the chances of successful resumption of spontaneous cardiac activity become less and less. If this state continues for longer than four to six minutes, irreversible brain damage results. The main objective of resuscitation is to break the vicious cycle of worsening hypoxemia and acidosis by taking over the heart's function with external cardiac massage and, thereby, improving tissue oxygenation. The delivery of an adequate supply of oxygen to the tissues will decrease anaerobic metabolism and the accompanying accumulation of acid metabolites. In addition, adequate oxygenation of the myocardium will make the heart more responsive to resuscitation and resumption of spontaneous cardiac activity.

CAUSES OF CARDIAC ARREST

The most common cause of cardiac arrest is hypoxia secondary to inadequate pulmonary ventilation. This is especially true in infants and children, where other major causes, such as myocardial infarction, are extremely rare. Common causes of inadequate ventilation are inadequate respiration during surgery, foreign bodies in the tracheobronchial tree, drowning, smoke inhalation, and most important of all, aspiration pneumonitis.

Hypovolemia secondary to blood loss or extracellular fluid depletion can result in profound cardiovascular collapse. Surgical or accidental trauma can lead to significant bleeding, and its inadequate replacement may result in cardiac arrest. Likewise, severe diarrhea in the infant can result in such large deficits in extracellular fluid volume that hypovolemia and subsequent cardiac arrest can occur.

Other causes of cardiac arrest are anesthetic agents and other toxic drugs, allergic reactions, air embolism, electrolyte imbalance (such as hyperkalemia, hypocalcemia, or both), and vasovagal reflexes.

DIAGNOSIS AND TREATMENT

Since irreversible brain damage will occur within a few minutes after the cessation of cardiac activity, the diagnosis must be made and the treatment started immediately and simultaneously. Resuscitative efforts should be started the moment one can no longer palpate a femoral pulse and no further efforts should be directed at verifying the diagnosis of cardiac arrest. Since the risks from external cardiac massage are small, it is safer to start resuscitation immediately, even if one is not sure that the heart has stopped beating. In the operating room and intensive care unit, the diagnosis is much more easily made since most patients are being monitored. In addition, if the chest or abdominal cavities are open, the surgeon can observe and palpate the aorta or heart.

As soon as the diagnosis has been made, cardiac massage is initiated. If the chest is open (e.g. during a thoracic procedure), open massage is begun by manual compression of the heart either against the spine or the sternum. Bimanual compression of the heart can also be used and may be more effective in the case of a small child or infant. In most situations, the chest will not be open and external cardiac massage will be the preferred method of treatment. In the older child, the physician presses against the lower one-third of the sternum with the base of his hand (thenar and hypothenar eminences), depressing it rhythmically 60–80 times per minute against the heart. The compression is held about one-half second with rapid release. There must be an adequate release between compressions so that the heart can fill with blood from the great veins. To accomplish adequate compression, the patient must be placed on a hard surface such as a plywood board. In infants and small children, effective cardiac massage can be accomplished by placing one's thumbs over the lower sternum and one's fingers along the spine and gently squeezing them together at a rate of 80–100 times per minute. One must be careful not to compress the sternum too forcefully, since various injuries such as rib and sternal fractures, liver and spleen lacerations, and gastrointestinal perforations can result. The effectiveness of external massage can be evaluated by having another person palpate the femoral pulse.

At the moment cardiac massage is started, restoration of pulmonary ventilation must be initiated in order to adequately oxygenate the blood. If equipment for endotracheal intubation is not available, this can be started with either mouth-to-mouth artificial respiration or with a face mask and a breathing bag. Prior to the initiation of any respiratory resuscitation, however, the mouth and pharynx must be examined for evidence of vomiting and must be adequately suctioned. As soon as possible, an endotracheal tube must be inserted and artificial ventilation continued with 100 percent oxygen. A rate of about one ventilatory effort for every two to four cardiac compressions is advisable depending upon a compatible respiratory rate for age.

Once adequate cardiac massage and artificial ventilation have been achieved, an intravenous route should be established, preferably via a cutdown. If possible, try to thread the catheter into a central position so that central venous pressure can be monitored. At the same time, arterial blood should be drawn for the determination of pH and arterial gases and the patient should be connected to an electrocardiogram machine. With the electrocardiogram, the type of cardiac arrest (i.e. ventricular fibrillation or asystole) can be determined and the appropriate measures taken.

In the case of *ventricular fibrillation,* cardiac defibrillation should be carried out as soon as possible. Since most hospitals have direct-current defibrillators, no discussion of alternating current defibrillation will be presented. If the chest is open, paddles wrapped in saline-soaked sponges are applied to the heart and a direct-current shock of 20–60 watt-seconds is delivered. External defibrillation is carried out by placing one paddle over the apex of the heart (below the left nipple) and one at the base of the heart (right second intercostal space). A shock of 100–400 watt-seconds is delivered. Start with a low voltage and increase it until cardiac standstill occurs. Coarse fibrillation is much easier to defibrillate than is fine fibrillation; the fibrillation can be made more vigorous by the intracardiac or intravenous injection of 1–2 ml of 1:10,000 epinephrine. Once the heart has been successfully shocked into standstill, it will frequently begin beating in regular rhythm, as pulmonary ventilation and cardiac massage are continued.

In the case of *cardiac standstill,* correction of the associated metabolic insult will often result in resumption of spontaneous cardiac action. Myocardial oxygenation is improved by adequate external cardiac massage and pulmonary ventilation. The severe acidosis that is almost always present can be corrected by the administration of a buffer such as sodium bicarbonate. The ordinary ampules of sodium bicarbonate contain 44 mEq or 3.75 gm in 50 ml. In infants and small children, 5–10 ml aliquots can be given every 8–10 minutes. In older children, 20–50 ml aliquots are given. The administration of bicarbonate is monitored by following the arterial pH. If sodium bicarbonate is contraindicated, then the buffer Tham may be used. If the above measures are unsuccessful, the intravenous or intracardiac administration of calcium chloride or calcium gluconate can be tried. One ml in infants and around 3 ml in older children is usually given. Likewise, 1–2 ml of a 1:10,000 solution of epinephrine can be given intravenously or directly into the heart. Isoproterenol (Isuprel) may be used instead of, or in addition to, epinephrine in a dose of 1 μg/kg/per minute either as a single intravenous or intracardiac dose or in a continuous intravenous drip. Occasionally, digitalization is required to improve myocardial contractility.

EQUIPMENT

In most hospitals, it is desirable to have a resuscitation cart or box available on each floor, in the operating room, and in the emergency room. The resuscitation cart should contain the following equipment: laryngoscopes and endotracheal tubes of various sizes, an oxygen supply, face masks of various sizes, an electrocardiograph and direct current defibrillator, syringes and needles of various sizes, a venous cutdown set, a tracheostomy set, a set for chest tube insertion, a plywood board, and the following drugs: epinephrine, sodium bicarbonate, isoproterenol, and calcium gluconate (or chloride). In addition, sterile catheters and a suction source must be available for aspiration of secretions in the mouth, larynx, and trachea. Periodic inventories should be made to ensure the presence of all equipment, supplies, and drugs.

POSTRESUSCITATION CARE

Once the patient is resuscitated and has an effective heartbeat and adequate pulmonary ventilation, he must be followed very closely since the myocardium, which is irritable, is still susceptible to further cardiac arrests.

The patient should be transferred to an intensive care unit and certain hemodynamic and metabolic parameters should be carefully monitored. (See Chapter 11.) An arterial catheter should be inserted if possible to monitor blood pressure and follow arterial pH and blood bases. Central venous pressure should be followed in order to detect early hypovolemia or impending heart failure. A catheter should be inserted into the bladder and urine output should be measured as an additional index of intravascular and extracellular fluid volume. Serum electrolytes should be periodically measured to detect dangerous abnormalities such as hypo- or hyperkalemia. Especially in infants, temperature should be continuously monitored with a rectal probe. Neurological status should be followed to determine if any serious brain damage has occurred. If significant cerebral edema is suspected (secondary to hypoxia from the cardiac arrest), the administration of glucocorticoids should be considered.

If the above measures are taken, the majority of infants and children will be resuscitated from a cardiopulmonary arrest relatively easily and successfully. Because of the very low incidence of permanent neurological damage after a cardiac arrest in childhood, these young patients can then look forward to a normal existence.

REFERENCES

1. Hardy, J.D.: Cardiac arrest. In Randall, H.T., Hardy, J.D., and Moore, F.D., eds: *Manual of Preoperative and Postoperative Care*. Philadelphia: W.B. Saunders, 1967.
2. Jude, J.R.: Cardiopulmonary arrest and resuscitation. In Gibbon, J.H., Jr., Sabiston, D.C., Jr., and Spencer, F.C., eds: *Surgery of the Chest*. Philadelphia: W.B. Saunders, 1969.
3. Kouwenhoven, W.B., Jude, J.R., and Knickerbocker, G.G.: Closed chest cardiac massage. *JAMA* 173:1064–1067, 1960.
4. Riker, W.L.: Cardiac arrest in infants and children. *Ped Clin N Amer* 16:661–669, 1969.

Section III

Infections

14

Nosocomial
Infections

Joseph W. St. Geme, Jr., M.D.

The dramatic developments of the past 30 years in the advance of potent antibiotics, effective vaccines, and uniform public health procedure have erased and significantly harnessed a host of serious infections in man. Infectious diseases which proliferated abundantly in community populations in the past are either infrequent at present or quickly aborted by appropriate antimicrobial therapy. In the wake of this progress there has evolved increasing concern about virulent, persistent bacterial, viral, and fungal infections which erupt in the tissues of the hospitalized individual. By definition, these infections arise from within the hospital environment. In fact, many of these infections arise from within the host who is confined for medical processing within the hospital. Such an individual, whose biologic and physiologic functions are subjected to the most striking perturbation, is often a surgical patient. It is our impression that the pediatric surgical patient is less often the focus of nosocomial infection than the adult.

ENVIRONMENTAL FACTORS

History suggests that the hospitals of the past, teeming with sick patients with uncontrolled lethal contagious infections, were unequivocal pest houses. Is this true today? Most modern community hospitals are clean, uncrowded, and well ventilated. These conditions afford a lower concentration of microbes on flat surfaces and in airstreams within a structural facility.

Microbes, particularly bacteria, and frequently antibiotic-resistant bacteria, have found sanctuary in certain areas within a hospital. Gram-negative bacilli of several species have been detected in hexachlorophene and benzalkonium solutions, in soothing hand lotions, and the fixed dispenser units for all of these topical agents. Plumbing fixtures and inadequately cleansed incubators have harbored nonfermentative gram-negative bacilli, the so-called "water bugs" with unique taxonomic nomenclature familiar only to laboratory microbiologists, and frequently Pseudomonas species.

There is no doubt that the hospital flora has changed and the principal nosocomial pathogens of today are gram-negative bacilli. Instead of the once-abundant staphylococcus aureus, one finds E. coli, Klebsiella, Enterobacter (Aerobacter), Proteus species, Pseudomonas aeruginosa, Serratia marcescens, Bacterioides species, and many other elegantly identified, but obscure, gram-negative rods. Whether these organisms are more abundant in the environment or only the patients within that environment is unclear.

It is true, however, that some of these same pathogens have been distributed to patients as neatly packaged and purified inocula in urinary catheter kits, cardiac catheter packets, polyelectrolyte solutions, whole blood, food, and ice. Hospital personnel may also serve as conduits for the transmission of pathogens to patients. Such transmission is far more frequent by direct manual contact than by the airborne spread of infected droplet nuclei. Although highly suspect, in total perspective, hospital personnel have not been clearly delineated as playing an important role in the evolution of nosocomial infection. It has proved difficult to detect the incriminated pathogens under the fingernails of nurses, physicians, and the galaxy of other hospital workers.

In summary, the hospital environment is where nosocomial infections occur, but, with few exceptions, the environment plays a passive role in the process.

PERMISSIVENESS OF THE HOST

The major threat to survival of the burned child is overwhelming Pseudomonas bacteremia. Although strains of gentamicin-resistant Pseudomonas may spread from burn units using topical gentamicin therapy to other patients in the hospital, a very serious nosocomial hazard, the original Pseudomonas organisms probably arise from the damaged tissues of the burn site rather than from the immediate environment of medical care. Similar phenomena occur in the recipient of an organ homotransplant. The microbial flora of the patient's respiratory and gastrointestinal tracts represent the major source of potential nosocomial pathogens. Antimicrobial therapy does not offer the only explanation for the shift in the patient's flora from a populace of mixed, ordinarily nonpathogenic microbes to the spectrum of aforementioned gram-negative bacilli. Physiologic functions of pulmonary ciliary action, alveolar phagocytosis, and gastrointestinal motility may have significant impact on the natural drainage of the respiratory tract and the composition and quantity of the bacteria in the gut.

One may anticipate invasive nosocomial infection in the surgical patient with protracted illness and convalescence when the flora of the respiratory tract shift to the gram-negative bacillary spectrum. The surgical patient who has been prepared for gastrointestinal operative procedures by enteric antimicrobial therapy may incur an added risk of subsequent invasive infection with pathogenic gram-negative organisms.

Neonatal surgery, so often executed in the preterm or very young fullterm infant, challenges a host with acknowledged limitations in natural bactericidal and phagocytic function. Restricted anatomical dimensions further compromise pulmonary and gastrointestinal convalescence and restoration of normal function. While, at present, the predominant problem with nosocomial superinfection of neonates involves gram-negative organisms, the discontinuation of routine hexachlorophene bathing of newborn infants may lead to the resurgence of staphylococcal complications of neonatal surgery.

Finally, the innate immunosuppression which enshrouds the burn patient and the induced immunosuppression of the homotransplant recipient, with particular attenuation of cellular immunity, must play a major role in conditioning these surgical hosts for potential and often realized nosocomial infections.

SURGICAL MANIPULATION

As mentioned above, surgical intervention may interfere with normal anatomical and physiological function. This is poignantly true for neonatal thoracic and abdominal surgery. The thoracic incision and chest catheters impair full ventilation. Delayed restoration of normal gastrointestinal function precludes adequate nutrition and the stabilization of the gut flora. The host is thus rendered permissive for potential nosocomial superinfection.

Neurosurgical procedures, most notably the insertion of ventricu-

lojugular shunts as an indwelling foreign body in the midst of ventricular and cardiovascular flow, may be followed by persistent, indolent
bacterial infection. During the recent years, we have witnessed a greater
percentage of gram-negative bacillary infections of these shunts.

Infants and children seem to be less susceptible to the complication of necrotizing aspiration pneumonitis. Nevertheless, aggressive
and prolonged endotracheal or nasotracheal intubation perturb normal
tracheobronchial toilet and disrupt the delicate epithelium of the respiratory tract. These events render the surgical host more susceptible
to the acquisition of nosocomial pulmonary infection and subsequent
bacteremia.

INFLUENCE OF PATIENT MONITORING

The umbilical catheter may be employed as a component of postoperative monitoring of the very young neonate who has experienced
a thoracic surgical procedure. The umbilical artery may be used to
sample blood chemistries and gases and provide a portal for infusion
therapy. The umbilical vein allows parenteral therapy, but umbilical
vein samples are inadequate for the evaluation of blood gases. When
carefully cultured, almost 50 percent of umbilical vein catheter tips
yield bacteria. However, only four to five percent of infants with implanted catheters experience true bacteremia. Since the umbilicus is
a superb environment for bacterial growth, the syndrome of the positive catheter tip may represent significant proliferation of organisms
at the tip or the accumulation of bacteria around the tip as it is withdrawn. One cannot elude the impressive percentage of infants with
true bacteremia. For several reasons, therefore, the preferred umbilical
catheter site is one of the two arteries. Bacteremia is less common
and with careful implantation, vascular accidents can be avoided
also.

The urinary bladder catheter poses a less significant problem for
the ordinary pediatric patient than for the adult. There is no doubt
that immature as well as mature bladders become infected following
the insertion of an indwelling catheter. In our experience, such infections are ordinarily minimal and transient. The innate resistance of the
bladder tissue of the child may be greater than that of the adult, particularly the much older adult. Nevertheless, the urinary tract may serve
as a focus for disseminated infection and the protracted use of a catheter to quantitate urinary flow is unnecessary in the vast majority of
surgical settings. Short of serious thermal burns, severe cranial and
abdominal trauma, extensive hemorrhage, a directly damaged bladder,
and vesical obstruction, there seems little need for an indwelling
catheter.

IMPACT OF THERAPEUTIC PROCEDURES

Because of the greater likelihood of bacteremia and pylephlebitis the umbilical vein is being used less as a portal for intravenous therapy in the neonate. Although the umbilical artery cannula is a suitable site for biochemical monitoring and parenteral infusion of corrective fluids, there is increasing enthusiasm for return to the use of the small-caliber needle, swatched onto a catheter, and inserted into a peripheral vein, as the preferred technique for parenteral therapy in the neonate.

Intensive parenteral nutrition with very concentrated glucose solutions and protein hydrolysates or amino-acid mixtures requires the meticulous implantation of a catheter usually into the superior vena cava. The parenteral solutions must be aseptically constituted and a millipore filter interposed between the access line for changing fluids and the distal venous inflow catheter. The risks of bacteremia are real and these catheters must be inserted and maintained with great care. For less intensive peripheral parenteral therapy a smaller needle-catheter unit may be employed to infuse less-concentrated glucose solutions.

As seems to be true for other sources of nosocomial infection, the venous cutdown imposes a less significant risk of bacteremia for the child than the adult. This is fortunate, for it would be difficult to comply with the recommended shift of the cutdown site every 72 hours in the child as is necessary with the adult. It is preferable to infuse routine fluids via a needle whenever possible. It does not seem right to insert a routine venous cutdown into every child simply because they are scheduled for a surgical procedure.

The potential hazard of contaminated parenteral fluids has been clearly documented during the past few years. Improper aseptic procedure in packaging and capping by the manufacturer, improper mixing of fluids by nurses and physicians, and careless addition of medications to parenteral fluids are the explanations for subsequent bacteremia.

Whole blood may be an occasional source of nosocomial viral infections, including serum hepatitis virus, cytomegalovirus, and Epstein-Barr virus. These infections become more significant when many units of blood are used for either severe hemorrhage or the extracorporeal circulatory systems of intracardiac surgery. On rare occasions, bacteria may gain access to cardiopulmonary pump units. These organisms may be "water bugs" and, indeed, some strains of Pseudomonas actually multiply at the blood storage temperature of 4°C. Bacteria are also able to multiply within packaged, concentrated platelets.

Protracted use of broad-spectrum antibiotics will alter the flora of the respiratory and gastrointestinal tracts and invite nosocomial in-

fection with resistant organisms. There is no reason to employ antibiotics to prevent contamination of a tracheostomy or a catheterized
bladder. Precise techniques will prevent many of these potential infections, whereas antibiotics will only insure infection with resistant
microbes. Intensive circumoperative antibiotic therapy may be essential for complicated, prolonged procedures. The opportunity for serious
intraoperative infection is significant. If one assumes infection, then
vigorous therapy becomes important and should be instituted immediately prior to surgery, and continued for 48 hours after the surgery.
Prolonged preoperative therapy simply conditions the bacterial population of the patient for potential invasion by resistant organisms and
is to be condemned.

There is continuing evidence that the nebulizing units of respirators are an awesome source of rapidly proliferating gram-negative bacilli. Severe gram-negative pneumonitis may follow the protracted use
of poorly decontaminated respiratory equipment. Oxygen tents laden
with mist may threaten the respiratory tract of the exposed patient
with the same gram-negative bacilli if the fluid reservoirs are not
changed and cleaned frequently. This is particularly true if the oxygen-
mist tents are used for more than 48–72 hours. The humidified atmosphere alone is not the sole factor because prolonged oxygen therapy
by mask or catheter may dessicate the entire respiratory tract, thus disturbing natural mechanisms of tracheobronchial debridement, and may
also depress alveolocyte surfactant production and phagocytic function
in the most peripheral segments of the lung. All of these events render
the host more susceptible to nosocomial pulmonary infection, primarily bacterial and occasionally mycotic in nature.

REMEDIAL STEPS

Hospital infection control committees have an enormous task in sustaining continued surveillance of potential sources of nosocomial infection. The issues of concern include soap and antiseptic dispensers,
hand lotions, vascular and bladder catheter kits, foods, ice, parenteral
fluid preparations, whole blood and blood products, inhalation therapy equipment, isolettes and oxygen tents, and indiscriminate use of
broad spectrum antibiotics. Modern surveillance techniques demand
both periodic bacteriologic sampling of these medications, adjuncts,
and items of equipment and the use of the hospital diagnostic bacteriology laboratory to investigate clusters of infection with nosocomial
pathogens.

Since most of the nosocomial pathogens arise from the patient,
the obviously crucial steps are those which maintain the host in good
nutritional balance and adequate immunologic competence, and ab-

breviate invasive therapeutic and monitoring manipulations. Effective surgical and anatomical drainage, minimized disturbance of the normal physiologic function of the entire respiratory tract, and the retention of the host's balanced microbial flora are the important goals.

Transfusions and antibiotics should be used with constraint and only when absolutely indicated.

The skin should be prepared for infusion with vigorous soap scrubs, the application of iodine, and final ablution with alcohol. These procedures may be crucial for even simple venesection in the patient immunosupressed by therapeutic design or because of fundamental disease process. Parenteral hyperalimentation should be executed with meticulous attention (see Chapter 9).

Respirator units should be changed every day, cleaned thoroughly, and decontaminated with gas sterilization. Water reservoir bottles for oxygen-mist tents should be replenished with fresh distilled water every 8 hours. Isolettes should be substituted every week and carefully cleaned and decontaminated.

Hospital personnel must practice the simplest of infection control technique, namely VIGOROUS HANDWASHING before and after the manipulation of every patient. Mask, gowns, and caps are of secondary importance despite their ritualistic attractiveness.

The medical and nursing care setting for critically ill patients, the prime candidates for nosocomial infection, should be clean and un-cluttered, with simple, free-flowing traffic patterns for the multitude of individuals of *all* disciplines who must attend such patients. One should strive for abundant open space which maximizes visual care and minimizes the number of personnel necessary for careful patient monitoring. Housekeeping personnel must also have adequate space in which to perform their important daily tasks of cleaning and de-contamination. But for the most unique of patients, life islands and isolation cubicles seem unnecessary and emotionally deprivational.

CONCLUSION

Hospitals must continue to monitor microbial morbidity, nursing techniques, physician practice, and structural sanitation. Despite increasing emphasis on ambulatory health care, hospitals will continue to be the scene of crisis care, much of it prolonged. Care, cleanliness, and cere-bration will go far in the attenuation of the alarming parameters of nosocomial infection. Teamwork on the part of all the professional disciplines within the hospital environment is essential.

15

Infections in the
Surgical Patient

Morton M. Woolley, M.D.

Infections frequently play a significant role in the clinical course of the pediatric patient who is hospitalized for surgical therapy. To facilitate rational therapy, such patients may be broadly categorized as follows:

1. The patient whose disease process is primarily inflammatory and infectious, and is treated definitively by a surgical procedure, i.e. an abscess which is treated by surgical incision for drainage of purulent exudate.
2. The patient who has an infection as a direct consequence of a surgical procedure, i.e. a surgical wound infection.
3. The "surgical" patient whose basic disease and/or age predispose him to infection, i.e. meconium ileus in a neonate with cystic fibrosis.
4. The patient who has acquired a disease or an injury which results in an infection requiring surgical therapy, i.e. severe thermal injury to the skin and subcutaneous tissues.

This classification is rather broad in its scope and the categories are not mutually exclusive. As an example, a patient with cystic fibrosis who is inherently predisposed to pulmonary infection, can receive a severe thermal injury resulting in burn wound sepsis, enhancing the propensity for pulmonary infection.

INFECTIONS TREATED DEFINITIVELY BY SURGICAL THERAPY

Cervical Abscess

Once a pyogenic cervical abscess has become well-established, it will require surgical drainage for cure. Such abscesses are most commonly due to suppurative staphylococcal adenitis following tonsillopharyn-gitis by several days or weeks. Although appropriate antibiotic therapy may abort the formation of an abscess, once the abscess has been well-established, antibiotic therapy may only delay the "pointing," thus pro-tracting the illness. Adequate drainage is curative.

The possibility of tuberculous adenitis can be excluded by chest x-ray and tuberculin skin test. Where geographically applicable, coc-cidiodin and histoplasmin skin tests are also advisable. A specimen of the exudate is submitted for bacteriological and fungal examinations to define the etiological agent and to exclude the possibility of actino-mycosis ("lumpy jaw").

Congenital Cervical Lesions Which May Become Secondarily Infected

Congenital lesions of the face, head, and neck which predispose the individual to infection include thyroglossal duct cyst, branchial cleft cyst, epidermal inclusion cysts, and preauricular sinuses. Thyroglo-glossal duct cysts are in the midline and overlie the hyoid bone. Epi-dermal inclusion cysts are commonly in the midline, but can present in a lateral position and frequently are located at the upper-outer margin of the eyebrow. Branchial cleft cysts and sinuses characteristically are located anterior to the sternocleidomastoid muscle, but lateral to the midline. Any of these lesions can become infected, under which cir-cumstances incision and drainage should be followed by definitive excision after the inflammatory process has subsided. Since excision prior to infection is always more desirable, such lesions should be excised when first discovered.

Of particular interest is the infected preauricular sinus. The ab-scess presents anterior to the ear and many such lesions have been re-peatedly drained without recognizing the presence of the sinus. The sinus opening is regularly present at the anterior extremity of the helix and is commonly found in numerous members of a family complex. Most such sinuses are innocous, but once infection occurs, the entire sinus must be removed. Otherwise the patient is beset with recurrent abscesses and an ugly granulating lesion anterior to the ear (Figure 15–1).

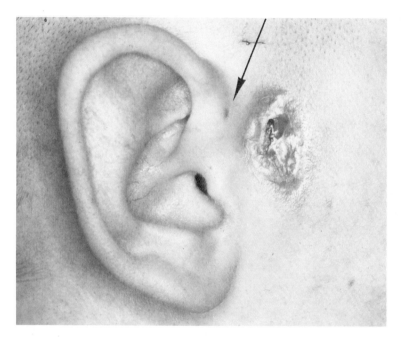

Figure 15–1
Infected preauricular sinus.

Appendicitis

The inflammatory involvement of the appendix is secondary to obstruction of its lumen, most commonly by an appendiceal fecalith. Lymphoid hyperplasia, secondary to viral infections such as measles, may also cause obstruction resulting in appendicitis. The time from onset of symptoms to full wall necrosis and perforation is rarely longer than 24 hours in infants and children and may be much shorter. Twenty-five to 35 percent of such patients have a calcified appendiceal fecalith which is visible by x-ray and aids in early diagnosis. If the appendix can be removed prior to necrosis and perforation, the patient should recover without significant complication. If the infectious process has traversed the appendiceal wall, resulting in localized or generalized peritonitis, the clinical course is significantly complicated by blood volume deficit, systemic sepsis, and the possibility of secondary abscess formation as well as wound infection and intestinal obstruction. When acute appendicitis is seriously suspected, it is in the patient's best interest to have an appendectomy performed promptly. With careful consideration of history, physical findings, and laboratory work, approximately 75–80 percent of such patients will have appendicitis. The other 20–25 percent of patients may have a variety of diseases causing abdominal pain. It is advisable to keep an open mind because we have seen such patients who subsequently were proved to have malignant tumors of the kidney, obstructive uropathies, specific intestinal infections such as salmonella and shigella, as well as Crohn's disease and ulcerative colitis. Specifically, we do not accept the diagnosis of "mesenteric adenitis" without bacteriological and histopathological proof.

If the patient has progressed to perforation (this will be the case in approximately 50 percent of the patients in the pediatric age group), preoperative preparation with appropriate fluids, colloid, blood, and antibiotics (see Chapter 16), is necessary to insure a safe course through anesthesia and through the early postoperative period. *Blood volume deficit is the most serious threat to the life of the patient with perforative appendicitis, particularly during the course of general anesthesia.* In addition to removal of the appendix, drains are left in the peritoneal space to allow exit of any remaining exudate. Such drains are left in place for ten days or longer to minimize the incidence of secondary abscesses. Intraperitoneal abscesses are most apt to occur in the pelvis or subphrenic spaces and should be suspected if the patient's temperature begins an upward trend after a postoperative defervescence. Since pelvic abscesses are easier to drain than subphrenic abscesses, it is logical to place the patient in a sitting position so that pus will collect in the pelvis rather than in the subphrenic space postoperatively. Pelvic abscesses are palpable by rectal examination. Subphrenic abscesses usually cause a reactive pleural effusion on the side of the abscess and commonly air-fluid levels develop in such an abscess due to gas-forming bacteria. Pelvic abscesses may be drained either through the incision or through the anterior rectal wall depending upon the proximity of the abscess. Subphrenic abscesses can be drained extraperitoneally from an anterior, posterior, or lateral approach depending upon the location.

Extremity Abscesses

An unexplained abscess located on an extremity must be considered to be osteomyelitis until proved otherwise. Many extremity abscesses will not show x-ray evidence of osteomyelitis during the initial phase of osteomyelitis. After adequate drainage of an extremity abscess, follow-up x-rays should be taken at biweekly intervals until the patient is asymptomatic so that underlying osteomyelitis will not be missed. Suppurative infections around the fingernails (paronychia), in the pulp of the finger tips (felon), and in the various palmar spaces are all treated by adequate surgical drainage in addition to antibiotics. Such abscesses are most commonly staphylococcal in origin.

Para-anal Abscess

Rarely does an abscess occur adjacent to the anus without a subjacent fistula-in-ano. Following the drainage of such an abscess, the patient should be followed in anticipation of demonstrating a fistula-in-ano. Once well-established, the fistula-in-ano should be excised to preclude the possibility of recurrent para-anal abscesses. Fistula-in-ano and para-anal abscesses are commonly associated with more proximal gastrointestinal disease processes such as ulcerative colitis and/or granulomatous enterocolitis (Crohn's disease). If the patient's illness appears to be out of proportion to the para-anal abscess, gastrointestinal studies should follow to exclude the possibility of diffuse intestinal inflammatory disease processes.

INFECTIONS OCCURRING AS A SEQUEL TO A SURGICAL PROCEDURE

Wound Infections

The majority of surgical incisions should and do heal *per primam* without significant inflammation and without suppuration. Unfortunately, some surgical wounds do become infected resulting in appreciable morbidity and in extreme circumstances, mortality. By careful observation, and with foreknowledge of predisposing factors, wound infections can frequently be anticipated, diagnosed early, and treated adequately and appropriately. If a wound infection is predicted, drains should be left in the incision or the incision can be left open, to avoid infection.

Routine, indiscriminate "prophylactic" use of antibiotics does not prevent wound infections and should be discouraged as it may encourage the emergence of resistant strains of bacteria and overgrowth of pathogenic bacteria in the gastrointestinal tract.

If there is no known bacteriological contamination of the wound, it is considered a "clean" wound and wound infection is not anticipated. If such a wound does suppurate, it is imperative that all technical aspects of the operating room function be reviewed to be certain that there is no break in surgical technique. This includes sterility of all equipment, appropriate preparation of the skin, scrubbing technique by all personnel, and the proper utilization of masks and control of ambient air currents to prevent excessive airborne bacteria.

The patient himself may be harboring pathogenic bacteria in the nose and throat, eyes, ears, or gastrointestinal tract and if an unexplained wound infection does occur, it is advisable to examine and culture all of these areas in an attempt to determine the source of the pathogenic organism. If the incision has been contaminated during an operative procedure, wound infection can be anticipated and the type of organism can be predicted depending upon the mechanism of contamination. For instance, if the gastrointestinal tract is opened for any reason during the operation, the wound is considered to be contaminated and if an infection ensues, one would anticipate flora residing in the intestinal tract. Cultures should be made of the contents of any opened bowel.

Since infections are much more apt to occur in tissues with poor blood supply, the individual with excessive subcutaneous adipose tissue poses a greater risk for a wound infection than an otherwise thin, muscular individual because the adipose tissue has poorer blood supply. The longer a wound is opened to the ambient air, the greater number of bacteria will be found in the wound, increasing the probability of infection. Shock with decreased tissue perfusion increases wound susceptibility to infection. Similarly, patients with cyanotic heart disease whose tissues are less well oxygenated have increased susceptibility to wound infection.

During necrosis and slough of the umbilical cord, the umbilical area may harbor a combination of pathogenic bacteria. If an abdominal operation is necessary during this period of time, it is impossible to completely sequester the umbilical area from the abdominal incision and one can anticipate an increased incidence of wound infection. If it is imperative that an operation be performed during the period of time when the umbilical area is infected, it may be of help to culture the umbilical area, then treat it with liberal amounts of silver nitrate, and sequester the umbilicus from the incision during the operative procedure.

Treatment of Wound Infections

A wound infection manifested by spreading erythema and edema within 8–12 hours after the operation, may be due to a virulent streptococcal infection. This infection can be best aborted by an appropriate intravenous antibiotic. If the wound becomes edematous, erythematous, and fluctuant, suppuration has occurred and the primary and most important therapeutic measure is adequate drainage. The temptation to open such a wound only slightly, hoping that a smaller opening will heal more quickly, should be resisted because adequate drainage results in earlier wound healing than does inadequate drainage. Commonly, suture material will extrude from such an incision and until it is all extruded or removed, the wound will continue to suppurate, granulate, and drain.

The advisability of ancillary antibiotic therapy for treatment of wound infection depends upon several factors. During early infancy, the immune mechanisms are less well developed and it is usually advisable to utilize antibiotics to prevent systemic infections. If the patient has another debilitating disease such as leukemia, nephrosis, or cystic fibrosis, or is on immunosuppression, antibiotics may be indicated. If the patient is otherwise normal and is well into the childhood years, antibiotics are of little benefit.

Pulmonary Infections

The neonate with any one of the forms of esophageal atresia or tracheoesophageal fistula is particularly prone to pneumonitis. An early gastrostomy is beneficial in preventing gastric reflux through a tracheoesophageal fistula. An indwelling catheter in the upper esophageal segment is helpful in preventing spill-over of saliva into the trachea. Postoperatively, such patients frequently require direct tracheal suction to stimulate adequate coughing to expand the lung and also to remove excessive secretions. The weak neonate cannot adequately clear secretions from the trachea without mechanical assistance.

Vomiting and aspiration of vomitus resulting in pneumonitis, can generally be avoided by a gastrostomy after major gastrointestinal surgery in the neonate. This is much better than an indwelling nasogastric tube because it functions better and it does not cause irritation of the nasopharynx which discourages adequate coughing and clearing of secretions.

Patients with cystic fibrosis are constantly at risk from pulmonary infection. If such a patient requires an operation and this can be performed with a noninhalation technique, such as ketamine, this would obviate the increased risk of pulmonary infection. If inhalation anesthesia is necessary, then careful tracheal toilet during and after surgery is mandatory.

If the patient is otherwise healthy, pulmonary complications are not as common in the childhood age group as in the adult population. Atelectasis can commonly be corrected by having the child blow up balloons.

Intravenous Therapy/Thrombophlebitis

If intravenous fluids and/or intravenous medications are given postoperatively, thrombophlebitis at the site of the intravenous needle or cannula is an ever-present danger. *If a patient develops a high fever during intravenous therapy, and this is out of proportion to his clinical toxicity, thrombophlebitis at the intravenous site is the common cause.*

In the later stages of thrombophlebitis, there will be erythema, edema, and marked tenderness at the site, but early, such physical findings may be minimal or absent. Under such circumstances, the best policy is to simply change the intravenous cannula site and usually the temperature will drop to normal in a precipitous fashion. The tip of the cannula should be submitted to the bacteriology laboratory for culture and antibiotic sensitivity studies. On rare occasions the thrombophlebitis may have progressed to frank suppuration, and it may be necessary to surgically excise the offending vein to control the infection. It is usually possible to avoid thrombophlebitis by routinely changing the intravenous site at least every three days.

Infections Associated with Total Intravenous Nutrition

Patients who are unable to take food or fluids via the gastrointestinal tract for prolonged periods of time, are now commonly "fed" by vein (see Chapter 9). Because this technique requires that a foreign body be left in the superior vena cava for prolonged periods of time, and since such patients are usually inherently debilitated, systemic infections do occur. Such infections are commonly monilial and/or bacterial and are not uniformly preventable by the use of systemic antibiotics. If such an infection does occur, it is necessary to remove the cannula. Scrupulous aseptic technique in handling such cannulas does minimize infection. The filter in the system should be changed every three days and cultured each time it is changed to ascertain the sterility of the system.

Leaking Gastrointestinal Anastomosis

The infant or child who develops a leak in a gastrointestinal anastomosis postoperatively may present a confusing clinical picture. If there is sudden appearance of abdominal distention and an x-ray reveals a large amount of free intraperitoneal gas, this is obviously due to a leaking gastrointestinal anastomosis. After appropriate replacement of fluids, such a patient should be promptly reoperated upon.

Quite commonly, however, the clinical presentation is much more subtle. The patient may gradually become lethargic, jaundiced, mildly febrile, and mildly distended. When moved or examined, he will usually be manifestly irritable. If appropriate laboratory studies are performed, it will be discovered that the bilirubin is elevated, particularly in the unconjugated fraction and the patient will have depression of one or more of the blood-clotting factors. Since the diffuse intravascular coagulopathy is secondary to sepsis caused by anastomotic leak, the leak must be corrected otherwise the D.I.C. will continue. Heparin therapy may be necessary but only if the primary cause is controlled and the D.I.C. continues.

DEFECTIVE IMMUNITY STATES

Age

The defense mechanism to infection in the neonate is poorly developed. He resists infection less well than his older counterpart and he reacts to infection in the clinical setting in a different fashion. Instead of a febrile "toxic" response that one sees in the older child, the infant may simply appear lethargic, jaundiced, hypothermic, and poorly responsive to painful stimuli. Once established, an infection spreads much more rapidly in the neonate than in the older child. Therefore, diagnostic studies and therapy are rationally instituted at an earlier time and with less "proof" of infection. The neonate who has undergone an extensive surgical procedure is rationally placed on "prophylactic antibiotics" and if this policy is not followed, the indications for antibiotics should be liberalized. In the clinical setting, one cannot afford to wait for the report of positive blood culture because, by that time, the patient's life may be unduly endangered.

Both phagocytosis and antibody formation appear to be less well developed in the infant than in the older child. However, in some individuals, adequate white blood cell phagocytosis and/or immune globulin antibody formation remains deficient into the childood age group. If the patient does not seem to be responding appropriately to infection, it is desirable to evaluate phagocytosis as well as immunoglobulin levels.

Splenectomy

Although the existing reports of infection following splenectomy are contradictory, there appear to be some general guidelines which are helpful in determining which patients will be at "risk" of increased incidence of significant infection after splenectomy. There are patients whose basic disease subjects them to increased infection prior to splenectomy and probably this postoperative predisposition is enhanced by splenectomy. One such syndrome is the Weskott-Aldrich syndrome, in which the immunoglobulins are decreased. After splenectomy, rapid, overwhelming infections occur. Any patient who is to undergo splenectomy for idiopathic thrombocytopenic purpura should have the Weskott-Aldrich syndrome excluded by history and determination of immunoglobulins. Since all patients under two years of age who have splenectomy appear to have an increased incidence of significant infection, splenectomy should be delayed until after age two years whenever possible.

Nephrosis

Patients with nephrosis, who present to the physician with abdominal pain require careful evaluation prior to recommendation of surgical therapy. Such patients are always subject to primary peritonitis, usually of pneumococcal origin. If such a patient does have primary pneumococcal peritonitis, he should be treated with appropriate antibiotics. On the other hand, these patients are usually being treated with steroids which makes them hypercoagulable and they do, on occasions, thrombose mesenteric veins resulting in segmental intestinal gangrene requiring surgical therapy. Patients with nephrosis can also develop appendicitis. In evaluating such patients, it is helpful to differentiate between the patient who has controlled nephrosis with little or no albumin in the urine and with little or no ascites compared to the uncontrolled nephrotic who has albuminuria and is ascitic. If ascites is present, the peritonitis is much more apt to be primary. If the patient has signs and symptoms of appendicitis and is urine albumin-free and does not have ascites, he is much more apt to have appendicitis and should be operated upon for such. The signs and symptoms of mesenteric vascular occlusion in nephrotic patients are the same as in others, i.e. shock, abdominal tenderness, and the development of a mass. Under these circumstances, the patient should be operated upon after the blood volume has been adequately replaced.

Pancreatitis is an ever-present possibility in all infants and children on steroid therapy.

Progressive Septic Granulomatous Disease of Infancy and Childhood

This is a disease which appears to be limited to males, is frequent in male siblings, and results in chronic, as well as acute, recurrent infections of lymph nodes, subcutaneous tissue, lungs, and other organs as the disease process progresses. It usually ends fatally prior to puberty. The exact etiology is not known and treatment is symptomatic both medically and surgically.

Lymphangioma

Since lymphangiomas are composed of lymphatic structures which are grossly dilated, these lesions do not handle infection as one would anticipate with normal lymphatic structures. Indeed, infection in lymphangiomas was a cause of death prior to the availability of antibiotics. If a large lymphangioma does become infected, intravenous antibiotic therapy in adequate dosage should be instituted immediately. To obviate infection, large lymphangiomas should be removed when technically feasible.

Diabetes Mellitus

Although diabetes mellitus is not commonly appreciated in infants or young children, it does begin to appear in the childhood age group (see Chapter 18). It is frequently quite brittle and infections in such patients should be treated as aggressively as they are in the adult population. It should also be recognized that a child without clinical diabetes, but who has a strong family history, may indeed develop diabetes during the stress of a severe illness. We treated one such patient with a severe burn who developed overt diabetes during the therapy and required insulin therapy. Once his burn had been taken care of by definitive skin grafting, his diabetic condition disappeared and the insulin was discontinued.

ACQUIRED DISEASES SUBJECTING THE PATIENT TO INFECTION

Thermal and Other Traumatic Injuries

The mechanism of tissue death in physical, thermal, or chemical injuries is interruption of the blood supply. The resultant necrotic tissue becomes a culture medium upon which a variety of organisms may thrive. If the tissue necrosis is well-established and the distribution of the necrosis is well-defined, excision of such tissue with wound closure either by suture or grafting will obviate secondary infection. This is most commonly possible in traumatic wounds where necrotic soft tissues may be debrided and viable wound edges coapted. In thermal injuries, this can occasionally be accomplished if the full thickness burn is well-established and the peripheral extent of the burn is well-delineated. If delineation is not clear, it is unwise to remove questionably third degree burn tissue because one may in fact be excising skin which is ultimately viable.

In all such injuries, hypovolemic shock should be avoided because poor tissue perfusion enhances tissue death and infection.

In thermal injuries, initial penicillin therapy is indicated to obviate early streptococcal invasive sepsis. This can be effectively achieved by three to five days of penicillin. Following this, it is generally advisable not to use systemic antibiotics for fear of overgrowth of more virulent strains. Sequential burn wound cultures will guide one in appropriate antibiotic therapy.

A variety of topical chemotherapeutic agents and antibiotics are available and are being used currently to prevent invasive sepsis. Among these are 0.5 percent silver nitrate, gentamycin, Sulfamylon, and silver sulfadiazine. When using any of these agents, one should be well-acquainted with their side effects and/or toxic propensities. It is important to recognize the possibility of marked fluid shifts which are an inherent result of thermal injuries and, when topical therapy is used, this may complicate the fluid shift either by electrolyte diffusion into the burn wound, as in the case of silver nitrate, or by carbonic anhydrase inhibition effect of Sulfamylon, causing diuresis. If one is not cognizant of these facts and does not make appropriate alteration in his fluid and electrolyte management, the patient may develop a severe electrolyte and fluid imbalance.

Purpura Fulminans

This rare, but devastating, disease process appears to be a delayed hypersensitivity reaction usually following a streptococcal or viral infection. The basic pathologic process is one of progressive, extensive, diffuse intravascular consumptive coagulation. Clinically, the disease begins with a small cutaneous hemorrhagic area which rather rapidly enlarges to ultimately involve necrosis of large areas of skin and subcutaneous tissue. Usually, it is bilaterally symmetrical in the lower extremities, but may involve any part of the body. Laboratory studies reveal extensive utilization of the clotting factor including platelets, prothrombin, Factors V and VIII, and fibrinogen, among others. Optimal therapy consists of early adequate heparinization to interrupt the progressive intravascular coagulation. If tissue necrosis has already occurred, the necrotic areas are treated the same as a thermal injury, i.e. by debridement and grafting.

A similar syndrome occurs in some patients with active infection, particularly meningococcus or pseudomonas. If the basic problem is active infection, it is then primarily treated with antibiotics, and heparinization is of value in interruption of the D.I.C.

Necrotizing Enterocolitis

A clinical entity, characterized by progressive necrosis of the mucosa of the intestine, invasion of the intestinal wall by gas, and eventual necrosis of a small area of the intestinal wall with perforation, or large segments of the full thickness of the intestine has been labeled "necrotizing enterocolitis." This entity has the following well-recognized, but poorly defined, evolutionary stages: an apparent inciting factor such as hypoxia, shock, or major electrolyte or blood-volute alteration. In the neonate, severe hypoxemia is a common antecedent factor. Exchange transfusions sometimes precede this entity. In the older infants, dehydration, shock, and major electrolyte abnormalities secondary to diarrhea are common historical events. In some patients, the enteritis follows immediately and in others there is a symptom-free interval. Next, the patient may have bloody stools, he becomes distended and has bile-stained emesis. At this time, he appears lethargic and "sick." X-rays will reveal intestinal distention and in some patients intraluminal gas, "pneumotosis intestinalis." Gas may be apparent in the portal venous system and, although in the past this was thought to be indicative of a fatal outcome, there are now patients who have survived with x-ray evidence of portal venous gas.

The last phase is that of full thickness intestinal wall necrosis with perforation. This may be in one or two small areas or it may involve the major portion of the small and large bowel.

All physicians and surgeons caring for infants and children must recognize that this entity can follow any one of the inciting causes. It is axiomatic that, whenever possible, the inciting factors should be avoided and, if they do occur, that they should be treated expeditiously to minimize the chances of subsequent necrotizing enterocolitis. Once necrotizing enterocolitis has been established, the therapy is specifically directed at combating infection and in correcting blood volume and electrolyte abnormalities. The bacteria involved with this entity vary from one patient to another, but usually it is a gram-negative bacillus.

The indication for surgical intervention is intestinal perforation. Since surgical intervention should follow perforation as soon as possible, abdominal x-rays should be taken at least every eight hours until the patient recovers or until surgical intervention is indicated. The presence of intrahepatic portal vein gas portends a guarded prognosis, but is not necessarily a lethal complication.

If one could anticipate perforation, it would seem logical to operate and excise obviously necrotic tissue before perforation occurs. At this time, we know of no way to make this judgment and since we have had patients survive this entity with medical therapy, we are hesitant to add the risk of surgery prior to frank perforation of the intestinal tract.

Since the disease entity is associated with some of the findings of diffuse intravascular coagulopathy, the question of heparin therapy is ever-present. We have used heparin therapy in selected cases and it appears to have been of some benefit. At the present time, if the patient has laboratory evidence of consumptive coagulopathy, we may use heparin, otherwise not.

MEDICAL-SURGICAL COOPERATIVE EFFORTS MANDATORY

Due to the complexity of medical and surgical therapy of infections in infants and children, it is evident that close communication and cooperation between medical, laboratory, and surgical specialists is of paramount importance in the care of the infant and child with a surgically treatable disease precipitated by or complicated by infection. The preparation for surgery is just as important as the anesthetic management which is just as important as the timing and technical aspects of the operation. Antibiotic therapy must be adequate, specific, and not overdone. The evaluation of the response of the blood to infection, particularly the clottting factors, is increasingly important and must be given proper interpretation. The interpretation of these findings is critical and it is no longer rational to simply treat deficient coagulation component parts by replacement, because the underlying process may require surgical therapy as well as medical therapy by either anticoagulation or replacement of coagulation component parts. By close, personal communication between pediatrician, surgeon, and anesthesiologist, optimal care can be provided for the little patients who are the victims of disease entities described in this chapter.

REFERENCES

1. Blaese, R.M., Brown, S.R., Strober, W., Waldman, T.A.: Wiskott-Aldrich syndrome. *Lancet* 1:1056–1061, 1968.
2. Carson, M.J., Chedwick, D.L., Brubaker, C.A., Clelland, R.S., and Landing, B.H.: Thirteen boys with progressive septic granulomatosis. *Pediatrics* 35:405–412, 1965.
3. Infection control in the hospital, *American Association Publication,* 1970.
4. Dudgeon, D.L., Woolley, M.M., and Gilchrist, G.S.: Purpura fulminans *Arch Surg* 103:351–358, 1971.
5. Weiser, Myrvik, and Pearsall: *Fundamentals of Immunology.* Philadelphia: Lee and Febiger, 1969.
6. Roback, S.A., et al: Chronic granulomatous disease of children: Surgical considerations. *J of Ped Surg* 6:601–611, 1971.
7. Stevenson, J.K., et al: Aggressive treatment of neonatal necrotizing enterocolitis: Thirty-eight patients with twenty-five survivors. *J of Ped Surg* 6:28–35, 1971.
8. A.J. Eraklis, et al: Hazard of overwhelming infection after splenectomy in childhood. *New Eng J Med* 276:1225–1229, 1967.

16

Antimicrobial Therapy

Benjamin M. Kagan, M.D.

The immediately preceding chapter has implied that, at the time of surgery, pediatric patients may have an infection whether or not it is related to the actual surgery itself; or that they may have unusual susceptibility to infections, a susceptibility possibly intensified by the condition necessitating the surgery. Furthermore, we must be aware that these patients might acquire clinical infections postoperatively. Some of the latter are nosocomial (see Chapter 14) and some are due to organisms carried by the individual which in the presence of reduced resistance, perhaps related to the surgery itself or to anesthesia or to some related situation, develops into clinical infection. In this chapter, we will discuss basic principles and their practical application in handling such situations. A table is provided for preliminary selection of antimicrobial agents and there is also a table giving dosages.

Bacteria are in a constant state of change, and some of these variations have clinical significance. Their growth rates may change in either direction, and their degrees of sensitivity to antibacterial agents may change. The latter can be due to a number of different mechanisms. Thus, there may be changes in the bacterial chromosomes, changes which are passed on only to the daughter cells of a mutant. In addition, genetic material in bacteria may be extrachromosomal; it may be carried in the cytoplasm and replicate independently of the chromosome. To make matters more complicated, both chromosomal and cytoplasmic genetic information can be transferred between different strains, different species, or even different genera of bacteria.

Several mechanisms for this transfer are known. Desoxyribonucleic acid (DNA) from cells of one strain can induce an inheritable change in cells of another strain (transformation); viral DNA can infect bacterial cells, resulting in production of a complete virus (transfection); virulent bacteriophage can multiply in and disrupt host cells, releasing numbers of virus particles which in turn infect and disrupt more host cells (transduction); there may be genetic exchange by sexual conjugation with cell-to-cell contact by a cytoplasmic bridge or tube between mating bacteria (sex factor Hf). When the exchanged material in such mating is extrachromosomal, it is called an F factor. It and other autonomous genetic elements which replicate independently in the cytoplasm are called episomes. This factor has been shown to occur in both gram-positive and gram-negative cells, although, thus far, the mechanism of transfer of episomal elements in the staphylococcus appears to be mediated by bacteriophage. The resistance (R factor) which is transferred by episomes is often a resistance not only to one but to many antibodies.

One can anticipate, therefore, the need for a continuing search for newer antimicrobial agents and never-ending reevaluation of the ever-changing relations between microbes, antimicrobial agents, and man. Fortunately, there has been an ever-increasing number of available antibiotics, although in recent years the rate of development has slowed. Some of the older antimicrobial agents have been dropped, either because they became relatively less effective or because greater toxicity was observed.

Thus streptomycin, once a widely used antibiotic, is now generally useful in only a few specific areas, such as tuberculosis, bubonic plague, tularemia, and enterococcal infections. Dihydrostreptomycin has lost its clinical role completely because of the associated deafness. In 1965, at least 24 antibacterial agents were reported for which there was some reason to hope there would be clinical application. Only three of these are available: methacycline, hetacillin, and doxycycline. All of these are derivatives of previously well-known antibiotics. Of six new antibiotics described in 1958, only two have survived: vancomycin and erythromycin propionyl ester (Ilosone). Of eight described in 1959, only four have survived: colistimethate (Coly-Mycin), paromomycin (Humycin), alphaphenoxyethyl penicillin (Syncillin), and demethylchlortetracycline (Declomycin). Two of these are similar to older agents, and the other two were derived from older agents.

Important additions have been modifications of penicillin: methicillin, oxacillin, nafcillin, cloxacillin, and dicloxacillin. Methicillin, oxacillin, cloxacillin, dicloxicillin, and nafcillin are penicillinase-restistant. A most important modification of penicillin has been added—ampicillin. Two entirely new antibiotics—cephalothin and lincomycin and their derivatives are also significant. Cephalothin is a different molecule from that of penicillin. The spectrum and effectiveness of cephalothin are very similar to those of penicillin, and in some ways similar to ampicillin. Patients sensitive to penicillin are thus far, with a few exceptions, able to tolerate cephalothin. Because of these apparently rare exceptions, and until more experience is available, penicillin-sensitive patients who must be given cephalothin should be observed closely, especially at the time of initial dose. Lincomycin is still a different molecule. It concentrates in bone. *In vitro* tests show that lincomycin has a high degree of effectiveness against staphylococcal L forms. Some studies suggest that it is effective in some patients with previously stubborn chronic osteomyelitis.

Knowledge of the pharmacology of these drugs is extremely helpful. For example, in the presence of staphylococcal enterocolitis or empyema of the gallbladder, erythromycin (Ilotycin, Erythrocin, Pediamycin) is particularly useful because it is excreted in large amounts into the gut through the biliary tree and is excreted in that area in larger amounts than is the propionyl ester (Ilosone) or its derivatives. On the other hand, the propionyl ester of erythromycin (Ilosone) provides higher blood and tissue levels elsewhere in the body. Similarly, in urinary tract infection, it is important to be aware that streptomycin, kanamycin, neomycin, and gentamicin are more active in an alkaline medium, whereas the tetracyclines are generally more effective in an acid medium. Gentamicin was found to be 100 times more active *in vitro* at pH 8.5 than at pH 5 against most strains of gram-negative bacilli. Erythromycin is also more potent in alkaline urine against gram-negative organisms and against enterococci.

The therapy of choice for infections depends more upon the nature of the microorganism involved than upon the area of the body affected. Nevertheless, it is still important to determine the site of the infection because, in the first place, the site gives us a lead as to what the most probable causative organism is likely to be and, in the second place, the tissue in which the infection resides influences, to some extent, the choice of drug. The reason for this is that some drugs concentrate better in certain tissues than do others.

Once the clinical diagnosis has been made and the site of the infection is determined, a tentative working etiologic diagnosis can often be made before there has been time for the bacteriologist to report on the cultures. If the infection is postoperative or nosocomial, it may be helpful to know what other infections may have occurred in recent days in the same hospital or area. Whenever possible, a smear stained with Gram stain should be examined. By utilizing such information which is available without undue delay, the physician may save many vital hours (Table 16–1).

Table 16–1
Tentative Choice of Antimicrobial Agent in Common Infections

Infection	Antimicrobial Agent
Aerobacter (Enterobacter) (variable)	Gentamicin Kanamycin Polymyxin
Achromobacter (*Alcaligenes faecalis*) (variable)	Polymyxin Kanamycin Tetracycline Chloramphenicol
Actinomyces	Penicillin Tetracycline Erythromycin Chlorlincomycin Chloramphenicol
Bacterioides fragilis	Chloramphenicol Chlorlincomycin Erythromycin Tetracycline Vancomycin
Bacterioides melaninogenicus (*nigrescens*) *Sphaerophorus*	Penicillin Chlorlincomycin Tetracycline Chloramphenicol
Brucella	Tetracycline ± Streptomycin Erythromycin Chloramphenicol Kanamycin
Clostridium perfringens (*welchii*)	Penicillin Tetracycline Chloramphenicol
Clostridium tetani	(Antitoxin) Penicillin Erythromycin
Coccidioidomycosis (if very ill or susceptible to dissemination)	Amphotericin B
Diphtheria (*Corynebacterium diphtheriae*)	(Antitoxin) Penicillin Erythromycin Cephalothin Chlorlincomycin

Table 16–1 (continued)

Infection	Antimicrobial Agent
Escherichia coli	Kanamycin Gentamicin Ampicillin Cephalothin Tetracycline Chloramphenicol Polymyxin
Fusobacterium (Vincent's fusospirochaeta)	Penicillin Chlorlincomycin Tetracycline Erythromycin
Gonococcus (*Neisseria gonorrhoeae*)	Penicillin Tetracycline Spectinomycin Erythromycin
Hemophilus influenzae	Ampicillin Chloramphenicol ± Streptomycin Tetracycline Streptomycin
Histoplasmosis (*Histoplasma capsulatum*)	Sulfonamide (primary lesions only) Amphotericin B (systemic disease)
Klebsiella (*Klebsiella pneumoniae*) (variable)	Cephalothin Kanamycin Gentamicin Chloramphenicol Tetracycline
Listeria monocytogenes	Tetracycline Ampicillin Penicillin Erythromycin
Meningococcus (*Neisseria meningitidis*)	Penicillin Ampicillin Chloramphenicol Erythromycin Tetracycline Sulfadiazine
Moniliasis (*Candida albicans*)	Amphotericin B Nystatin
Mycobacterium unclassified (atypical)	Ethambutol Ethionamide Kanamycin Isoniazid PAS Streptomycin

Table 16–1 (continued)

Infection	Antimicrobial Agent
Mycobacterium tuberculosis	Isoniazid Rifampin Ethambutol Streptomycin PAS Ethionamide
Nocardia	Sulfonamide Chlorlincomycin Erythromycin Amphotericin B
Pasteurella (*pestis* or *tularensis*)	Streptomycin + Tetracycline or + Chloramphenicol
Pneumococcus	Penicillin Cephalothin Erythromycin Chlorlincomycin
Pertussis (*Bordetella pertussis*)	Ampicillin Tetracycline

Proteus (indole-positive)
   Proteus morgani
Proteus rettgeri
   Proteus vulgaris
	Kanamycin
	Gentamicin
	Cephalothin
	Nitrofurantoin (renal)
	Tetracycline
	Chloramphenicol

Proteus (indole-negative) *Proteus mirabilis*	Ampicillin Penicillin Cephalothin Kanamycin Gentamicin Tetracycline Chloramphenicol Nitrofurantoin (renal) Nalidixic acid (renal)

Pseudomonas aeruginosa
   (*Bacillus pyocyaneus*)
   (variable)
	Gentamicin
	Polymyxin
	Carbenicillin
	Oxytetracycline

Salmonella (not typhosa)	Ampicillin Chloramphenicol Tetracycline Cephalothin
Salmonella typhosa	Chloramphenicol Ampicillin

Table 16–1 (continued)

Infection	Antimicrobial Agent
Serratia marcescens (variable)	Gentamicin Kanamycin Chloramphenicol
Shigella	Sulfonamide Ampicillin Tetracycline Cephalothin Chloramphenicol
Staphylococcus aureus (*Micrococcus pyogenes*)	Penicillin (if sensitive) Methicillin, oxacillin, cloxacillin, dicloxacillin or nafcillin (if penicillin-resistant) Penicillin + Methicillin Cephalothin Chlorlincomycin Vancomycin
Streptococci, anaerobic, microaerophilic	Penicillin Chlorlincomycin Erythromycin Chloramphenicol Vancomycin
Streptococcus, beta-hemolytic (*pyogenes*) Group A	Penicillin Cephalothin Erythromycin Chlorlincomycin
Streptococcus faecalis (Enterococci)	Ampicillin ± Streptomycin Penicillin + Streptomycin Chloramphenicol Penicillin + Kanamycin Vancomycin Tetracycline (for *S. liquifaciens*)
Streptococcus viridans	Penicillin Vancomycin Cephalothin Chlorlincomycin
Syphilis (*Treponema pallidum*, *Spirochaeta pallida*)	Penicillin Erythromycin Tetracycline

A culture, taken ideally before any drug is started, may be the next step in determining whether the drug or drugs first selected should be continued. The result of the culture, however, should be generally of less importance than is the clinical response. By the time the report of a culture becomes available, clinical response can often have been estimated. If the clinical response has been good, treatment can often be continued as initiated regardless of the results of the culture. However, if the clinical response has not been satisfactory, the culture can help the clinician avoid another blind guess and can help make the difference between final success or failure.

In addition to the culture, sensitivity tests are valuable, especially in serious infections due to organisms such as Proteus, whose species vary greatly in susceptibility to the different agents. If the patient has not responded to initial therapy, information obtained from the sensitivity tests may prove helpful in the choice of more effective therapy. On the other hand, if the response is favorable, the initial therapy may usually be continued even though the report on sensitivity suggests that the drug used appears to be among the least effective or, *in vitro,* was even without effect. In such cases one should generally be guided by the clinical response rather than the laboratory report. Less often, the patient appears to be clinically better, but the reasons for this are clearly unrelated to the antibiotic given. Under such circumstances (from the nature of the identified organisms), it can sometimes be anticipated that deterioration of the patient may be expected. The culture, and possibly the sensitivity tests, will guide the physician to new therapy. An example of such a situation is the patient with an abscess and septicemia who may seem better clinically after drainage and 24 hours of I.V. methicillin. The patient may seem to be better for a variety of reasons such as the drainage, bed rest, improved fluid, and electrolyte balance. However, the report reveals a pure culture of *E. coli* from the blood and the abscess. It is resistant to methicillin. It would seem prudent, in spite of the improved condition of the patient, to change to an antibiotic which is likely to be more effective.

The bases for choice among the antimicrobial agents are, except for the newborn, basically the same for infants and children as they are for adults. It must be remembered, however, that there are differences in the causative agents of disease in different age periods and that this important factor must be considered. The clinician must make a presumptive etiologic diagnosis based upon probability and must begin therapy with the most promising drug or drugs. One cannot, at present, hope to treat for every possibly causative organism, and the use of too many drugs may do more harm than good.

In the newborn, most sepsis is due either to *E. coli* or to the staphylococcus. Bacterial pneumonia in children under 1 year of age is today most often due to the staphylococcus. Most osteomyelitis also is due to the staphylococcus (although in sickle cell disease, osteomyelitis is often due to salmonella). An otitis media which has not responded to an adequate dosage of penicillin, sulfonamide, or tetracycline is likely to be due to a resistant staphylococcus or to pseudomonas. A severe throat infection which has not responded to penicillin is not likely to be due to a Group A beta-hemolytic streptococcus (which might lead to rheumatic fever or acute glomerulone-phritis). One must search for another cause and, of course, different therapy. In various situations in which, wisely or not, prophylactic drugs have been used and during which time fever has appeared, it is unlikely that the superimposed infection is one which will respond to the usual doses of those drugs which have already been given. Super-imposed infections are often difficult to treat, because, unfortunately, they tend to be caused by resistant staphylococci or by such organisms as Pseudomonas, Proteus, or Monilia.

Persistent fever following dental extractions and not due to local causes suggests bacterial endocarditis. However, fungal disease, es-pecially actinomycosis, nocardiosis, and cryptococcosis, may also follow dental extraction. Patients with fever who have a local lesion and regional lymphadenopathy may have cat scratch disease, rickettsial-pox, tuberculosis, anthrax, tularemia, or plague. Persistent fever fol-lowing cardiac operation suggests endocarditis, most commonly due to *Staphylococcus aureus,* Pseudomonas, or Candida. Peripheral gan-grene during the course of fever suggests pneumococcal, meningo-coccal or pseudomonas septicemia, endocarditis, cholera, or Rocky Mountain spotted fever. In the course of tetracycline therapy, the most likely superinfections are due to *Staphylococcus aureus, Strepto-coccus hemolyticus,* Monilia, Pseudomonas, or Enterococci.

The best judgment depends upon adequate evaluation of the total situation. This includes a tentative or final etiologic diagnosis, knowl-edge of the tissue affected, and pharmacology of the drug. This under-standing enables one to give a large enough amount of the drug to which the causative microorganisms are susceptible, by the proper route, as early as possible and to continue such treatment for an ade-quate time to ensure eradication of the infection.

A single bactericidal agent is generally preferable to a single bacteriostatic one. A well-chosen narrow-spectrum antibiotic is more desirable than a less specific broad-spectrum antibiotic.

Antibiotic combinations should be reserved for mixed infections, for delaying the emergence of resistant strains, or for cases in which the evidence is substantial that combined therapy will be better than either agent of a pair. Combinations are also justified in an acute in-fection when temporary cover is necessary while awaiting bacterio-logic diagnosis, or when laboratory investigations fail to isolate a pathogenic organism and the etiologic agent remains obscure. Selec-tion and wise use of combinations are important, but these should not be used as short cuts or as devices to avoid responsibility for establish-ing an accurate diagnosis and initiating specifically directed antibiotic therapy.

The usefulness of a combination of drugs may be estimated by testing the antibacterial effect of the patient's serum against the spe-cific infecting organism. In very serious infections, it should be pos-sible to dilute the patient's serum 16 or more times and obtain a bactericidal effect against the infecting organism. Unless one can obtain this effect with a dilution of at least four times, a favorable clinical response may not result.

Use of commercially prepared mixtures should be avoided as much as possible. With these, inadequate amounts of the effective drug are often used, the fixed ratios are rarely likely to be appropriate even if the individual components are, and some mixtures include inferior drugs. Claim for synergism can be made only for a specific strain of a bacterium, and none of the available combinations has been proved to be more effective than the best of the individual components. Fortunately, many of these have been removed from the market.

There is some clinical, as well as theoretical, evidence and there are also laboratory data which suggest that, on occasion, bacteriostatic agents, such as tetracycline, may reduce the effectiveness of bactericidal agents, such as penicillin. Mixtures tend to increase the development of sensitivity by the patient, increase the incidence of side effects and confuse the clinical picture and the management. Furthermore, their use unfortunately often leads to a false sense of security, to the development of resistant infections or superinfections, and to delay in efforts toward a specific diagnosis.

The goal should be the proper dose for the correct length of time. Sometimes information about exact dosage is lacking. The tetracyclines tend to accumulate in the body if the dose is only a little higher than that recommended. The toxicity of polymyxin B given intramuscularly is closely related to larger doses. It seems to be minimized, for example, by giving smaller doses at shorter intervals of time. On the other hand, when penicillin is given far in excess of that needed for therapeutic effect, freedom from toxicity is remarkable. This may be due to the fact that penicillin does not readily pass through the wall of human cells, whereas it enters susceptible bacterial cell walls; or it may be due to inactivation of the penicillin within the human cell. The sodium or potassium content of a penicillin compound, on the other hand, may limit the total amount which can safely be given within a stated period of time. Convulsions and central nervous system complications have been related especially to prolonged intravenous drip of high doses of penicillin, such as 40 million units per day or more, in the adult with reduced renal function. There is some suggestion that when such high doses are being given, "push" doses may be preferred to continuous drip. On the other hand, very high doses given over a short period of time can be fatal. One authority estimates that 20 million units given in less than five minutes may kill two out of three human adults.

Antimicrobial agents may fail to give expected favorable results:

1. When they are used to treat undiagnosed fever or distress, e.g. connective tissue disease, malignancy, drug fever, infectious mononucleosis;

2. When they are used to treat culture reports rather than patients, or when there is overdependence on sensitivity tests;

3. When there is poor choice of drug or poor choice of route, inadequate or improper dosage, improper intervals between doses, or the mixing of interfering drugs, such as kanamycin with methicillin in the same syringe or giving tetracycline with aluminum hydroxide;

4. When there is failure to obtain adequate concentration at the site of infection, especially when circulation is poor or in a well walled-off abscess, chronic leg ulcer, fibrotic lesion or cavity, malignancy or foreign body;

5. When there is delay in starting proper treatment;

6. When insufficient attention is given to host resistance as through control of hematologic status, diabetes, fluid and electrolyte balance, shock, agammaglobulinemia, and so forth;

7. In the presence of a mixed infection;

8. When there is failure to recognize need for surgical drainage or debridement;

9. When there is lack of judgment in considering risk to the patient from the drug as against the seriousness of the disease;

10. When the same therapy is continued in an acute infection, (a) in spite of failure to respond after three to four days of adequate dosage, (b) in the presence of recurrence of fever, or (c) when the illness recurs after improvement had clearly begun and while the patient is still receiving the same drug;

11. When there is lack of frequent reevaluation of patients receiving such therapy and consideration is not given to the fact that new, persistent, or recurrent disease may be easily masked, e.g., mastoiditis, appendicitis, or even meningitis, something which occurs especially in patients receiving either steroids or antibiotics;

12. When fever is due to failure to lose body heat, as in extensive skin disease, dysautonomia, congenital absence of sweat glands, ichthyosis, or eczematoid dermatitis;

13. In the mild elevations of temperature that may accompany congestive heart failure and which may be due to poor heat dissipation because of decreased cardiac output, decreased cutaneous blood flow, the insulating effect of edema or increased heat production secondary to increased muscular activity associated with dyspnea. Fever may result from poor heat loss due to atropine or antihistamines or from increased muscular activity, as in tetanus. It is dangerous to consider these possibilities unless such conditions as the following have been excluded: endocarditis, rheumatic fever, thromboembolic disease, myocardial infarction or myocardial infection, and urinary tract infection.

There are real hazards as well as benefits in the use of the antibiotics. Although in general, untoward effects are less common in children than in adults, they are so frequent that these must always be kept in mind. Their incidence can be reduced by not giving the drugs for minor ailments, by avoiding local application of systemically useful ones, by avoiding depot types unless needed, by giving preference to the oral route whenever feasible, and by avoiding simultaneous administration of other possible antigens. The first point probably is the most important, i.e. to avoid giving the drugs when they are not necessary. Much of the sensitivity to antibiotics is avoidable. Most of the antibiotics used are wasted. Between 20 and 50 tons of penicillin are sold in this country each year. It is estimated that one out of every four people in the United States received penicillin in one year and that 90 percent was wasted. Fortunately, not more than 25 out of every 10,000,000 penicillin injections leads to serious consequences. Of these, however, three may be fatal.

After an injection of penicillin, it has been estimated that some reaction may be expected in 2.5 percent of children, in 5 percent of nonallergic adults, and in 15 percent of persons with an allergic diathesis. The risk with oral administration is less, estimated as about 0.2 percent. Reaction rates are said to be increasing by 1 percent each year, possibly because of prior sensitizing doses of penicillin. Reactions, however, also occur in persons not known to have received penicillin previously.

There is as yet no readily available, reliable, and safe test to enable one to anticipate the most dangerous kind of penicillin reaction, anaphylaxis. A history of any allergy should be of some warning. Once a patient has had a reaction to one form of penicillin, it should be assumed that he is just as likely to have a reaction to any of the other derivatives of penicillin. Especially when allergy is suspected, it is wise to inject the drug into the arm at a level low enough so a tourniquet may be applied if a severe reaction ensues. For example, with a syringe prepared with 1 cc of 1:1000 epinephrine on hand, along with a tourniquet to block absorption if anaphylaxis should occur, one might inject 10 units of penicillin G intradermally into the forearm of such a person. If no reaction ensues, one can at 30-minute intervals, proceed with 100 units subcutaneously low in the triceps area, then 1000 units subcutaneously low in the triceps area, then 10,000 units intramuscularly low in the triceps area, and following that, 100,000 units intramuscularly low in the triceps area. At such a time, it is incumbent on the physician to be prepared to meet any emergency. In addition to the tourniquet and epinephrine, sterile syringes should be available as well as an antihistaminic for parenteral use and, if possible, oxygen. Should a reaction occur, the epinephrine and antihistaminic should be given intravenously, the airway should be kept open, and oxygen administered. These immediate measures should be followed by intravenous administration of hydrocortisone or by intramuscular or oral administration of cortisone.

Most antibacterial agents are derived from molds, and there may be a cross allergy between them. This may explain the reactions observed in some individuals with athlete's foot or those who are allergic to moldy basements, bread molds (beer or wine), and so forth.

Some so-called anaphylactic reactions may be due to accidental intravenous injection of the commonly used aqueous suspension of procaine penicillin. Withdrawal of the syringe plunger to avoid intravenous injection is thus essential. It is fortunate that for patients known to be allergic to penicillin, cephalothin, which is a distinctly different molecule, may often be effectively and safely substituted. It should be appreciated, however, that a patient allergic to penicillin is an "allergic patient" and therefore may react badly to any drug, including, of course, cephalothin.

Persistence, and often recurrence, of fever during therapy may be due to the drug itself or to superinfection occurring as a result of the antibiotic. This calls for reevaluation of the patient, not merely continuation of the therapy or increasing the dosage.

Toxicity due to drugs such as chloramphenicol is well known. Chloramphenicol, the sulfonamides, novobiocin, and nitrofurantoin (Furadantin) should be avoided whenever possible in the newborn.

Severe neuritis in which sensory losses or disabling motor paralyses followed intramuscular injection of penicillin, streptomycin, or tetracycline has been described in infants and in adults. In some cases, the disabilities persist for months, and in a few seem permanent. The sciatic nerve has been involved most frequently after intragluteal injections, though the deltoid region was affected in some. The immediate onset of symptoms in some instances suggests a more or less mechanical injury or perhaps intraneural injection rather than intramuscular. In others, notably after injection of penicillin, the symptoms appear only after several days, leading one to believe that the effect may be related to the known toxicity of penicillin for nerve tissue. The complication is of infrequent occurrence, but the consequences may be disabling. Because of this, injection in the anterior outer aspect of the thigh has been suggested, especially in infants and young children.

There is often a lag between discovery and application. There appears to be a similar lag between application and adequate appreciation of toxicity. The story of chloramphenicol in this regard is one which most can recall. The tetracyclines were once considered to be among the safest drugs. Yet now we know that they can cause sudden death with hepatic necrosis if given intravenously to patients with renal impairment. Also they can cause unattractive brown staining and hypoplasia of teeth during the formative stages of tooth development; retardation of growth in low–birth weight infants; when degraded, as may occur through aging, a reversible Fanconi-like syndrome (nausea, vomiting, acidosis, proteinuria, glycosuria and gross amino-aciduria); photosensitivity, especially with demethylchlortetracycline; and anaphylactoid reaction. Even the oral use of poorly absorbed agents may result in untoward effects. For example, the oral use of agents of the desoxystreptamine group (neomycin, kanamycin, gentamicin, paromomycin) may cause a malabsorption syndrome, which fortunately is temporary.

Antibiotic prophylaxis against the bacterial world at large is not practical, and, in fact, may induce more infection than it aims to prevent. In one study, 130 patients with measles received antibiotics prophylactically. About 30 percent developed superimposed bacterial infections, whereas superimposed infection occurred in only about 15 percent of 298 patients who did not receive antibiotics. Of 165 patients with bulbar poliomyelitis, superimposed infection developed in only 16 percent not receiving drugs, but they did develop in 53 percent of 63 similar patients given so-called prophylactic antibiotics. Such "prophylaxis" does little more than ensure that the superimposed infections will be resistant to the antibiotics used. One survey showed that two-thirds of all patients admitted, exclusive of the obstetric and newborn services, received antibiotics, most of which were given "prophylactically" before operations. In another study, bacterial complications in clean operations were five times as high in "prophylactically" treated patients as in patients not given antibiotics "prophylactically." Similar results have been reported in other studies of the "prophylactic" use of antibiotics in surgical cases.

There are a few situations in which prophylactic antibiotics are effective. Some legitimate indications for prophylaxis are the use of penicillin against Group A beta-hemolytic streptococci, sulfadiazine against meningococcus (penicillin, if a sulfonamide-resistant strain), penicillin against pneumococcus and streptococcus, particularly in the presence of agammaglobulinemia, prevention of endocarditis in susceptible patients having dental work, penicillin against gonococcus and *Treponema pallidum,* selected drugs before surgical treatment for infected areas, such as tuberculous lung, sulfonamides or other agents for shigella dysentery in a closed population, or neomycin in an outbreak of diarrhea due to type specific *E. coli* in a nursery.

Although used commonly in the following situations, the value of such prophylaxis is doubtful: women with prolonged and difficult labor, surgery involving division of a bronchus, bowel sterilization before bowel surgery, and contaminated wounds of violence.

In the following situations in which "prophylaxis" is often used, it is not only valueless, but also sometimes dangerous: virus infections, routine preoperative or postoperative care, comatose patients, bulbar poliomyelitis, tracheotomized patients, very ill patients with noninfectious diseases and patients receiving steroids (except to prevent a specific disease in a high-risk group, such as in an outbreak of streptococcal illness in a community, or in patients with tuberculosis or sarcoidosis).

The value of cephalothin, cephaloridine, cephaloglycin, and cephalexin was reviewed recently.[1]

Carbenicillin [2] is one of the newer derivatives of penicillin. In large doses, it has been found effective in some cases of Pseudomonas, Proteus, and enterococcal infections. Resistance tends to develop during therapy. It is often synergistic and is used effectively together with gentamicin, especially in severe Pseudomonas infections.

A new antibiotic, rifampin, may exceed isoniazid and streptomycin in efficacy, rapid action, and low toxicity. It can be given orally and is of special importance when the organisms are resistant to the other agents.

Chlorlincomycin, a derivative of lincomycin, is better absorbed, produces high blood levels, and appears to be less toxic. These agents have been found to be effective against some anaerobic pathogen and also against norodia. Lincomycin was reported to control actinomycoses in four patients allergic to penicillin.

Most postsurgical infections are abscesses and thus require drainage or excision of necrotic tissue; this is often more useful and necessary than antibiotics. However, a Gram stain and culture should *always* be done. Sometimes the abscess is in an obscure area such as subdiaphragmatic, subhepatic, or retroperitoneal. The most common operation to precede these is an appendectomy for a perforated appendix.

In postoperative infections, the time of onset of the fever may be a helpful clue. A fever which appears first within 48 hours after surgery suggests bronchopulmonary infections; one that starts three to five days after surgery suggests a urinary tract infection. Fever due to wound infections appear at variable times after surgery, but most often between the fourth and ninth postoperative day.

Since "prophylactic" use of antibiotics has been used much less often, there has been a concomitant drop in frequent serious postoperative endocolitis due to staphylococci. On the other hand, serious infections due to staphylococcus and to Monilia are now seen with long-term use of centrally placed catheters for nutritional supplementation.

Table 16-1 lists "Tentative Choice of Antimicrobial Agent in Common Infections." It was assumed that if the infection is serious and warrants the most effective agents that a parenteral route is required. Obviously, in less serious infection, an agent lower on the list, but which can be given orally might be preferred. Some drugs are in the list primarily because the concentrations obtained in the urine are so high that they are effective in urinary tract infections even though less effective elsewhere. Whenever polymyxin is listed, colistimethrate could be substituted unless the drug were to be given intravenously or

Table 16–2

Antimicrobial Agents: Dosages, Routes of Administration, and Preparation Procedures for Parenteral Therapy*

Drug	Daily Dosage Schedule for Premature and Fullterm Infants		
	Oral	Intramuscular	Intravenous
Bacitracin		900†–1000‡units/kg in 2–3 doses	
Carbenicillin§		(same as iv)	100 mg/kg 1st dose then 225 mg/kg in 3 doses‡ or 300 mg/kg in 4 doses‡
Chloramphenicol‖	25†–50‡‡ mg/kg in 4 doses	25†–50‡‡ mg/kg in 3–4 doses**	15†–25‡ mg/kg in 3–4 doses
Colistin (Coly-Mycin)	3–8 mg/kg in 3–4 doses	1.5–5.0 mg/kg in 2–4 doses	
Erythromycin	20–40 mg/kg in 4 doses	10 mg/kg in 2 doses	10–20 mg/kg in 2–4 doses
Gentamicin§		3–6 mg/kg in 2–3 doses	
Kanamycin	50 mg/kg in 4 doses	15 mg/kg in 2–3 doses	
Neomycin	50 mg/kg in 4 doses	4 mg/kg in 2–4 doses	
Nystatin	200,000–400,000 units in 4 doses		
Penicillin G††	50,000 units/kg in 4 doses	20,000–50,000 units/kg in 2–4 doses	20,000–50,000 units/kg in 2–4 doses

Penicillin derivatives:			
ampicillin	50–100 mg/kg in 3–4 doses	100–200 mg/kg in 3–4 doses	50–200 mg/kg in 3–4 doses
methicillin		100–200 mg/kg in 3–4 doses	50–200 mg/kg in 3–4 doses
nafcillin oxacillin	25–50 mg/kg in 4 doses	20–50 mg/kg in 3–4 doses	
Polymyxin B	10–15 mg/kg in 4 doses	1.5†–2.5‡ mg/kg in 2–4 doses	
Streptomycin		10–40 mg/kg in 2–3 doses	
Tetracyclines‖	20–40 mg/kg in 4 doses	6–12 mg/kg in 2 doses	6–12 mg/kg in 2 doses (1 mg/ml)

* Adapted from article by Levin, H.S. and Kagan, B.M., in B.M. Kagan, *Antimicrobial Therapy*, W.B. Saunders Co., Philadelphia, 1970, and published with the permission of the authors and publisher.

† Premature

‡ Fullterm

§ Dosage not well established nor approved by FDA

‖ Avoid if possible

Some authorities advise using 25 mg/kg for fullterm infants

** Intramuscular use not currently advised

†† Potassium penicillin G is preferred to procaine penicillin G in the newborn

‡‡ Dose may be doubled in severe infections

§§ Intracavitary refers to intraperitoneal, intraarticular, or intrapleural administration

‖‖ Not to be used in conjunction with anesthetic and muscle-relaxing agents

Oral penicillins are best absorbed when given 1 to 2 hours before meals

*** Some authorities have advised 3 to 4 mg/kg in life-threatening situations

††† First dose should be doubled

Table 16-2 (continued)

Antimicrobial Agents: Dosages, Routes of Administration, and Preparation Procedures for Parenteral Therapy

Daily Dosage and Routes of Administration of Antimicrobial Agents

Drug	Oral	Intramuscular	Intravenous	Other Methods of Administration	Adult or Maximum Dose
Amphotericin B (Fungizone)			1.0 mg/kg (0.1 mg/ml); Begin with smaller dose	*Intrathecal:* 0.5–0.75 mg every 1 to 2 days (0.3 mg/ml in 5% dextrose water)	1.5 mg/kg/day
Bacitracin		1000 units/kg in 3–4 doses (10,000 units/ml in 2% procaine)		*Intrathecal:* 500–10,000 units/day (1000 units/ml) *Intraventricular (CNS):* 250–10,000 units/day (1000 units/ml) *Aerosol:* 20,000–50,000 units/ml *Intracavitary:* ‖ 1000 units/ml	*Intramuscular:* *Child:* 50,000 units/day *Adult:* 100,000 units/day
Cephalexin (Keflex)	25–50 mg/kg in 4 doses				1–4 gm in 4 doses
Cephalothin (Keflin)		40–80 mg/kg in 4 doses	40–80 mg/kg in 4–6 doses	*For peritoneal dialysis:* 6 mg/100 m¹	12.0 gm/day

Drug				
Cephaloridine (Loridine)	30–50 mg/kg in 4 doses	30–50 mg/kg|| in 3–4 doses	30–50 mg/kg|| in 3–4 doses	4.0 gm/day
Chloramphenicol (Chloromycetin succinate)	50–100 mg/kg in 4 doses	50–100 mg/kg in 3–4 doses (25–40% solution)**	50–100 mg/kg in 3–4 doses (10% solution)	*Child:* 3.0 gm/day *Adult:* 4.0 gm/day
Colistin (Coly-Mycin)	6–8 mg/kg in 3 doses (5 mg/ml)	1.5–5.0 mg/kg in 2–4 doses		300 mg/day
Cycloserine (Oxamycin) (Seromycin)	10 mg/kg in 2–3 doses			500 mg/day first 2 weeks (Drug may be cautiously increased to 1.0 gm/day but should be used with pyridoxine to minimize neurotoxicity.)
Erythromycins: Erythromycin salts (Erythrocin) (Ilotycin) (Pediamycin)	30–50 mg/kg in 4 doses	10–20 mg/kg in 3–4 doses	40–50 mg/kg in 4 doses	*Oral:* 2.0 gm/day *IM:* 600 mg/day *IV:* 2.0–4.0 gm/day
Erythromycin estolate (Ilosone)	25–40 mg/kg in 4 doses			2.0 gm/day
Gentamicin sulfate (Garamycin)		3–5 mg/kg in 3 doses (7 to 10 days)	3–5 mg/kg in 3 doses Conc. should not exceed 1 mg/ml. Each dose should infuse over 1–2 hours.	5 mg/kg/day

Table 16–2 (continued)

Antimicrobial Agents:: Dosages, Routes of Administration, and Preparation Procedures for Parenteral Therapy

Daily Dosage and Routes of Administration of Antimicrobial Agents

Drug	Oral	Intramuscular	Intravenous	Other Methods of Administration	Adult or Maximum Dose
Griseofulvin (Fulvicin) (Grifulvin) (Griseofulvin-Ayerst)	20 mg/kg in 2–3 doses				1.0 gm/day
Griseofulvin microcrystal-line (Fulvicin-U/F) (Grifulvin V) (Grisactin)	10 mg/kg in 2–3 doses				0.5 gm/day
Isoniazid (Nydrazid)	15–20 mg/kg in 3 doses	10–20 mg/kg in 2 doses			*Child:* 500–600 mg/ day *Adult:* 7 mg/kg/day
Kanamycin (Kantrex)	50 mg/kg in 4 doses	15 mg/kg in 2–4 doses	15–30 mg/kg in 2–3 doses (2.5 mg/ml)	*Intrathecal:* 1 mg/day for 3 days (newborn period only) *Aerosol:* 2 ml. q.i.d. (125 mg/ml) *Intracavitary:*§§ (2.5 mg/ml)	*Oral:* 4.0–6.0 gm/day *IM:*} *IV:*} 1.0–1.5 gm/day *Aerosol:* 1.0 gm/day *Peritoneum:*|||| 0.5 gm/day

Drug				
Lincomycin (Lincocin)	30–50 mg/kg in 3–4 doses	10–20 mg/kg in 2–3 doses	10–20 mg/kg in 2–3 doses	Oral: 2.0 gm/day IM:} IV:} 1.2–1.8 gm/day
Clindamycin	8–20 mg/kg in 3–4 doses			Oral: 1.8 gm/day
Methenamine mandelate (Mandelamine)	<5 yrs: 1.0 gm in 4 doses; >5 yrs: 2.0 gm in 4 doses			4.0 gm/day
Nalidixic acid (NegGram)	50 mg/kg in 4 doses			4.0 gm/day
Neomycin (Mycifradin)	50–100 mg/kg in 4 doses	7.5–15 mg/kg in 4 doses (limit to 10 days)	Intraperitoneal:‖‖‖ 20 mg/kg (5–10 mg/ml) Aerosol: 2 ml q.i.d. (50 mg/ml)	Oral: 4–6 gm/day IM: 1.0 gm/day Peritoneal: 1.0 gm/day
Nitrofurantoin (Furadantin)	5–7 mg/kg in 4 doses		6.0 mg/kg in 2 doses	Oral: 400 mg/day IV: 360 mg/day
Novobiocin (Albamycin) (Cathomycin)	20–45 mg/kg in 4 doses	15–40 mg/kg in 2–3 doses	15–40 mg/kg in 2–3 doses	Oral: 2.0 gm/day IM:} IV:} 1.0 gm/day
Nystatin (Mycostatin)	<2 yrs: 0.4–0.8 million units; >2 yrs: 1–2 million units in 3–4 doses			3.0 million units/day

Table 16-2 (continued)

Antimicrobial Agents: Dosages, Routes of Administration, and Preparation Procedures for Parenteral Therapy

Daily Dosage and Routes of Administration of Antimicrobial Agents

Drug	Oral	Intramuscular	Intravenous	Other Methods of Administration	Adult or Maximum Dose
Oleandomycin (Triacetyl [TAO]—oral only) (Cyclamycin —oral only)	<8 yrs: 30 mg/kg in 4 doses >8 yrs: 0.5–1.0 gm/ day in 4 doses	30–50 mg/kg in 3–4 doses	30–50 mg/kg in 3–4 doses		Oral: Child: 1.0 gm/day Adult: 2.0 gm/day IM:} 800 mg/day IV:} 3.0 gm/day
Para–amino-sali-cylic acid (Pamisyl) (Para-Pas) (Parasal)	250–300 mg/kg in 3–4 doses				12.0 gm/day
Paromomycin (Humatin)	25–60 mg/kg in 4 doses				4.0 gm/day
Penicillin G Potassium or Sodium	0.5–2.0 million units in 4–6 doses ½–1 hr. a.c.	20,000–50,000 units/ kg in 4–6 doses	20,000–500,000 units/ kg in 4–6 doses	Aerosol: 2 ml q.i.d. (50,000 units/ml) Intracavitary:§§ 10,000–20,000 units/ml	20–60 million units/ day (in selected cases, 100 million units/day)
Procaine		100,000–600,000 units/dose in 2–4 doses			

Drug	Dosage
Benzathine (Bicillin) (Permapen) (Duapen)	600,000–1.2 million units single injection q. 15–30 days
Penicillin, phenoxymethyl‡‡ (Compocillin V) (Pen-Vee) (V-Cillin) 1 mg = 1695 units	25,000–50,000 units/kg in 4 doses (25–50 mg/kg in 4 doses)
Penicillin, potassium phenoxymethyl‡‡ (Compocillin-VK) (Pen-Vee K) (V-Cillin K) 1 mg = 1600 units	
Phenethicillin, potassium‡‡ (Darcil) (Maxipen) (Syncillin) 1 mg = 1600 units	3–4 gm/day (6.0 million units/day)

Table 16–2 (continued)

Antimicrobial Agents: Dosages, Routes of Administration, and Preparation Procedures for Parenteral Therapy

Daily Dosage and Routes of Administration of Antimicrobial Agents

Drug	Oral	Intramuscular	Intravenous	Other Methods of Administration	Adult or Maximum Dose
Semisynthetic Penicillins‡‡ Ampicillin (Amcill) (Omnipen) (Penbritin) (Polycillin) (Principen)	50–200 mg/kg in 4 doses	100–300 mg/kg in 4 doses	100–300 mg/kg 4–6 doses		*Oral:* 4.0 gm/day *IM:* ⎱ 8–14 gm/day *IV:* ⎰
Carbenicillin		50–400 mg/kg/day in 4–6 doses	200–500 mg/kg in 4–6 doses or continuous drip		8–40 gm/day
Cloxacillin‡‡ (TegoPen)	50 mg/kg in 4 doses				4–6 gm/day
Dicloxacillin (Dynapen) (Pathocil) (Veracillin)	12.5–50 mg/kg in 4 doses				2–3 gm/day

Drug				
Methicillin (Dimocillin-RT) (Staphcillin)		100–300 mg/kg in 4 doses	100–300 mg/kg in 4–6 doses	12.0 gm/day
Nafcillin‡‡ (Unipen) Oxacillin‡‡ (Prostaphlin) (Resistopen)	50–100 mg/kg in 4 doses	50–100 mg/kg in 4 doses	50–100 mg/kg in 4–6 doses	6.0 gm/day
Polymyxin B (Aerosporin)	10–20 mg/kg in 4 doses	2.5 mg/kg*** in 4–6 doses	2.5 mg/kg*** in 2–3 doses (0.4 mg/ml in 5% dextrose in water for endocarditis) *Intrathecal:* Administer for 3–4 days, then every other day. <2 yrs: 2 mg/day >2 yrs: 5 mg/day (0.5–1.0 mg/ml in NaCl)	*Oral:* 400 mg/day *IM:* } *IV:* } 200 mg/day
Rifampin	10–20 mg/kg/day in one dose			600 mg/day
Streptomycin		20–40 mg/kg in 2–3 doses	*Intrathecal:* 1.0 mg/kg (5 mg/ml) *Aerosol:* 2 ml q.i.d. (150 mg/ml) *Intracavitary:*† 50 mg/ml	*IM:* 2.0 gm/day *Intrathecal:* 20 mg/day

Table 16–2 (continued)

Antimicrobial Agents: Dosages, Routes of Administration, and Preparation Procedures for Parenteral Therapy*

Drug	Daily Dosage and Routes of Administration of Antimicrobial Agents				
	Oral	Intramuscular	Intravenous	Other Methods of Administration	Adult or Maximum Dose
Sulfonamides Sulfadiazine††† Sulfisoxazole††† (Gantrisin) Triple sulfona- mides††† (oral)	120 mg/kg in 4 doses		120 mg/kg in 4 doses (50 mg/ml)	*Subcutaneous:* 120 mg/kg in 2–4 doses (25 mg/ml)	6.0 gm/day
Phthalylsulfathia- zole (Sulfathalidine)	125 mg/kg in 4–6 doses				8.0 gm/day
Succinylsulfa- thiazole (Sulfasuxidine)	250 mg/kg in 4–6 doses				12.0 gm/day
Salicylazosulfa- pyridine (Azulfidine)	75–125 mg/kg in 4–6 doses				*Adults:* 8–12 gm/day *Children:* >7 yrs: 6.0 gm/day 5–7 yrs: 3.0 gm/day

276

Drug				
Tetracyclines				
Tetracycline (Achromycin) (Panmycin) (Polycycline) (Steclin) (Sumycin) (Tetracyn) (Tetrex)	20–40 mg/kg in 4 doses	12 mg/kg in 2 doses	10–15 mg/kg in 2 doses (1.0 mg/ml)	Oral:⎫ IV:⎬ 2.0 gm/day ⎭ IM: 500 mg/day
Chlortetracycline (Aureomycin) Oxytetracycline (Terramycin)	20–40 mg/kg in 4 doses	12 mg/kg in 2 doses	10–20 mg/kg in 2 doses (1.0 mg/ml) Aerosol: (oxytetracycline only): 1 ml b.i.d. (50 mg/ml) in 10% propylene glycol	Oral:⎫ IV:⎬ 2.0 gm/day ⎭ IM: 500 mg/day
Demethylchlortetracycline (Declomycin)	6–12 mg/kg in 2–4 doses			600–900 mg/day
Methacycline (Rondomycin)	6–12 mg/kg in 2–4 doses			600 mg/day
Doxycycline (Vibramycin)	2–4 mg/kg in 2 doses			200 mg/day
Vancomycin (Vancocin)	2–4 gm/day in 4 doses (for adults)	40 mg/kg in 2–4 doses or continuous iv (2.5–5.0 mg/ml)		IV: 4.0 gm first day; 2.0 gm/day thereafter

injected into the spinal fluid, in which case polymyxin (which is free of dibucaine) is preferred. Also, whenever cephalothin is listed, any one of the cephalosporin derivatives could be considered, i.e. cephalothin itself or cephaloridine, cephaloglycin or cephalexin.

The remarkable effectiveness of antimicrobial therapy should not obscure the great importance of host resistance. Even with bactericidal agents, host resistance can be the decisive factor. Measures to augment host resistance should always be considered either instead of or in conjunction with the use of antimicrobial drugs. Before the "antibiotic era," lives were saved from serious infectious diseases by the judicious use of whole blood, plasma or serum, and gamma globulin, and by attention to such essentials as nutritional status, fluid and electrolyte balance and control of diabetes or other coexisting disease states.

REFERENCES

1. E.J. Benner, et al, eds.: Symposium on cephalosporin antibiotics. *Postgrad Med J* 47:Supplement, 1971.
2. Kirby, W.M., ed.: Symposium on carbenicillin: A clinical profile. *J Infect Dis* 122: Supplement, 1970.
3. Kagan, B.M., ed.: *Antimicrobial Therapy.* Philadelphia: W.B. Saunders Co., 1970.

Special Problems

17

Preoperative Hematologic Evaluation and Management

Gerald S. Gilchrist, M.B., B.Ch., D.C.H.

It is considered good medical practice to perform a complete blood count routinely on all patients scheduled for a surgical procedure in a hospital. Similarly, depending on the nature of the surgical procedure and the circumstances, a preoperative laboratory evaluation is often indicated in patients undergoing office procedures. Measurement of the hemoglobin concentration or hematocrit value, leukocyte count, and differential cell count and estimation of platelet number on the routine blood smear provide a minimum in the way of hematologic evaluation. The increasing use of electronic equipment inevitably will lead to the inclusion of the erythrocyte count, red cell indices, and even the absolute platelet count on all reports from the laboratory. These could be useful in some situations. For example, when an unexpected decrease in hemoglobin concentration is found, the automatic availability of indices will allow for earlier definition of the type of anemia and thus expedite diagnosis and treatment. Similarly, a report of decreased platelets on a routine blood smear would inevitably have to be substantiated by an absolute platelet count, so that its routine inclusion would be of help to the physician and would obviate repeated sampling, decrease the attendant discomfort to the patient, and prevent delay in further diagnostic evaluation.

A good medical history is essential and must take into account the patient's age, the presence of underlying disorders which may or may not be directly related to the surgical procedure, and an awareness of the hematologic complications of any underlying disease. The operation may be undertaken to alleviate the underlying condition (for example, when splenectomy is performed for relief of the hemolytic state in hereditary spherocytosis) or it may be for treatment of a complication of the underlying disorder (as in hemophilia complicated by a subdural hematoma).

This chapter will outline an approach to the patient in whom an unexpected hematologic abnormality is detected at the "eleventh" hour by history or routine laboratory studies, review some of the situations in which an operation is indicated for relief of a hematologic disorder, and provide a basis for managing the patient in whom such a disorder is diagnosed.

DISORDERS OF HEMOSTASIS

History

A history of a bleeding tendency should be sought in all patients about to undergo operation. This could be in the form of a questionnaire to be completed by the patient's parents; the completed questionnaire is then reviewed by the responsible physician in order to evaluate the significance of any positive responses. This requires that the physician obtain information on age at onset, sites of hemorrhage, nature of the bleeding episode, precipitating factors, whether or not bruising or bleeding was out of proportion to the traumatic insult, severity of bleeding, what measures were necessary for control of the bleeding (whether transfusion of blood or blood products was required), and whether there was any relationship to the ingestion of drugs. Common sense will dictate whether or not the bleeding was significant, and a detailed chronologic history will allow one to distinguish a lifelong (and therefore probably inherited) disorder from an acquired one. A history of uncomplicated tooth extraction or other operation is invaluable in assessing hemostatic status.

The nature of the bleeding is helpful in determining etiology. Petechial eruptions suggest a defect related to platelets or small blood vessels; hemarthroses are virtually diagnostic of hemophilia. Recurrent nosebleeds which are relatively easily controlled are rarely related to a disorder of hemostasis or coagulation unless associated with other bleeding manifestations.[1] A history of bleeding from the umbilical stump is suggestive of Factor XIII deficiency,[2] whereas the presence or absence of bleeding associated with circumcision cannot be construed as evidence for or against the diagnosis of even severe hemophilia. Baehner and Strauss [3] reviewed the histories of 107 severe hemophiliacs with either Factor VIII or Factor IX deficiency and found that less than 50 percent had had abnormal bleeding at circumcision. On the other hand, depending on technique, age at circumcision, and hemostatic measures, bleeding can occur in apparently normal newborns unrelated to underlying coagulation factor abnormalities.

A family history should be obtained, particularly when one is dealing with a young patient who has not been subjected to the stresses likely to bring to light an abnormal bleeding tendency. Naturally, if there is a history of bleeding in the patient, the family history must be reviewed to assist in diagnosis. This requires questioning about aunts, uncles, and cousins in addition to the immediate family members. In this way, a pattern of sex-linked autosomal recessive transmission can be elucidated and would be suggestive of hemophilia A or B; an autosomal dominant pattern would be consistent with von Willebrand's disease. But it must be stressed that information similar in detail to that obtained from the patient must be sought in assessing the significance of the familial bleeding tendency. Particularly with the sex-linked recessive disorders, a negative family history does not exclude this possibility. As many as 40 percent of hemophiliacs report no family history.[4] This is explained by a high rate of mutation, but it is just as likely to be a reflection of genetic transmission by clinically normal females through a number of generations.

Laboratory Studies

In selecting laboratory studies to determine whether or not the patient has a bleeding tendency, one must take into account the personal and family histories. For example, if the patient is being evaluated purely because the mother's brother has classic hemophilia (Factor VIII deficiency), it would seem unnecessary to perform any tests other than those designed to detect such a deficiency in the patient at risk. On the other hand, when one is not certain of the nature of the suspected defect on the basis of history, one is obligated to arrange for an appropriate set of laboratory investigations. Dependence on normal bleeding and clotting times as evidence of intact hemostasis must be deplored. Even with the Lee and White whole blood coagulation time, many severe hemophiliacs fail to exhibit any abnormality. With the less sensitive and less well controlled capillary tube clotting time, many major defects in coagulation certainly would be missed.[5] Similarly, the Duke bleeding time is often within normal limits in the presence of documented qualitative or quantitative platelet disorders.[5]

Conversely, one cannot justify the use of sophisticated laboratory tests as a routine preoperative procedure in the absence of a reasonable suspicion based on the history or the presence of disease having hemostatic complications. Such an approach results in unnecessary expense for the patient and, unless one orders a complete hemostatic survey, the surgeon is lulled into a false sense of security by isolated normal laboratory values.

Figure 17–1 summarizes the sequence of events which results from damage to small blood vessels. First, platelets adhere to the collagen exposed by damage to the endothelium. Soon thereafter, a platelet plug forms as a result of release of adenosine diphosphate (ADP) from platelets themselves and from erythrocytes in the area. Simultaneously, the coagulation mechanism is triggered through activation of the surface contact factors, Factors XI and XII, resulting in thrombin generation (Figure 17–2). The small amounts of thrombin thus generated cause further platelet aggregation, increase intrinsic thromboplastin generation by activating Factor VIII, and, most importantly, convert fibrinogen to fibrin. This fibrin clot enmeshes the cellular elements, thus consolidating the platelet plug. Thrombin also activates another plasma factor (Factor XIII) which is responsible for stabilizing the fibrin clot by cross-linking the fibrin monomer molecules with covalent bonds.

Lysis of the clot is the physiologic response which occurs after the deposition of fibrin. Plasminogen, a normal constituent of plasma, is deposited with the fibrin, and substances present in the vascular endothelium activate it to plasmin, a proteolytic enzyme capable of digesting fibrin and fibrinogen. Except in rare instances, this fibrinolytic response is localized to the area of fibrin deposition, so there is no effect on the circulating fibrinogen.

Based on the patient's history and a knowledge of the various stages of hemostasis, a relatively simple series of tests will suffice to evaluate the competence of each stage (Table 17–1).

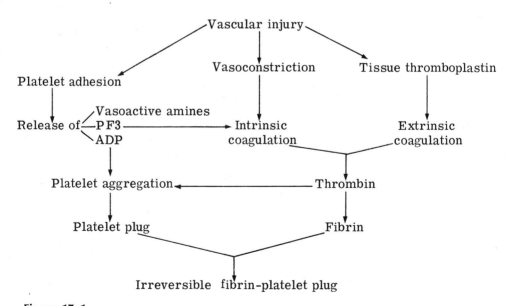

Figure 17–1
Sequence of events resulting from damage to small blood vessels. (Modified from Owen et al [2].)

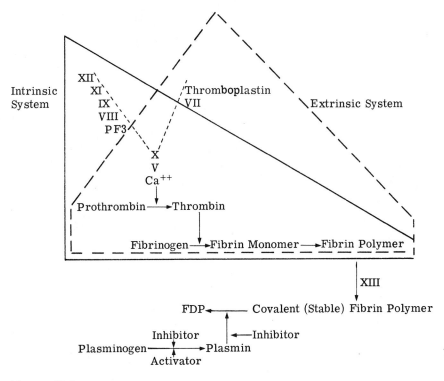

Figure 17–2
Coagulation mechanism, showing intrinsic system (within solid lines), extrinsic system (within broken lines), and steps common to both.

Table 17–1
Tests for Detecting Disorders of Coagulation and Hemostasis*

Inherited disorders
    CBC and platelet count
    Ivy bleeding time (if platelet count >50,000/cu mm)
    Activated partial thromboplastin time
    Quick prothrombin time
    Thrombin time (or screening test for fibrinogen)
    Factor XIII screening test
Acquired disorders
    CBC and platelet count
    Ivy bleeding time (if platelet count >50,000/cu mm)
    Activated partial thromboplastin time
    Quick prothrombin time
    Thrombin time
    Screening test for fibrinogen
    Fibrinolytic profile
    Serum fibrin degradation products

* These procedures can be expected to detect virtually all significant disorders of coagulation and hemostasis. More specific assays of individual coagulation factors and tests of platelet function may be necessary to define the exact nature of the disorder.

Platelet Count

The majority of laboratories report a normal range of 200,000 to 400,000/cu mm, but normal hemostasis can be achieved with as few platelets as 50,000/cu mm. In view of the technical error inherent in platelet counting, for practical purposes a platelet count less than 100,000/cu mm should be considered abnormal and worthy of further study.

Thrombocytopenia may be the result of decreased platelet production, as in leukemia, invasion of bone marrow by tumor, or aplastic anemia. Decreased platelet numbers also may reflect shortened platelet survival in the presence of normal or accelerated production, as in the various immunologic thrombocytopenic purpuras (ITP) complicating viral infections and in lupus erythematosus. Increased utilization of platelets in clot formation, as occurs in localized or disseminated intravascular coagulation, also leads to thrombocytopenia. Redistribution of platelets in an enlarged spleen would be reflected in a decreased whole blood platelet count.

Ivy Bleeding Time

This is a much better test of platelet-vessel interaction than is the Duke method, but it requires standardization. Two recently described modifications of this technique provide reproducible results,[2,6] but the test has not been standardized in infants. This procedure provides the only true test of the first stage of hemostasis. The bleeding time is prolonged in the presence of thrombocytopenia (less than 50,000 to 80,000/cu mm), qualitative platelet defects, and von Willebrand's disease.

It would seem appropriate at this point to stress the effect of drugs on the bleeding time. The ingestion of 300 mg of acetylsalicylic acid (ASA) by an adult can, in sensitive individuals, prolong the bleeding time well into the abnormal range,[6] and other drugs, such as the antihistamines, have a similar effect. The effect of aspirin may last up to a week, thus making it difficult to interpret the prolonged bleeding time in many patients. While aspirin certainly does have a profound effect on in vitro tests of platelet function, only relatively few individuals can be considered to be compromised hemostatically as a result of aspirin ingestion. On the other hand, analysis of blood loss after tonsillectomy and adenoidectomy has revealed a significant increase in patients receiving acetylsalicylic acid.[7] It would seem prudent, therefore, to withhold all compounds containing acetylsalicylic acid for one week preceding elective surgery in order to minimize this risk. Other conditions in which qualitative platelet disorders have been observed include chronic uremia,[8] glycogen storage disease,[9] and hyperbilirubinemia,[10] but it is unusual for serious bleeding to be encountered in affected pediatric patients.

Von Willebrand's disease is characterized by prolonged bleeding time, variable decrease in Factor VIII, decreased platelet retention by glass beads, and an exaggerated Factor VIII increase after infusion of normal or hemophiliac plasma.[11] It is transmitted as an autosomal dominant, and the severity of the bleeding tendency appears to be related in the main to the Factor VIII level.[11] Many patients with von Willebrand's disease, but with normal Factor VIII levels, have undergone major surgery without abnormal bleeding.

Activated Partial Thromboplastin Time (PTT)

This test is a measure of the intrinsic system of coagulation [12] and is sensitive to levels of various procoagulants less than 20–25 percent of normal. Thus, the PTT would be prolonged in the presence of any significant decrease in levels of Factors XII, XI, IX, VIII, X, V, or II (prothrombin) or fibrinogen (Figure 17–2). It would be expected to be normal, however, in many hemophiliac carriers and in patients with von Willebrand's disease in whom levels in the range of 20–30 percent might be present. Since it is generally accepted that a Factor VIII or IX level of 30 percent is necessary to provide hemostasis for major surgery, a specific assay might be indicated in special situations even in the presence of a normal PTT. Because the partial thromboplastin acts as a platelet substitute, this test does not measure the procoagulant activity of platelets; in reality, an isolated deficiency of platelet factor 3 as a basis for a bleeding diathesis is extremely rare. It is of interest that, although Factor XII (Hageman) is essential for coagulation to proceed normally in the test tube, no clinical bleeding has been observed in patients deficient in this factor, even after major operations. This highlights the fact that the laboratory procedures must be used as an adjunct to clinical evaluation and not as a substitute.

The presence of circulating anticoagulants also could prolong the PTT. By its antithrombin action, heparin would have this effect, as would some of the acquired inhibitors such as in systemic lupus erythematosus.

Quick Prothrombin Time

In this test, a measure of the extrinsic clotting system, a normal result is dependent on adequate levels of Factors VII, V, X, and II and fibrinogen.[13] With the exception of Factor VII, all these factors also are required for the PTT (Figure 17–2). Thus, these two tests alone can be used to provide clues to the identity of a missing factor or factors. By modifying the Quick prothrombin time, one can make it a true measure of the vitamin K–dependent factors (Factors VII, X, and II). This is achieved by using a thromboplastin to which has been added adsorbed bovine plasma to provide an excess of Factor V and fibrinogen. In conjunction with the Quick prothrombin time, this modification, which is also known as the "P and P" (prothrombin and proconvertin) test, can provide further diagnostic assistance.

Thrombin Time

When dilute thrombin is added to plasma, the clotting time is dependent on fibrinogen concentration and the presence of heparin-like anticoagulants.[13] Thus, this test is an indirect measurement of clottable fibrinogen concentration. It is a rapid measure of the third stage of coagulation and is independent of the intrinsic and extrinsic systems.

Factor XIII

Since the fibrin-stabilizing action of this factor is not measured by any of the preceding tests, its presence can be evaluated only by testing the solubility of the clot in 5M urea, a relatively simple screening test.[13]

Fibrinolysis

Tests of fibrinolytic activity include the euglobulin lysis time, which is mainly a measure of plasminogen activator.[13] A shortened euglobulin lysis time is indicative of abnormal activation of plasminogen. The use of standardized fibrin plates allows for a more discriminating assessment of the fibrinolytic system components by measuring zones of lysis after incubation of the euglobulin fraction, streptokinase-treated plasma, and whole plasma.[14] Lysis by the latter is evidence of circulating plasmin, a potentially serious situation.

For practical purposes, particularly in pediatric practice, fibrinolysis is virtually always secondary to intravascular coagulation when widespread activation of clotting results in excessive consumption of platelets, fibrinogen, and various labile clotting factors. If the intravascular coagulation is acute and intense enough, circulating plasma is replaced by platelet-poor circulating serum.[15] More often, the body is able to compensate for the increased consumption, and normal or even increased procoagulant levels are found. In this situation, when one is dealing with the effects of thrombin *and* plasmin on fibrinogen and fibrin, it is sometimes possible to distinguish this from primary fibrinolysis by testing for the presence of early products of thrombin action on fibrinogen.[13] This fibrin monomer can be detected by ethanol gelation or addition of protamine sulfate; both of these substances cause paracoagulation of fibrin monomer, whereas they have no effect on the products of fibrin digestion. Primary fibrinolysis does occur occasionally in pediatric patients and is seen in patients with cyanotic congenital heart disease with exceptionally high hematocrit values [16] and in some patients with chronic liver disease. It is important to stress again that, in the majority of patients, fibrinolysis is secondary to intravascular clotting and that the use of an antifibrinolytic agent such as ε-aminocaproic acid (EACA; Amicar) may be extremely dangerous since it interferes with the body's attempt to lyse abnormal accumulations of fibrin. Under these circumstances, if treatment is indicated, anticoagulation with heparin is the therapy of choice although this may appear to be a drastic undertaking in the bleeding patient.[15]

Preparation for Operation

After the nature of the coagulation defect is determined—on the basis of appropriate screening tests and, if indicated, more sophisticated assays of individual coagulation factors or platelet function—it may be necessary to attempt to correct these if it is anticipated that hemostasis will not be adequate. One must take into consideration the nature of the underlying defect, the extent of the surgical procedure, and the patient's probable response to the operation.

Platelet Transfusion

The patient with thrombocytopenia (platelet count of less than 50,000/cu mm) should be considered a candidate for platelet transfusion, particularly if the thrombocytopenia is the result of decreased production of platelets. An increment of 12,000 to 13,000 platelets/cu mm can be expected for each unit of platelet concentrate transfused per square meter of body surface.[17] Thus, an infusion of 6 units of platelet concentrate per square meter should, in most circumstances, provide adequate coverage for a major operation. However, this response may be compromised by the presence of platelet antibodies, intravascular coagulation, or sepsis.[17] A trial of platelet therapy could be undertaken a few hours before operation to ensure that an adequate increment is obtained. Depending on the nature of the surgical procedure, platelet levels in excess of 50,000/cu mm should be maintained for at least five to seven days postoperatively. When the platelet count is marginal, it would be prudent to have platelet concentrates available and to evaluate the effectiveness of hemostasis during the early part of the surgical procedure. If it is obvious to the surgeon that there is excessive oozing, the platelets then can be infused.

One of the drawbacks to routine platelet transfusion is that, particularly in the patient who is not on immunosuppressant therapy, there is a strong likelihood that platelet antibodies will develop, thus compromising future responses to such replacement treatment. In the patient with immunologic thrombocytopenic purpura who is undergoing splenectomy as therapy for the primary disease, abnormal bleeding is an unusual complication since the marrow is hyperactive and, although not reflected in the peripheral blood, platelets are being produced and are presumably available for hemostasis. It has not been found necessary to transfuse such patients with platelets.

Correction of Coagulation Factor Deficiency

A number of concentrates are available, through blood banks and commercial sources, for replacement treatment of the various types of hemophilia. Since the concentrates are indicated only for specific plasma-factor deficiencies, it is essential to determine the exact nature of the underlying disorder before instituting replacement therapy. Hematologic consultation should be obtained, and laboratory support is essential for adequate monitoring of such patients. It is beyond the scope of this chapter to discuss surgery in patients with hemophilia but, with the availability of concentrates, major surgery is now a practical reality. However, there is an increased risk of hepatitis with concentrates made from pooled plasma.

Deficiency of the vitamin K–dependent factors (Factors VII, IX, and X and prothrombin) provides the basis for the bleeding tendency in the newborn.[18] In the majority of situations, it is prevented by the prophylactic administration of 1 mg of vitamin K_1 oxide, but the premature or sick newborn may not respond adequately. One should anticipate a return of the prothrombin time to within normal limits within 24 hours after administration of vitamin K parenterally to a newborn but, if the response is suboptimal, replacement therapy should be considered. Except in unusual circumstances, one should avoid the use of commercial prothrombin complex concentrates since the risk of hepatitis is high. Adequate improvement in the prothrombin time can be obtained by the use of fresh-frozen plasma, and this should be the first therapeutic attempt. The failure of the sick newborn to respond to vitamin K may be complicated by the presence of intravascular coagulation, particularly if there is bacterial or viral sepsis.[19] Doses of vitamin K larger than 1 mg are unnecessary and could be dangerous. Recently it has become apparent that vitamin K deficiency can recur during the first two to three months of life and it would be considered good practice to administer 1 mg of vitamin K to any infant who is to have an operation within the first three months of life, in order to obviate the possibility of this so-called delayed-onset hemorrhagic disease.[20]

Vitamin K deficiency also can complicate malabsorption syndromes and liver disease. The former should respond promptly to parenteral vitamin K, but in the latter situation one is often faced with an unresponsive patient in whom serum hepatitis is an even greater hazard than in the normal child. As in the newborn, fresh-frozen plasma should be tried, but, if there is no response and operation is urgently required, a prothrombin complex concentrate such as Konyne[21] or Proplex[22] could be used to correct the clotting factor deficiency.

Reference has already been made to the problem of intravascular coagulation, and there now is increased awareness of its presence in many disease states.[15] In a majority of situations in which there is compensated intravascular coagulation with the increased utilization of platelets and clotting factors being balanced by production, anti-coagulant therapy does not seem warranted. On the other hand, the severely ill bleeding patient who urgently requires an operation prob-ably should be given heparin for anticoagulation and then treated with appropriate replacement of platelets and coagulation factors.

ANEMIA

Anemia is defined as a below-normal number of erythrocytes per cubic millimeter of blood, concentration of hemoglobin, or volume of packed erythrocytes (PCV) per 100 ml of blood, and the examining physician must be aware of the variations of normal in determining whether anemia, in fact, exists and, if so, what the severity is. This is particularly pertinent in the pediatric age group where age-dependent variation in these parameters is at its maximum. At birth, the hemo-globin concentration is usually in the range of 19 to 20 gm/100 ml (19.8 ± 2.4) with parallel increases in packed cell volume and erythro-cyte count as compared to adult "normals."[23] By the end of the first month there is a significant decrease in hemoglobin and packed cell volume; the decrease in erythrocyte count is less marked. By the end of the second or third month, the nadir in erythrocyte values is reached, a reflection of the so-called physiologic hypoplasia of the bone mar-row. Thus, in the newborn a hemoglobin value of 13 gm/100 ml repre-sents severe anemia, whereas in the 5-month-old a value of 10 gm/100 ml is within the acceptable range of normal.[23] This provides the basis for using 10 gm/100 ml as the lower limit of normal between 1 and 18 months of age and 11 gm/100 ml in subsequent years. Naturally, factors such as birth weight, time of clamping the umbilical cord, nu-trition, and altitude will influence hemoglobin levels during the first years of life.

One must approach the diagnosis of anemia by determining first whether it is normochromic normocytic, hypochromic microcytic, or macrocytic[24] (Table 17–2). A reticulocyte count is essential for deter-mining the activity of the bone marrow in response to anemia; a de-creased reticulocyte count in the presence of moderate or severe anemia is indicative of bone marrow depression or absence of hemato-poietic factors such as iron. An increased reticulocyte count may in-dicate hemolysis or a response to acute blood loss. Evaluation of the blood smear is essential to assist in diagnosis, and other appropriate tests may be indicated once an initial categorization of the anemia is made on the basis of the hemoglobin concentration, red cell indices, reticulocyte count, and blood smear. If intravascular coagulation is suspected, erythrocyte morphology is often seriously disturbed, with burr cells, schistocytes, and other distorted cells appearing in the peripheral blood smear.

Table 17–2
Possible Diagnoses with Various Types of Anemia

Type of Anemia	Diagnostic Categories
Hypochromic microcytic	Iron deficiency
	Nutritional
	Blood loss
	Malabsorption
	Thalassemia
	Lead poisoning
	Sideroachrestic anemia
Macrocytic	Normal newborn
	Megaloblastosis
	Vitamin B_{12}
	Folate
	Liver disease
Normochromic	
Increased reticulocyte count	Hemorrhage
	Hemolysis
	Intracorpuscular defects
	Abnormal hemoglobin
	Enzyme deficiency
	Structural abnormality
	Extracorpuscular defects
	Antibody
	Hypersplenism
	Microangiopathy
	Combined defects
	Chemicals or drugs
	Unstable hemoglobin
	G6PD deficiency
Low reticulocyte count	Malignant infiltration
	Leukemia
	Metastatic tumor
	Aplastic or hypoplastic anemia
	Chronic renal disease
	Chronic infection

It is beyond the scope of this chapter to review all the causes of anemia and their treatment. Reference will be made to the more common situations encountered in pediatric surgical practice.

Neonatal Anemia

In the newborn, anemia usually is associated with hemorrhage or hemolysis. Serious blood loss from the infant's circulation can result from rupture of the umbilical cord or placental vessels, as a complication of placenta previa or abruptio placentae, or by hemorrhage into the maternal circulation.[25] If the hemorrhage is severe enough, the infant may be born in obvious shock, but, if bleeding is less massive, pallor may be the only presenting feature. With less severe bleeding, the physician may not be aware of anemia at birth, but the decreased hemoglobin mass may become evident later as a result of growth and increase in blood volume. A careful history will uncover overt causes of bleeding which might account for the loss of hemoglobin but, particularly toward the latter part of the first year, proof of blood loss into the maternal circulation cannot be substantiated because fetal erythrocytes would have disappeared from the maternal circulation by the third or fourth month.

Hemolysis in the newborn is usually the result of isoimmunization, most commonly resulting from Rh or ABO blood group incompatibility. Less commonly, structural or metabolic defects in the erythrocytes produce anemia.[25] Jaundice usually is a feature of hemolytic disease of the newborn, but this is dependent on the degree of maturation of the liver and the extent to which bilirubin can be conjugated and excreted. Thus, in the premature newborn with poor liver function, a relatively mild degree of hemolysis may result in severe jaundice whereas the otherwise normal premature newborn may be able to cope with massive hemolysis with only a minimal increase in the bilirubin level. Undetected hemolytic disease of the newborn often presents with anemia of varying degree between the second and 12th weeks of life. It is essential to keep this possibility in mind and to examine for isoimmunization, by Coombs' testing and determination of maternal and infant blood groups. This is particularly pertinent in the patient about to undergo operation because, if isoimmunization has occurred, blood for transfusion should be compatible with maternal serum, since the infant has passively acquired antibodies from her circulation. In many institutions, cross-matching is routinely performed against the maternal specimen for all infants requiring transfusion within the first three or four months of life. Treatment of anemia should be directed toward the underlying disorder but, as in many of the causes outlined above, no specific treatment can be undertaken and erythrocyte replacement may be indicated prior to a surgical procedure. Under these circumstances, packed or sedimented erythrocytes should be utilized in order to achieve an optimal hemoglobin level.

Iron-Deficiency Anemia

During the latter part of the first year of life the incidence of iron-deficiency anemia increases, and this is particularly noticeable in patients who were born with decreased hemoglobin mass as a result of either blood loss or prematurity. In particular, the premature infant, who may increase his birth weight six- or sevenfold within the first year of life, requires exogenous iron to maintain a reasonable hemoglobin concentration. For example, a 1.5-kg newborn has a blood volume of approximately 120 ml; assuming a hemoglobin concentration of 18 gm/100 ml, the total body hemoglobin would be 21.6 gm. By the end of the first year, this infant may have increased his weight to 9 kg, a sixfold increase. With no exogenous iron, his 21.6 gm of hemoglobin now has to be distributed in a blood volume of 630 ml; his hemoglobin concentration thus would be about 3.5 gm/100 ml. This extreme example stresses the importance of hemoglobin mass at birth and the lack of dietary iron in the development of anemia. These patients are iron deficient and would be expected to respond promptly to oral administration of iron. An increase in hemoglobin concentration of 1 to 2 gm/100 ml per week can be anticipated. Unless the need for operation is urgent, the patient should be allowed to regenerate his hemoglobin value to acceptable levels during a regimen of administration of exogenous iron.[24]

In an emergency situation, replacement by transfusions of packed or sedimented erythrocytes should be undertaken, taking into account that, with severe anemia, the cardiovascular system may be compromised. Too rapid or too large an infusion of erythrocytes may result in cardiac failure. As a rule of thumb, in a single transfusion one should not give more than 10 ml/kg of body weight over three to four hours. When the hemoglobin concentration is less than 5 gm/100 ml, it is safer to use smaller amounts for transfusion; a guide is the following formula:

$$2 \times \text{Hb (gm/100 ml)} \times \text{body weight (kg)} = \text{volume for transfusion}$$

There is virtually no indication for the use of whole blood except in the presence of acute blood loss. Not only is the use of packed or sedimented erythrocytes likely to provide less circulatory overload, but it also allows the plasma and platelets to be utilized for other patients who may require these components.[26]

Hereditary Spherocytosis

This is a classic example of a hemolytic anemia for which the primary therapy is splenectomy. In this condition, there is an inherited intrinsic defect in the erythrocytes which results in their premature sequestration and destruction in the normal spleen. Removal of the spleen does not cure the spherocytosis, but does remove the organ of destruction, thus alleviating the hemolysis and the potential complications of aplastic crisis and cholelithiasis.

Splenectomy is also undertaken in other hereditary erythrocyte disorders, in occasional patients with acquired or immune hemolytic anemia, and in selected children with hypersplenism. Splenectomy often results in a dramatic response and an increase in hemoglobin concentration so that a conservative approach to preoperative transfusion is indicated, particularly in hereditary spherocytosis in which one uniformly can anticipate an increase in hemoglobin immediately postoperatively. The degree of anemia and its effects must be weighed against the complications of transfusion, such as circulatory overload, sensitization, and transmission of disease.

Splenectomy should not be undertaken electively in a patient under 2 years of age, because of the apparent risk of overwhelming sepsis particularly with pneumococci or *Escherichia coli*.[27] In older children, the risk of overwhelming sepsis still might be a problem in patients with diseases in which there is decreased immunologic tolerance or resistance to infection.

Sickle Cell Disease

Approximately 8 percent of American blacks are heterozygous with respect to the gene for hemoglobin S, but the overwhelming majority of these persons are asymptomatic and have no detectable anemia.[28] However, when oxygen tension is decreased, sickle cell crises may occur. This is particularly pertinent during major operations, and therefore it is essential that all black patients be screened for sickle cell trait before surgical procedures. If the trait is present, steps must be taken to ensure adequate oxygenation during induction and maintenance of anesthesia and, most important, during the postoperative period. The goal is to decrease the risk of sickle cell crisis and infarcts which could result in permanent damage to major organs, particularly the brain.

The patient with sickle cell anemia presents a more complex problem. He will inevitably require blood transfusions since anemia is a significant feature of the disease. In these patients, it is even more essential to maintain adequate oxygenation. Attempts to suppress sickle cell production by hypertransfusion with normal erythrocytes for a few days preoperatively have met with variable success. One has to weigh the advantages of suppressing hemoglobin S production against the risks of repeated transfusion. With modern anesthetic techniques, it would seem reasonable to transfuse such patients to a hemoglobin value of 10 or 11 gm/100 ml and carefully monitor oxygenation well into the recovery phase after anesthesia. Maintenance of oxygenation will ensure against any major degree of sickling. Because of the associated hyposthenuria, there is a tendency for negative water balance to occur. Since dehydration can aggravate intravascular stasis and sickling, adequate hydration with maintenance of pH and electrolyte balance is mandatory.[28]

Glucose-6-Phosphate Dehydrogenase (G6PD) Deficiency

In this erythrocyte defect, patients are not anemic unless challenged by oxidant drugs.[28] Primaquine is the prototype for inducing hemolysis in these patients, but the number of incriminated compounds is considerable, making it essential that blacks and persons of Mediterranean origin, both male and female, be screened for G6PD deficiency prior to surgical procedures. In this way, drugs known to cause hemolysis in such patients can be avoided. Although the deficiency is transmitted as a sex-linked recessive disorder, some heterozygous females have sufficient deficiency to be at significant risk. A simple screening test is available for detection of G6PD deficiency in the erythrocytes.[29]

ERYTHROCYTOSIS

The newborn has an increased erythrocyte count compared to older children and adults. Erythrocytosis is not commonly seen in the pediatric age group, and most patients with increased hematocrit values have some form of cyanotic congenital heart disease or chronic pulmonary disease; the increased erythrocyte count represents a response to hypoxia and stimulation of the marrow to increase the oxygen-carrying capacity of the blood. With respect to cyanotic congenital heart disease, it should be mentioned that, with increasing hypoxia and erythrocytosis, a number of hemostatic defects become evident and these include thrombocytopenia, fibrinolysis, and some abnormalities of intrinsic and extrinsic clotting.[16] It is important to screen for abnormalities of hemostasis in patients with cyanotic congenital heart disease in order to plan for preoperative and postoperative management. Polycythemia vera is virtually unknown in children, but occasional examples of erythrocytosis secondary to renal cyst or neoplasm have been documented and benign familial erythrocytosis is a well-recognized, although rare, condition. Generally, treatment of erythrocytosis is not indicated except in the severely affected patient with cyanotic congenital heart disease in whom erythropheresis, by decreasing the hematocrit, results in improvement of various parameters of hemostasis and coagulation.

LEUKOPENIA AND LEUKOCYTOSIS

Evaluation of abnormalities in the leukocyte count also is dependent on a knowledge of normal values at various ages. The total leukocyte count tends to be higher at birth, ranging from 9000 to 38,000/cu mm (mean, 22,000/cu mm) during the first two days of life. There is a decrease during the first week to a mean of 12,000/cu mm (range, 5000 to 21,000/cu mm). Thereafter the total leukocyte count remains fairly stable during the first year of life, with gradual decrease to adult values by the fourth or fifth year. The percentage of neutrophils averages 60 percent at birth, but during the second week there is a reversal of the neutrophil:lymphocyte ratio and neutrophils then comprise about 40 percent. Between the fourth and sixth months, the percentage of neutrophils reaches 30 percent followed by a gradual increase so that by approximately 4 years of age, there are equal proportions of neutrophils and lymphocytes. From the fourth year onward there is a gradual increase in the percentage of neutrophils so that adult values are reached by the sixth or seventh year.[24] Thus, with the exception of the first week of life, relative lymphocytosis is the normal pattern during the first four years. Total leukocyte counts tend to be lower in the premature infant.

The finding of leukopenia should raise the question of infection and, except for certain specific bacterial and viral infections, the presence of leukopenia in a situation in which, under normal circumstances, leukocytosis might be expected should be considered of serious prognostic import.[24] Neutropenia also may result from isoimmunization or may complicate various other immune diseases such as lupus erythematosus. Constitutional or acquired aplastic anemia and leukemia of childhood have leukopenia and neutropenia as frequent components. In any event, any patient presenting with significant leukopenia and neutropenia should be studied in order to determine the nature of any underlying disease.

Leukocytosis with neutrophilia usually is evidence of bacterial infection but, early in the course of many viral infections, relative neutrophilia is the rule prior to the appearance of the relative lymphocytosis. Tuberculosis and most viral infections are characterized by relative or absolute lymphocytosis. Acute leukemia of childhood characteristically presents with normal or decreased total leukocyte count and blast cells may not be evident in the peripheral blood.

REFERENCES

1. Schulman, I.: The significance of epistaxis in childhood. *Pediatrics* 24:489–492, 1959.
2. Owen, C.A., Jr., et al: *The Diagnosis of Bleeding Disorders.* Boston: Little, Brown & Company, 1969.
3. Baehner, R.L. and Strauss, H.S.: Hemophilia in the first year of life. *N Eng J Med* 275:524–528, 1966.
4. Strauss, H.S.: The perpetuation of hemophilia by mutation. *Pediatrics* 39:186–193, 1967.
5. Diamond, L.K. and Porter, F.S.: The inadequacies of routine bleeding and clotting times. *N Eng J Med* 259:1025–1027, 1958.
6. Mielke, C.H., Jr., et al: The standardized normal Ivy bleeding time and its prolongation by aspirin. *Blood* 34:204–215, 1969.
7. Singer, R.: Acetylsalicylic acid, a probable cause for secondary post-tonsillectomy hemorrhage: A preliminary report. *Arch Otolaryngol* 42:19–20, 1945.

8. Eknoyan, G., et al: Platelet function in renal failure. *N Eng J Med* 280:677–681, 1969.

9. Gilchrist, G.S., Fine, R.N., and Donnell, G.N.: The hemostatic defect in glycogen storage disease, type I. *Acta Paediat Scand* 57:205–208, 1968.

10. Suvansri, U., Cheung, W.H., and Sawitsky, A.: The effect of bilirubin on the human platelet. *J Pediat* 74:240–246, 1969.

11. Bowie, E.J.W., and Owen, C.A., Jr.: Von Willebrand's disease. *Med Clin N Amer* 56:275–284, 1972.

12. Proctor, R.R., and Rapaport, S.I.: The partial thromboplastin time with kaolin: A simple screening test for first stage plasma clotting factor deficiencies. *Am J Clin Pathol* 36:212–219, 1961.

13. Bowie, E.J.W., et al: *Mayo Clinic Laboratory Manual of Hemostasis.* Philadelphia: W.B. Saunders Company, 1971.

14. Bishop, R., et al: The preparation and evaluation of a standardized fibrin plate for the assessment of fibrinolytic activity. *Thromb Diath Haemorrh* 23:202–210, 1970.

15. Abildgaard, C.F.: Recognition and treatment of intravascular coagulation. *J Pediat* 74:163–176, 1969.

16. Ekert, H., et al: Hemostasis in cyanotic congenital heart disease. *J Pediat* 76:221–230, 1970.

17. Karon, M., et al: Leukemia in children. *Calif Med* 114:31–43, 1971.

18. Aballi, A.J., and de Lamerens, S.: Coagulation changes in the neonatal period and in early infancy. *Pediat Clin N Amer* 9:785–817, 1962.

19. Hathaway, W.E., Mull, M.M., and Pechet, G.S.: Disseminated intravascular coagulation in the newborn. *Pediatrics* 43:233–240, 1969.

20. Nammacher, M.A., et al: Vitamin K deficiency in infants beyond the neonatal period. *J Pediat* 76:549–554, 1970.

21. Hoag, M.S., et al: Treatment of hemophilia B with a new clotting-factor concentrate. *N Eng J Med* 280:581–586, 1969.

22. Gilchrist, G.S., et al: Evaluation of a new concentrate for the treatment of factor IX deficiency. *N Eng J Med* 280:291–295, 1969.

23. Moe, P.J.: Normal red blood picture during the first three years of life. *Acta Paediat Scand* 54:69–80, 1965.

24. Smith, C.H.: *Blood Diseases of Infancy and Childhood,* ed 2. St. Louis: C.V. Mosby Company, 1966.

25. Oski, F.A., and Naiman, J.L.: *Hematologic Problems in the Newborn.* Philadelphia: W.B. Saunders Company, 1966.

26. Chaplin, H., Jr.: Packed red blood cells. *N Eng J Med* 281:364, 1969.

27. Horan, M., and Colebatch, J.H.: Relation between splenectomy and subsequent infection: A clinical study. *Arch Dis Child* 37:398–414, 1962.

28. Harris, J.W., and Kellermeyer, R.W.: *The Red Cell: Production, Metabolism, Destruction; Normal and Abnormal.* Cambridge: Harvard University Press, 1970.

29. Beutler, E.: A series of new screening procedures for pyruvate kinase deficiency, glucose-6-phosphate dehydrogenase deficiency, and glutathione reductase deficiency. *Blood* 28:553–562, 1966.

18

Surgery in the Child with Diabetes Mellitus

Howard S. Traisman, M.D., F.A.A.P.

There are approximately four million diabetics in this country, a prevalence rate of 20 per 1000 population. About forty percent of this number are undiagnosed.

Juvenile diabetes mellitus affects those individuals 15 years of age or less. These affected children comprise five percent of the total diabetic population. The sex distribution is equal.

The juvenile diabetic is insulin-dependent and poses more of a problem in regulation than the adult diabetic patient. There are more metabolic fluctuations in the day-to-day management of these children. Good control of the diabetic patient involves freedom from hypoglycemia and avoidance of marked hyperglycemia.

Surgical procedures occur no more often in the diabetic child than in the nondiabetic. The common operations not related to diabetes include hernia repair, tonsillectomy and adenoidectomy, appendectomy, and eye and dental surgery. This is in contradistinction to the adult diabetic patient whose surgery usually involves the gastrointestinal tract, treatment of abscesses and ulcers, amputations for compromised vascular supply to the specific extremity, and treatment of malignant disease. Except for acute appendicitis or severe trauma, the surgical procedures in juvenile diabetics are usually elective.

The surgical mortality rate of juvenile diabetics is no higher than that of the nondiabetic. The postoperative medical morbidity is no higher in the diabetic child than in the nondiabetic patient. The surgical morbidity in diabetic children is higher than the nondiabetic because of postoperative infections (especially if the diabetic control is not good) or, if there is a urinary tract infection from the use of an indwelling catheter. In most well-controlled diabetics, wound healing will proceed at a normal rate. With proper fluid, electrolyte and insulin administration, and the judicious use of antibiotics, postoperative morbidity in the juvenile diabetic is very low.

PREOPERATIVE MANAGEMENT

The juvenile diabetic is usually admitted to the hospital 36–48 hours before an elective surgical procedure. If his diabetes is poorly controlled, he may have to be hospitalized three to four days before surgery. Management of the surgical diabetic child should be a cooperative team effort involving the pediatrician, surgeon, and anesthesiologist.

In our hospital, the pediatric service is responsible for all insulin and fluid orders unless emergency conditions in the operating room require change. Appropriate antibiotic therapy, when required, is jointly discussed and decided upon by the pediatric and surgical staffs. The choice and route of anesthetic agent is primarily the prerogative of the surgeon and anesthesiologist, though the pediatrician is informed. When admitted to the hospital, a CBC, urinalysis, blood glucose, serum electrolytes, and CO_2 determinations are ordered. Other laboratory tests are performed when specifically indicated.

The patient's diabetic diet is ordered for him and his intermediate-acting insulin (lente or NPH), with or without unmodified insulin (regular), is administered. Insulin dosage is adjusted to achieve optimum control. A "second voided urine specimen" is tested immediately before meals and at bedtime utilizing Clinitest and Acetest tablets. The urine testing procedure that I am describing involves a complete emptying of the bladder thirty minutes prior to a scheduled feeding. A second specimen is collected thirty minutes after the first specimen which is immediately before the scheduled feeding.

Not infrequently, a 24-hour quantitative urine glucose determination is performed to aid in establishing good diabetic control. This may even be divided into four six-hour samples for greater accuracy. Blood glucose determinations can be done one to four times a day so as to observe the correlation between urine and blood glucose levels.

It is essential that the patient's diabetes be regulated so that there will not be any fluctuations from hyperglycemia, and even ketoacidosis, to hypoglycemia.

The diabetic patient and his parents should be informed about what the surgical procedure will entail, details of the postoperative period, and approximate duration of hospitalization. When indicated, enemas and/or local skin preps are done the evening before surgery.

THE DAY OF SURGERY

One-half hour before surgery, blood glucose, electrolyte, and CO_2 determinations are done as baseline studies in addition to a second voided urine specimen which is tested for glucose and acetone.

Insulin

Insulin is ordered. If the patient is having a surgical procedure that is of relatively short duration and minimal postoperative disability (i.e. herniorrhaphy, EENT, or dental surgery) and the diabetic child will be able to take oral feedings later on in the day, then his regular dose of intermediate-acting insulin (lente or NPH) and regular insulin (if he is taking same) is administered subcutaneously. If the patient has a history of hypoglycemic episodes, then I will reduce his insulin dosage by 10 or 20 percent.

Approximately thirty percent of my juvenile diabetic patients routinely take two injections of intermediate-acting insulin, with or without regular insulin daily. Two-thirds of the total dose of intermediate-acting insulin is given before breakfast, with or without some regular insulin, and the remaining third of the total dose of intermediate-acting insulin is given before supper. If this is the case, then I follow the same procedure preoperatively.

Regular insulin administration is recommended whenever a major surgical procedure such as cardiac, intraabdominal, retroperitoneal, orthopedic, genitourinary, or central nervous system is planned. The amount of regular insulin injected at this time is approximately one-quarter of the total dose of intermediate and regular insulin that is usually administered. As an example, if the patient is receiving 30 units of lente insulin and 10 units of regular insulin each morning, he would be given 10 units of regular insulin prior to surgery, and approximately the same amount every six hours.

Some physicians may wish to use regular insulin injections for any surgical procedure requiring a general anesthetic. This is acceptable except that it frequently causes a delay of about 24 hours in returning to the patient's standard diabetic diet and use of intermediate-acting insulin. Consequently, I prefer to continue with the use of unmodified insulin whenever possible.

Under no circumstances should regular (unmodified) insulin be put in an intravenous solution. It has been proven that as much as thirty percent of the insulin adheres to the intravenous bottle and tubing and never reaches the patient.

Fluid

An intravenous infusion of glucose is then started and six-hour management begins. We usually schedule surgery for our diabetic patients at 8:00 A.M. This allays patient and parent anxiety and allows us to begin six-hour management on our standard schedule.

Six-Hour Management

This regime consists of dividing each day into four periods of six hours each (8 A.M., 2 P.M., 8 P.M., and 2 A.M.) Parenteral fluid consisting of anywhere from 30 to 60 grams of glucose is administered over a six-hour period. One to two grams of glucose per kilogram of body weight is the basis for determining whether a patient receives 30, 40, 50, or 60 grams. This depends upon the patient's size and the physician's judgment. A large, adolescent, pubescent child or adult would receive 50 or 60 grams of glucose every six hours. No more than 10 grams of glucose per hour is given, or a maximum of 60 grams (even for an adult) per each six-hour period. If 40 grams of glucose are to be administered over a six-hour period, it can be 400 ml of 10 percent dextrose in water or 800 ml of 5 percent dextrose in water.

Second voided urine specimens are tested near the end of each period to determine the amount of the next dose of insulin. If a patient cannot void, a blood glucose determination can be done. Dextrostix (finger stick) can be utilized here. Juvenile diabetics having surgery are *not* routinely catheterized. An indwelling catheter is used postoperatively only if the patient cannot void. They are usually in use for only 12–24 hours.

If regular insulin is being used during this regime, it usually should not be omitted, even if there is no glucosuria. However, if the patient is hypoglycemic, then it may be omitted for 4–6 hours. The possibility of *hypoglycemia* occurring should always be kept in mind. This may occur with or without the classical signs and symptoms of hunger, irritability, tachycardia, pallor, perspiration, personality or nervous changes, and weakness. When intermediate-acting insulin is used, regular insulin can be used as a complement when there is glucosuria. Occasionally, there may be the need for blood glucose determinations and regular insulin administration every three to four hours during an especially stressful operation, such as open-heart surgery. Here we are not only dealing with stress as a cause of hyperglycemia, but also additional infused glucose. This is in the form of the dextrose component of citrated blood, and the 5 percent dextrose-Ringer's lactate solution that is used in a cardiac pump. Baum and associates reported decreased insulin response during anesthesia with hypothermia in nondiabetic children undergoing cardiovascular surgery. They cautioned that glucose infusions during hypothermia may cause hyperglycemia and hyperosmolarity. When the injection of regular insulin is three to four hours after a previous injection, then the time of the six-hour management should be adjusted. Regular insulin can be administered intravenously, if necessary, for a more rapid onset of action.

It is impossible to give a dosage schedule for regular insulin. This is dependent upon the age and size of the patient, duration of his diabetes, and clinical status. The last mentioned includes type of surgical procedure, degree of glucosuria and hyperglycemia, with or without ketoacidosis, or hypoglycemia. It is the pediatrician who knows his individual patient who is in the optimum position of ordering the proper amount of insulin. The insulin dose can vary from ¼ to ½ unit per kilogram of body weight if diabetic control is good, to two to four units of regular insulin per kilogram of body weight if diabetic control is poor or if the child is acidotic.

Proper amounts of the necessary electrolytes should be administered to keep the patient in electrolyte balance. Total fluid and electrolyte requirements can be calculated by a variety of methods (see Chapters 6 and 9), and all are gross approximations. Careful and frequent clinical evaluation of the patient is imperative. This allows for modification of treatment as is necessary. At our hospital we use the calorie expenditure system. The following outline is a plan that contains average values applicable to the majority of cases and problems encountered.*

MAINTENANCE REQUIREMENTS

Quantity

Based on the accepted premise that maintenance fluid requirements depend on caloric expenditure according to a relationship of 100 milliliters fluid per 100 calories expended, the requirements may be calculated according to the following formulas.

00 to 10 kg = 100 cal/kg of body weight
10 to 20 kg = 1000 cal + 50 cal/kg of body weight for each kg over 10
20 kg and up = 1500 cal + 20 cal/kg of body weight for each kg over 20
(1 gram of glucose = 4 calories
100 cc of 5% dextrose (glucose) in water =
5 grams of glucose or 20 calories)

* Reproduced through the courtesy of C.V. Mosby Co., St. Louis. As appears in Traisman, H.S.: *The Management of Juvenile Diabetes Mellitus*, ed 2, 1971.

These quantities allow 50 ml/100 cal for insensible water loss and 50 ml/100 cal for urinary loss; small amounts of fluid normally lost in stool are covered by these allowances.

Type of Solution

The requirements for electrolytes are less exactly established, but are approximately as follows:

Sodium (Na) 3 mEq/100 cal
Chloride (Cl) 2 mEq/100 cal
Potassium (K) 2 mEq/100 cal

The maintenance electrolytes can be approximated in 100 ml of fluid by mixing as follows:

3.0 ml molar Na lactate (18 ml M/6 Na lactate)
1.0 ml 2/M KCl
up to 100 ml 5% dextrose in water

It is emphasized that a potassium-containing solution is not given if there is renal insufficiency. Children with diabetic acidosis usually receive potassium three to six hours after insulin and fluid therapy have been started.

DEFICITS

Magnitude of Deficit

Fluid and electrolyte deficits are best considered in terms of weight loss, because these losses are not a function of energy metabolism. Deficits may vary from five to fifteen percent of the body weight with the usual clinically manifest state (moderately severe dehydration) representing ten percent and approximates 100 ml/kg of body weight. In general, *deficits greater than ten percent are replaced on the second day.*

Type of Solution

Immediate reexpansion of the extracellular fluid (ECF) compartment with an isotonic fluid will improve blood pressure, circulation, and renal output. Ringer's lactate is preferable in most instances (except in severe vomiting, i.e. diabetic acidosis, when physiologic saline is preferable) and is given the first hour in the amount of 20 ml/kg of body weight. The electrolytes given are included in the repair calculations. If shock is present, one should give five percent albumin solution

Table 18–1

Magnitude of Losses (per kg of body weight if 10–12% dehydrated):

	H_2O(ml)	Na(mEq)	K(mEq)	Cl(mEq)
Fasting and thirsting	100–120	5–7	1–2	4–5
Diabetic acidosis	100–120	8–10	5–7	6–8

or whole blood (if the patient is anemic) in a dosage of 10 ml/kg of body weight.

Rate of Administration

1. Dehydration: Rate is usually a function of the volume to be received.
    First twenty-four hours:
    a. Up to one hour: 20 ml/kg of body weight of Ringer's lactate, or physiologic saline.
    b. If the child has not voided or if shock remains, give 5 percent albumin solution—10 ml/kg of body weight. *Do not* give potassium solutions until patient has voided.
    c. Next eight to ten hours: deficit fluids.
    d. Next twelve hours or more: maintenance fluids.
    Second twenty-four hours:
    e. Additional deficit fluids over ten percent.
    f. Continuing losses.
    g. Maintenance fluids.
2. Maintenance: Calculate to run twenty-four hours. Instructions to nurses should be in terms of ml/hour.
3. Blood: Usual dose for whole blood is 10 to 15 ml/kg of body weight per twenty-four hours. Should not exceed 20 ml/kg of body weight except when active bleeding is present.
    Packed red blood cell (RBC) dosage is 10 ml/kg of body weight per twenty-four hours. With severe anemia, packed RBC may cause sufficient hypervolemia to produce congestive heart failure. Thus, the lower the hemoglobin, the smaller the transfusion (i.e. 3–5 ml/kg of body weight) at any one time.

Evaluation of Fluid Therapy

1. Weigh daily.
2. Physical examination.
3. Hematocrit.
4. Urine specific gravity.
5. Measure electrolytes, blood urea nitrogen (BUN), blood glucose, carbon dioxide content, and pH.

Hypotonic Deficit Calculation

Concentration desired: Actual concentration $\times$ factor of distribution $\times$ body weight (kilogram) equals the milliequivalents required.

140 − 120 $\times$ 0.6 $\times$ wt (kg)
20 $\times$ 0.6 $\times$ 10 kg = mEq Na required

Factors of distribution:

Na 0.6
Cl 0.3
HCO_3 0.5

Hypertonic Deficit Calculation

Free water loss can be estimated from the elevation of serum sodium —an increase of one mEq/L over 145 would indicate a free water loss of 4 ml/kg body weight. Thus, if 100 ml/kg body weight is lost (moderate dehydration) and the serum Na is 160 mEq/L, then:

4 ml $\times$ 160 − 145 = 60 ml/kg = free water deficit, and
40 ml/kg = water and electrolyte deficit

Water is not lost in the ECF/ICF (intracellular fluid) 60/40 ratio as in isotonic and hypotonic dehydration, but rather in ECF/ICF 50/50 ratio; thus, of the 40 milliliters, 20 milliliters equals ECF and 20 milliliters equals ICF lost.

20 ml or .02 $\times$ 140 mEq/L = 2.8 mEq Na loss/ kg body weight
.02 $\times$ 100 mEq/L = 2.0 mEq Cl loss/kg body weight
.02 $\times$ 150 mEq/L = 3.0 mEq K loss/kg body weight

Sodium concentration in the repair solution should not exceed 40 mEq/L, and 20 to 25 mEq/L is preferable.

Table 18–2
Oral Solutions

	Na (mEq/L)	K (mEq/L)	Cl (mEq/L)	HCO_3 (mEq/L)	Cal (per L)
Milk	22	36	28	30	670
Coke	0.4	13		13.4	435
Pepsi	6.5	0.8		7.3	480
Orange juice	0.2	49		50	540
Lytren	25	25	30	20	280
Ginger ale	3.5	0.1		3.6	360

Table 18–3
Parenteral Solutions

	Na (mEq/L)	K (mEq/L)	Cl (mEq/L)	HCO₃ (mEq/L)
Saline	154		154	
3% saline	513		513	
M/6 lactate	167			167
Ringer	147	4	155	
Ringer's lactate	130	4	109	28
Darrow KL	122	35	104	53
Plasma	146	5	105	25

It is recommended that an intravenous needle or catheter not remain in one site longer than 24 hours, so as to minimize the chance of infection.

Anesthesia

The type and mode of administration is primarily the decision of the anesthesiologist and surgeon. Inhalation anesthesia is used almost exclusively in pediatric surgery. Local anesthesia is used infrequently except for very minor procedures, and spinal anesthesia is rarely, if ever, used in children.

Halothane (Fluothane) is the most widely used inhalation anesthetic. Occasionally, nitrous oxide with oxygen is used for a short procedure. Ether and cyclopropane cause hyperglycemia due to stimulation of pituitary ACTH production. They cause an increased production of epinephrine and norepinephrine with a resultant hyperglycemia and decreased insulin sensitivity. Halothane has none of these effects and is also noninflammable, minimally irritating, and rapid awakening. Thiopental (Pentothal) and muscle relaxants may also be used at times.

POSTOPERATIVE MANAGEMENT

Immediately postoperative blood glucose, CO_2, and electrolytes should be determined. A blood glucose level of about 200 mg% is acceptable considering that parenteral glucose is being administered. The above determinations are made as frequently as the clinical condition of the patient dictates.

Six-hour management continues as long as necessary during the postoperative period. This may be 12 to 48 hours of parenteral fluid therapy followed by oral feedings which consist of the same number of grams of available glucose as was given parenterally. As an example, 400 ml of ginger ale or orange juice contain 40 grams of available glucose. This is equivalent to 400 ml of 10 percent dextrose in water or 800 ml of 5 percent dextrose in water. Progress is made from liquid to a solid diet—a 40-gram glucose solid feeding can consist of one egg, 40 grams of bread, and 150 grams of milk. Examples of these diets may be found in Colwell's and Traisman's books.

When the patient is retaining solid feedings with his six-hour regime and his glucosuria is controlled, and there is no acetonuria for 24 hours, he can then progress to his standard diabetic diet. Intermediate acting insulin, with or without regular insulin, is administered at this time.

Ambulation is started as soon as the patient's condition will permit. Antibiotics are not given routinely postoperatively. They are only prescribed when specifically indicated, such as after cardiac surgery, removal of infected teeth, or if there is evidence of a postoperative infection. If a urethral catheter has been used, it is imperative that a urine culture be obtained before discharge from the hospital. When an infection develops, antimicrobial therapy should be instituted.

SPECIFIC CONDITIONS

Acute Appendicitis

This common surgical condition in children poses a serious problem for the juvenile diabetic. Initially, it is important to differentiate the abdominal pain of acute appendicitis from that of diabetic ketoacidosis. The metabolic changes that occur in diabetic ketoacidosis due to an insufficient amount or ineffective utilization of insulin are impaired storage of glucose as glycogen, and increased glycogen breakdown with an increased production of glucose. There is also hepatic breakdown of protein and fat with resulting ketonemia and ketonuria. A metabolic acidosis then develops. At this time, there is an increased catabolic state with a resultant loss of electrolytes and fluid via the urinary system and from the lungs because of the Kussmaul respirations. As these events progress, there is a resulting dehydration and shock with hemoconcentration, drop in blood pressure, and decreased circulating blood volume. Tissue cellular damage occurs because of the increased metabolic state and acidosis. When acidosis occurs, there is an effect upon the smooth muscle of the gastrointestinal tract and the myocardium, as well as neuromuscular irritability.

In diabetic ketoacidosis, abdominal pain is generalized, and there may also be diffuse abdominal tenderness. Rigidity of the abdomen is rare. Peristaltic activity is present, but may be diminished. Headache, nausea, vomiting, malaise, glucosuria, and ketonuria accompany this condition. An important differentiating point is that in diabetic acidosis the nausea and vomiting precede the pain, whereas in the acute surgical abdomen, the reverse is usually true. An elevated white blood cell count with a shift to the left is not diagnostic, as it can occur in both conditions.

It is not unusual for the pain and vomiting of acute appendicitis in the juvenile diabetic to cause ketoacidosis. Such a patient should have surgery delayed for four to six hours to correct this metabolic derangement by the proper administration of fluids, sodium bicarbonate, electrolytes, and the administration of regular insulin. The ketoacidotic patient is a bad surgical and anesthetic risk due to the hemodynamic changes that occur, and the ultimate effect upon the cardiorespiratory system.

Other conditions that can produce an acute surgical abdomen in children and confuse the clinician are severe gastroenteritis, peptic ulcer, steroid therapy, and rarely, acute pancreatitis, and familial hyperlipidemia with secondary pancreatitis.

Burns

Nondiabetic patients with large surface-area burns may have hyperglycemia and glucosuria. In the diabetic child, his disease will be more difficult to control and he will require additional insulin. There is an increased release of cortisol and epinephrine, shortly after the burn occurs, which is associated with a decreased glucose utilization by the peripheral tissues. During recovery, hyperglycemia, with or without ketosis, dehydration, and coma may ensue. This condition is known as *hyperglycemic, hyperosmolar diabetic coma,* and has also been reported to occur in thyrotoxicosis, pancreatitis, carcinoma of the pancreas, administration of certain drugs, and after hemodialysis and peritoneal dialysis. It is a result of increased nitrogen catabolism, inadequate insulin, high carbohydrate feeding, and loss of body fluids. This can be prevented if one is aware of its occurrence in any patient receiving high carbohydrate feedings.

Treatment of hyperosmolar diabetic coma is not standardized. The essentials of therapy consist of adequate insulin, hypotonic electrolyte solutions for hydration, and potassium replacement when renal function is satisfactory. Sodium bicarbonate is used for the correction of marked acidosis (serum carbon dioxide levels below 10 mEq/L) if it is present. Insulin dosage should be less than is usually prescribed for the treatment of diabetic acidosis because of an increased sensitivity to insulin in patients with hyperosmolar diabetic coma. Where an initial dose of three to four units of regular insulin per kg of body weight might be given in diabetic acidosis treatment, one to two units of regular insulin per kilogram of body weight is recommended for the child with hyperosmolar diabetic coma. The hypotonic electrolyte solution should *not* contain glucose. Normal saline diluted with equal parts of distilled water, or Ringer's lactate solution diluted with distilled water to give a sodium concentration of 76–80 mEq/L is recommended. Rubin and associates administered 140 ml of parenteral fluid per kilogram of body weight during the first twelve hours of treatment, but their patients were not well hydrated until the second day of treatment. Cerebral edema may result from too-rapid administration of parenteral fluid. Unexplained fever may be an early sign of this complication and therapy with steroids and/or mannitol should be considered.

Skin Infections, Abscesses, Calluses, and Warts

These problems are no more prevalent in the well-controlled juvenile diabetic than in his nondiabetic contemporary. However, skin infections (bacterial and monilial) and subcuticular abscesses are seen more frequently in the poorly regulated diabetic child. Appropriate treatment for the skin infection and good diabetic control will yield successful results. Occasionally, prompt incision and drainage and antibiotic treatment of an abscess is necessary to reestablish a satisfactory metabolic state; waiting for better regulation of the diabetes may only compound the problem. Calluses, warts, and corns in the juvenile diabetic can be treated as in the normal child, if there is proper control of his disease.

Subclinical Diabetes Mellitus

Individuals with this form of diabetes usually have a normal glucose tolerance test, but an abnormal cortisone tolerance test. Impaired carbohydrate tolerance is noted during periods of stress, such as surgery, trauma (emotional and/or physical), infections, and endocrinopathies. Diabetes is precipitated by these stressful conditions because of an increased release of growth hormone and an epinephrine-induced suppression of insulin secretion.

Here, stress in an apparently normal child can cause glucosuria and mild hyperglycemia (approximately 200 mg%). There may or may not be symptoms of diabetes mellitus. Usually the glucosuria is discovered on routine urinalysis. A blood glucose level is determined which is elevated. I would not prescribe insulin under these circumstances, but would observe the patient closely. After the period of stress, the patient's impaired carbohydrate metabolism returns to normal. The performance of a glucose tolerance test, and even a cortisone tolerance test, when the patient has recovered, may reveal that this child has subclinical diabetes. This is the first stage of future islet cell decompensation. He should be watched for the development of overt diabetes mellitus.

Infrequently, subclinical diabetes may present postoperatively or after severe trauma, as diabetic ketoacidosis. If the patient is severely ill, that is, a serum CO_2 level of less than 15 mEq/L, and the blood glucose is usually over 300 mg%, three to four units of regular insulin per kg of body weight should be administered. One-half of the dose is given intravenously, and the other half subcutaneously. Subsequent injections of regular insulin will be needed every four to six hours. The subsequent doses of regular insulin will vary from ½ to 1 unit per kg of body weight. Fluid and electrolyte therapy with added sodium bicarbonate should be instituted. 0.058 gm of sodium bicarbonate per kg of body weight will raise the CO_2 content 1 mEq. Never correct for more than a 10-mEq deficit in a 24-hour period. Also, do not give the whole calculated amount of sodium bicarbonate at one time as it may cause a rapid shift of potassium ions into the intracellular compartments causing hypokalemia. There are 3.75 grams of sodium bicarbonate (44.6 milliequivalents) per 50 ml ampule, or 0.075 gm per ml of solution.

If the CO_2 content is 15–20 mEq/L, and the blood sugar is under 300 mg%, sodium bicarbonate is not necessary, and one to two units of regular insulin per kg of body weight is the usual initial insulin dose. Appropriate fluid and electrolyte therapy is necessary. Subsequent regular insulin injections are given every four to six hours in a dose of ¼ to ½ unit per kg of body weight. This individual may be insulin-dependent for a short period of time after the stress situation, or even permanently. Details of the treatment of diabetic ketoacidosis may be found in the writings of Guest, Shirkey, and Traisman.

SUMMARY

The basic principles and a scheme for the management of the juvenile diabetic surgical patient have been explained. A cooperative effort on the part of the pediatrician, surgeon, and anesthesiologist will improve the management of these patients.

REFERENCES

1. Baum, D., Dillard, D.H., and Porte, D., Jr.: Inhibition of insulin release during hypothermic cardiovascular surgery. *New Eng J Med* 279:1309–1314, 1968.
2. Beaser, S.: Surgical management *in* Ellenberg and Rifkin, *Diabetes Mellitus: Theory and Practice.* New York: McGraw-Hill, 1970, pp 746–759.
3. Colwell, A.R.: *Types of Diabetes Mellitus and Their Management,* ed 1. Springfield, Illinois: Charles C. Thomas, 1950, pp 81–92.
4. Danowski, T.S., and Nabarro, J.D.N.: Hyperosmolar and other types of non-ketoacidotic coma in diabetes. *Diabetes* 14:162–165, 1965.
5. Guest, G.M. and West, C.D.: Fluid therapy in diabetic acidosis. *Pediat Clin N Amer* 11:903–910, 1964.
6. Holvey, S.M.: Surgery in the child with diabetes. *Pediat Clin N Amer* 16:671–679, 1969.
7. Rosenberg, S.A., et al: The syndrome of dehydration, coma and severe hyper-

glycemia without ketosis in patients convalescing from burns. *New Eng J Med* 272:931–938, 1965.

8. Rubin, H.M., Kramer, R., and Drash, A.: Hyperosmolality complicating diabetes mellitus in childhood. *J Pediat* 74:177–186, 1969.
9. Shirkey, H.C., ed.: *Pediatric Therapy.* St. Louis: C.V. Mosby, 1968, pp 803–809.
10. Traisman, H.S.: *The Management of Juvenile Diabetes Mellitus,* ed 2. St. Louis: C.V. Mosby, 1971, pp 29, 30, 39, 40, 105, 111–122, 208–211.
11. Wheelock, F.C., Jr. and Marble A.: Surgery and diabetes in A. Marble, et al, eds, *Joslin's Diabetes Mellitus,* ed 11. Philadelphia: Lea-Febiger, 1971, pp 599–620.

19

Surgery in the Allergic Child

Sheldon L. Spector, M.D.

Percy Minden, M.D.

Richard S. Farr, M.D.

DEFINITIONS AND SCOPE

Allergy is currently defined as "a broad spectrum of untoward physiologic responses which are mediated by a variety of fundamentally different immunologic mechanisms."[1] This definition is permissive in that it recognizes that most organ systems of the body can become involved in an allergic response. On the other hand, this definition is very demanding in that it requires identification of the immune mechanism causing the problem. Immunologic mechanisms that cause symptomatic allergic states have been classified into four types by Gell and Coombs.[2] Type I reactions, those mediated by homocytotropic antibody (reagins), are the most common and are often responsible for hay fever symptoms and sometimes asthma. Type II reactions involving cytotoxic antibody are responsible for Goodpasture's disease

This publication was supported in part by the U.S. Public Health Service Grant A1-09841 and by the Allergy Disease Center Grant A1-10398.

and certain hemolytic anemias. Type III or Arthus reactions involve antigen-antibody complexes and are seen in such conditions as Farmer's lung, systemic lupus erythematosus and serum sickness reactions. Type IV reactions are cell mediated and largely responsible for contact sensitivities, poison ivy, transplantation, and tumor rejections. A stepwise procedure to identify the immune mechanism involved in a particular allergic patient is often possible and worthwhile.[3]

Celiac disease and disaccharidase deficiency states may resemble allergies, but are not immunologically mediated and are referred to as pseudoallergies. Sometimes it is difficult to tell whether certain entities are allergies or pseudoallergies, but a careful history will usually dictate avoidance of a presumed etiologic stimulus on an empirical basis.

A detailed description of how to develop a comprehensive management program for the treatment and prevention of symptoms in an "allergic" child as broadly defined above is beyond the scope of this chapter, and the reader may wish to refer to other texts for this purpose.[3-6] The following discussion will be oriented toward preparing the child with asthma for elective or emergency surgery. Many of the principles that apply to the management of asthma also apply to the treatment of other symptomatic allergic states such as contact sensitivity, eczema, and rhinitis.

PREPARATION OF THE ALLERGIC CHILD FOR ELECTIVE SURGERY

In most cases, a pediatrician or allergist will have seen the patient and the surgeon and his consultant will have already outlined a management approach for the child. However, consideration by the surgeon of some aspects of the child's past history and current health status will frequently be of great value.

Environmental History

A child with allergic rhinitis or reversible bronchospasm (asthma), can spend a more comfortable hospitalization if environmental factors which cause symptoms are eliminated. For example, feather pillows, plants, and certain stuffed toys should be removed and the hospital room dust-proofed. The child should not be exposed to tobacco smoke, cleaning chemicals, fresh paint, strong hair sprays, or deodorants. Strong odors have the potential of provoking an asthmatic attack, probably by means of autonomic nervous system stimulation. Other environmental factors such as heat, cold, barometric pressure, and humidity also affect some individuals and these factors should be kept as constant as possible. Electrostatic air cleaners may generate ozone which can serve as an irritant.[7,8]

Diet

Foods which are thought to induce symptoms should be avoided. However, should this list be excessive or lead to an unbalanced diet, the entire question of the role of "food allergy" in that patient should be reevaluated.

Drug History

A history of reactions to antibiotics, especially to penicillin, is important. A positive skin test with benzylpenicillin may indicate the existence of penicillin allergy, especially when the history is unclear. However, a negative skin test to benzylpenicillin does not exclude a potential problem. With the use of major and minor penicillin determinant mixtures, it is usually possible to predict which individuals are likely to have an immediate or anaphylactic type reaction to penicillin.[9] Unfortunately, these skin test reagents are not available for general use and a convincing history of penicillin allergy is cause to use a substitute antibiotic. Penicillins may cross-react with the cephalosporins.[10,11] In unusual circumstances, desensitization to penicillin may be necessary as in cases of bacterial endocarditis when it is essential to give this drug.[12] Ideally, surgery should be delayed when entities such as acute sinusitis, secondarily infected eczema, or beta hemolytic streptococcal infections are present.

The anesthetic halothane should be used with caution.[13] The pathogenesis of the occasional ensuing hepatitis or hepatic necrosis is thought to be secondary to a Type IV or delayed hypersensitivity reaction.[14] Anyone with a history of jaundice or fever following this anesthetic should not receive it again.[15]

A history of aspirin intolerance is important because of the high incidence of untoward reactions to these drugs among asthmatics.[16] Until more is known about the pathogenesis of aspirin intolerance, children with asthma, rhinitis, or sinusitis should be given a substitute for aspirin.[17]

Blood for transfusions should be obtained from fasting nonallergic donors because it is known that donor blood containing reagins to an allergen such as horse dander can sensitize an individual to a subsequent attack of asthma following exposure to the allergen.[18] Also, it is conceivable that a donor's blood can contain food antigens to which an allergic individual may be sensitive. Blood transfusions as a source of lymphocytes and transfer factor can induce a positive tuberculin skin test in a previously nonreactive patient.[19] Other types of transfusion reactions are discussed in detail in Chapter 10.

With the wide availability of human tetanus antitoxin, it is now inexcusable to use horse antitoxin with its potential to cause reactions. Reactions to tetanus toxoid are rare, but have also been described.[20]

A careful history of allergy or pseudoallergy to contrast media should be obtained. Although the etiology of these sometimes serious reactions remains unknown, they do occur more frequently among allergic subjects.[21] Like any other procedure, the need for the examination must justify the risk. Iodine-containing substances for bronchography can be substituted with barium-carboxymethocellulose. Premedication with diphenhydramine HCL (Benadryl) is thought to reduce the less severe reactions, but has had no effect on reducing severe reactions and death.[22] In the event that an intravenous pyelogram is deemed essential in a child in whom iodide sensitivity is suspected, we would recommend premedication with antihistamines, corticosteroids, an intravenous drip to keep the vein open, and emergency standby equipment. The initial dose of contrast media should be 0.01 ml injected into the iv tubing and the amount gradually increased if no untoward reaction occurs. If an iv "push" of the entire bolus of contrast media is required, this should be done only after the above procedures have been accomplished safely.

Other Factors Important in the History

Corticosteroid usage within the previous year should alert the surgeon for the need of supplemental hormone for surgical or other kinds of stress.

A history of chronic cough often means the child is having subclinical episodes of bronchospasm and suggests the need for spirometric or peak flow determinations.

A history of rheumatic fever or a heart murmur consistent with mitral stenosis should alert the surgeon to the possibility that wheezing may have a cardiac etiology. Appropriate diagnostic studies such as cardiac catheterization and barium swallow may be indicated.

A travel history may suggest wheezing associated with certain parasitic infections. However, parasitism is not a very frequent cause of wheezing in the United States.[23]

Emotional History

A chronic illness such as asthma fosters feelings of dependency and fear. We know of two worthwhile books that can be read to the child prior to hospitalization.[24,25] It may be comforting for the child to bring his "Linus blanket" or pacifier to the hospital. A few kind words from the hospital staff, especially nurses, the anesthesiologist, and the surgeon can be very reassuring. Simple verbal explanations of the procedures involved may also help alleviate the child's anxiety. If possible, the mother should be allowed to "live-in" with the child before and after surgery. This important topic is covered in greater detail in Chapters 1, 3, and 7.

Family History

Although the family history of allergies is emphasized in many textbooks, it is of limited value in an individual case since the absence of a positive family history in no way invalidates the exstence of allergy in that patient. Conversely, a careful inquiry into possible nonallergic causes of asthma should be pursued in the presence of a positive family history. Hereditary angioedema is now known to be due to C'l-esterase deficiency inherited as an autosomal dominant and is not an immunologic problem. However, patients with this enzyme deficiency sometimes present as an "acute abdomen" which has occasionally prompted an unnecessary surgical exploration.[26]

Physical Examination

Certain findings during the physical examination suggest that an allergic evaluation be made prior to elective surgery. In young children it is important to make certain that eczema is not a manifestation of agammaglobulinemia, phenylketonuria, or Wiskott-Aldrich syndrome. A child who repeatedly rubs or wrinkles his nose or one with conjunctival redness or tearing may have allergic rhinitis. The presence of nasal polyps or nasal deviation may be especially pertinent if one is contemplating nasotracheal intubation. An asymmetrical chest should alert the surgeon to possible cardiac or pulmonary problems. Abdominal muscle hypertrophy may be present in a severe asthmatic who uses his auxiliary muscles for breathing. Cyanosis of the extremities or mucous membranes requires further investigations, including blood gases. If inspiratory or expiratory wheezes are heard in the chest, appropriate round-the-clock bronchodilator therapy, as outlined below, should be instituted to achieve a "wheeze-free" state prior to surgery.

Laboratory Information

Eosinophilia in the peripheral blood, sputum, or nasal secretions is frequently seen in symptomatic allergic states. However, steroid therapy may cause an eosinopenia, an absolute lymphopenia, and an elevated total white blood count. Serum electrolytes, especially potassium values, should be determined prior to surgery for all patients taking steroids and/or high doses of xanthines. An elevated erythrocyte sedimentation rate may indicate the presence of chronic or unsuspected infection, and, in certain circumstances, it is wise to delay surgery in order to correct the underlying cause.

A child with repeated or chronic respiratory infections merits special laboratory evaluation. Sweat chloride determinations may rule out mucoviscidosis. Quantitative immunoglobulins and isohemagglutinin determinations may help to rule out humoral antibody deficiency syndrome. Intramuscular gamma globulin should not be given unless a true hypogammaglobulinemia of the IgG class exists. Administration of intravenous gamma globulin is to be avoided and has been associated with anaphylactic-type reactions.[27] The presence of Type IV skin reactions to monilia, trichophyton, mumps, or vaccinia may rule out defects of the delayed type hypersensitivity defense system. Alpha 1 antitrypsin deficiency most often presents in the adult, although cases manifesting at a younger age have been described.[28]

A chest x-ray of an asthmatic child may show signs of air trapping, hyperinflation, or atelectasis. It may also reveal other conditions that may cause wheezing such as a foreign body obstruction of the trachea or bronchi, pneumonia, bronchiectasis, Loeffler's syndrome, or Type III allergic pulmonary infiltration. It excludes the diagnosis of Kartagener's syndrome. Sinus x-rays may help diagnose an air fluid level or retention cyst in acute or chronic sinusitis. Older children and teenagers with asthma should have routine sinus x-rays because they can have significant sinus disease without the usual symptomatology.

Pulmonary function tests are essential for the evaluation of the preoperative status of the severe asthmatic patient. A considerable amount of information can be obtained about the degree of obstruction from the FEV_1 and vital capacity after a simple forced expiratory effort. These determinations can best be followed in children over 3 years of age where one can expect fairly good cooperation. The peak flow test provides somewhat less information, but is easily performed and well suited for repetitive measurements in the younger child.[29] If possible, elective surgery should be postponed if parameters of pulmonary function are less than the maximum values previously observed for the particular patient. Appropriate round-the-clock bronchodilator therapy should be instituted to achieve the best possible pulmonary function values. Depending on the extent of the surgical procedure contemplated, more elaborate pulmonary function data, as well as adequate blood gas information, including acid-base studies may be desired.

PREOPERATIVE MEDICAL MANAGEMENT FOR ELECTIVE SURGERY

Many children with allergic states will be asymptomatic prior to admission for surgery as a result of a previously established medical management program. In such cases, preparation for surgery may simply be a matter of substituting parenteral or rectal routes of administration for medications usually taken orally.

Elective surgery should not be performed on a child with symptomatic allergic states. Instead, these conditions should be brought under good control prior to surgery, either on an outpatient basis or possibly during a few days of presurgical hospitalization. Patients should not only be given immediate relief of symptoms, but a program of medical

management should be started to prevent recurrence of an acute episode during the postsurgical period. Two broad principles of drug
therapy should be the basis for such a program:

(1) *The allergic child usually has a chronic illness.* The rationale
of administering pharmacologic agents is to raise a patient's stimulation
threshold so that he is less likely to have symptoms when confronted
with a surgical, antigenic, infectious, or otherwise noxious insult. To
be effective for this purpose, medication should be prescribed on a
regular round-the-clock basis. Orders of the "p.r.n." type should be
avoided. Regular maintenance doses of medication should be administered as long as there is objective evidence of a symptomatic allergic
state.

(2) *All phases of the medication program should be adjusted to
the needs of the individual child.* Doses of medication supplied by
manufacturers and those referred to below are average doses that do
not necessarily represent the optimal dose for an individual child. If
undesirable side affects occur, a recommended dose should be reduced
to eliminate them, and in many instances a therapeutic response is still
achieved. If a poor response follows a recommended dose, it frequently
can be gradually increased until the desired benefit occurs.

A great variety of drugs have been promoted for the symptomatic
relief of allergic symptoms in children, and it is almost impossible for
one physician to be well acquainted with them all. Familiarity and
experience with a few drugs of each type is preferable to a superficial
knowledge of many.

Drug Therapy

Xanthines

Theophylline and its derivatives such as aminophylline (theophylline
ethylenediamine) are probably the most valuable group of drugs for
bronchodilitation. Aminophylline is available in tablet or elixer form
and should be given in round-the-clock doses between 4–10 mg/kg of
body weight every four to six hours. Sustained release preparations of
aminophylline for smaller children (Aerolate Jr., 130 mg) and for
larger children and teenagers (Aerolate Sr., 260 mg and Aminodur
Dura-Tab-300 mg) are available to maintain blood levels at night. For
patients having severe or acute bronchospasm, the intravenous route
is preferred. Although 4 mg/kg of intravenous aminophylline is the
usual dose, up to 7 mg/kg may be necessary to reach the therapeutic
levels. Our method of administering these relatively high doses of
aminophylline is discussed in detail in connection with parenteral corticosteroid therapy. Fleet's theophylline enema can be given up to
7 mg/kg repeated every six hours. Toxic effects, usually preceded by
nausea and vomiting, consist of central nervous system stimulation
including convulsions or coma, pallor, hematemesis, cyanosis, and

albuminuria and dehydration. Theophylline preparations should be administered with utmost caution if any of these conditions exist before therapy. Specifically, a child with a history of convulsions should also be given appropriate doses of phenobarbital or diazepam (Valium) every 6 hours.

Sympathomimetic Drugs

Ephedrine is useful in some children, especially in a round-the-clock manner along with xanthines. For older children, up to 25 mg every four hours can be used. This drug should be individualized and discontinued if relief of asthma above and beyond that obtained with xanthines alone does not ensue. Sustained release capsules (Ectasule, Jr., 30 mg ephedrine with and without 15 mg amobarbital, and Ectasule, Sr., 60 mg ephedrine with and without 30 mg amobarbital) are available to maintain effects through the night.

Epinephrine is the most rapidly effective and potent of the sympathomimetics, but its period of action is relatively short and it is not effective when given orally. Its systemic use is likely to produce tachycardia, palpitations, headache, excitement and nervousness. These side effects may be serious with children with heart disease, hyperthyroidism, or hyperreactivity to sympathomimetic amines, but in the otherwise healthy child they are more unpleasant than dangerous. Because of its prompt action, epinephrine is one of the most useful drugs for the relief of acute asthma, anaphylactic shock, severe generalized atopic reactions, acute urticaria and angioedema. The dose will vary greatly with the severity of the symptoms being treated. Except in the most severe emergencies, it is wise to use a relatively small dose of the 1:1000 solution initially, 0.1 to 0.2 ml subcutaneously, which may be repeated every 10 minutes for two or three doses until the desired effect is obtained.

Sus-Phrine is an aqueous suspension of epinephrine tannate 1:200. It is somewhat slower in action, but effects persist for six to eight hours. It may be used to supplement and sustain the effects of an aqueous solution. Dosage is 0.05 to 0.2 ml subcutaneously every four to six hours.

Isoproterenol has an effect similar to that of epinephrine. Similar to ephedrine, it also stimulates myocardial action and may cause palpitation, but it is not as vasopressive as epinephrine. It is administered chiefly by inhalation, but is sometimes effective when administered sublingually using 5 mg and 10 mg tablets.

Sedatives and Tranquilizers

These may be needed to reduce anxiety, to control purposeless and extensive crying among infants, and to counteract the stimulatory effects of sympathomimetic drugs. Chloral hydrate, 15 mg/kg at six-to-eight hour intervals by mouth or by rectum is recommended for sedation, but in the presence of respiratory difficulties should be used with great caution to avoid hypoventilation. When children are taking high doses of xanthines and sympathomimetic drugs, appropriate doses of phenobarbital or diazepam (Valium) are our drugs of choice.

Antihistamines

Although these drugs tend to dry mucous membranes, they are occasionally useful when there is concomitant allergic rhinitis, pruritis of eczema, contact dermatitis, or the dermatitis of drug reactions. There are some children who experience relief from asthma with anti-histamines. Hydroxyzine (Atarax and Vistaril), with its many pharma-cologic effects, including its antihistaminic properties, is a very useful drug for the treatment of urticaria.

Expectorants

The best expectorant is adequate hydration and this can be ac-complished by urging liquids *per os* or by intravenous fluids. Humid-ification by a mist tent is no longer recommended.[30] Saturated solution of potassium iodide is occasionally useful,[31] but glyceryl guaiacolate is of questionable value.[32]

Mixture of Drugs

Many preparations are available that combine ephedrine, a xan-thine, a barbiturate, an expectorant, or an antihistamine. The physician should be aware of the possible disadvantages of such preparations because they frequently do not contain the appropriate dose of each ingredient for the patient being treated.

Aerosols with and without Bronchodilators

Isoproterenol, epinephrine, and isoetharine—phenylephrine—thenyldiamene (Bronkosol) are frequently used as aerosolized broncho-dilators. They are helpful additions to oral medication in severe asth-matic conditions, especially in conjunction with postural drainage when the child is productive of sputum. Inhaled bronchodilators should not be the primary medication for the control of asthma. They are fre-quently administered by means of freon-propelled pressurized can-nisters or an intermittent positive pressure breathing apparatus (IPPB). There is recent evidence to suggest that the freons may contribute to cardiac arrhythmias and we do not use the pressurized cannisters. Also, the overuse of an IPPB machine can cause or contribute to pneumothorax, subcutaneous emphysema, subdiaphragmatic or medi-astinal emphysema,[33] or pneumatosis cystoides intestinalis.[34] In most circumstances, hand or bulb nebulizers, or other compressor-driven nebulizers, e.g. Maxi-myst, are usually adequate to deliver an aerosol. Nebulizers should be frequently cleaned to prevent the patient from being reinfected by bacteria or fungi which can grow in them.

Whether in a pressurized cannister or a hand nebulizer, aero-solized bronchodilators tend to be abused because of their convenience and rapid action—and because asthmatic children have difficulty waiting the additional 15–20 minutes for the relief obtained from additional doses of xanthines and/or ephedrine by mouth. Overuse can be harmful and actually cause bronchoconstriction. In the case of isoproterenol, the mechanism may be related to a breakdown product which has bronchoconstrictive activity.[35,36] Another group of asthmatics have a paradoxical response even when isoproterenol is used for the first time.[37] These individuals may not be identified routinely because of a deceptive initial response of bronchodilatation which is then followed by bronchoconstriction and even coma. There are other compounds (metaproterenol and salbutamol) available in Britain, but still under investigation in the United States. Their advantages over isoproterenol are longer lasting bronchodilatation and fewer side effects. Salbutamol has also proved effective in two out of two "isoproterenol-droppers" recently tested at our hospital.[38]

The use of ultrasonic nebulizers is somewhat controversial, especially in the young infant where overhydration may occur.[39] Such compounds as acetylcysteine (Mucomyst) may produce bronchospasm in the asthmatic and in general should be avoided.

Antibiotics

The use of antibiotics is discussed in detail in Chapter 16. As concerns the asthmatic, however, it has been our experience that broad-spectrum antibiotics such as ampicillin or erythromycin sometimes are useful in the treatment of bronchitis with purulent sputum, even in the absence of specific pathogenic organisms.

Corticosteroids

The indications for corticosteroids in the treatment of allergic states are severe symptoms which cannot be satisfactorily controlled by maximum tolerated doses of previously discussed medications. Corticosteroids should be the last medication added to the type of medical program described above, and, after control has been attained, should be the first to be tapered and discontinued if possible.

Corticosteroids may suppress the tuberculin reaction. Thus children should receive a tuberculin test prior to the time the need for corticosteroids may arise.

If a patient has been on maintenance doses of corticosteroids or has taken them during the previous year, an increased dose should be given the day prior to surgery, the day of surgery, and the day after surgery. It is then usually possible to resume the preoperative schedule. It is hazardous to omit or reduce steroids at the time of surgery. It has been our experience that patients on even large doses of steroids have little or no trouble with wound healing.

We prefer shorter acting preparations such as prednisone, prednisolone, and methylprednisolone. We do not ordinarily use corticotropin (ACTH) since there is risk of an allergic reaction to it and its use presumes that the adrenal glands have a normal functional capacity to produce cortisol. This is frequently not the case in patients who have received previous corticosteroid therapy.

Corticosteroid therapy can begin with relatively high doses such as 10–25 mg of prednisone orally every six hours each day for the first three or four days. For more severe symptoms, an alternative plan is to use equivalent or higher doses of intravenous or intramuscular methylprednisolone (Solu-Medrol) in association with intravenous aminophyllin and fluids. We prefer to administer aminophyllin over a 30-minute period every four to six hours by means of a second intravenous set inserted into the tubing of the primary set. The patient is usually "symptom-free" following this type of intensive therapy and is then ready for surgery. Following surgery and depending on the patient's condition, a single dose of prednisone may be administered every other morning in order to minimize adrenal suppression. The patient should be carefully observed on the alternate days when corticosteroids are withheld. Steroids should not be stopped abruptly, but the dose should be tapered and discontinued according to the patient's clinical condition. If an exacerbation of symptoms occurs, it may be necessary to resume corticosteroids on a daily basis, preferably as a single morning dose.

PREOPERATIVE MEDICAL MANAGEMENT FOR EMERGENCY SURGERY

Most of the general principles previously outlined for elective surgery are applicable to emergency surgery. Conceivably, an asthmatic under poor control might be involved in an automobile accident or develop an acute surgical emergency such as appendicitis. Ideally, the patient should be in an intensive care unit and an experienced anesthesiologist should be called since the decision to place the child on a ventilator is important and difficult. Aside from the surgical indications for intubation or tracheostomy, assisted ventilation is required when the asthmatic child has barely audible breath sounds and/or arterial pCO_2 of greater than 65 mm mercury. Nasotracheal intubation should be performed and the child then placed on a volume respirator. The stomach should be emptied prior to intubation with a nasogastric tube. If the child fights the ventilator, sedation and/or paralysis may be necessary. Although curare and morphine are both histamine releasers, in actual practice these agents have been used in asthmatics on respirators without much difficulty. Muscle paralysis should not be attempted by individuals unfamiliar with these potentially hazardous drugs.

There may be an advantage in intubating a child while he is awake. Once skeletal muscle paralysis has been induced, there is no second chance if one cannot intubate quickly. Since the asthmatic may generate airway resistance great enough to potentially produce pneumothoraces while on the ventilator, one should ventilate only to the threshold volume and pressure to produce adequate blood gases.

There is rarely an indication for tracheostomy on a short-term basis since intubation will provide an adequate airway. Tracheostomy can be a hazard in a patient who may require many such operations. The inherent risk of bronchoscopy in an asthmatic is decreased if it is done when the child has reached a deeper level of anesthesia rather than during the lighter phases of anesthesia.

An indwelling arterial catheter is often useful in following the patient's progress with serial blood-gas determinations, and sufficient oxygen should be administered to prevent ·hypoxemia. Sodium bicarbonate or similar base should be used in situations where the pH is low subsequent to carbon dioxide retention. Acid-base imbalance may contribute to an "epinephrine-fast" state.[40] Management is complex and is best done in a center where trained nursing staff and auxiliary personnel are available.

In an emergency situation, vigorous use of bronchodilators is mandatory, aiming for an endpoint of as few obstructive symptoms as possible prior to the actual operation. Intravenous fluids, aminophylline, and epinephrine, as discussed above, are the mainstays of therapy. Large and frequent doses of corticosteroids may also be necessary together with the bronchodilators. Potassium supplementation should be given empirically if the patient has been on high-dose steroid therapy for prolonged periods and has adequate renal function. Appropriate doses of these drugs are discussed earlier in this chapter under "Preoperative Medical Management for Elective Surgery" and in Chapters 9 and 11.

Anaphylaxis is an acute medical emergency and occasionally may require tracheostomy. The mainstay of medical therapy is epinephrine which may be repeated every 10 minutes if necessary. Corticosteroids and antihistamines may also be used, but mainly for their delayed benefit.

PREVENTION OF COMPLICATIONS

The asthmatic child should be placed in a respiratory intensive care unit, when available. This is the optimal setting for follow-up care and often for preoperative care as well. Please refer to Chapters 3 and 12 for details, but we would like to stress here that a nasotracheal tube should not be left in place for longer than three days or there is risk of inducing subglottic stenosis.[41] If there is a complication such as pneumonia that might require its more prolonged use, a tracheostomy should be considered.

Blood-gas determinations and serum electrolyte values should be carefully monitored. Special attention should be paid to potassium levels and the child should be weighed frequently and/or put on "intake and output" in order to help monitor the state of hydration. This is especially important in an asthmatic since the diuretic action of aminophylline can contribute to dehydration. Oxygen therapy may be used when appropriate, but its overuse can also lead to complications of oxygen toxicity.[42,43]

Pneumomediastinum is another complication of asthma that occurs especially in children. Although many of these cases are idiopathic, overuse of an IPPB machine or a volume respirator can be contributory or etiologic.[33] An equally disturbing finding in pre- and postsurgical asthmatic children is the right middle lobe syndrome characterized by partial atelectasis of the right middle lobe with bronchitis or pneumonia. This diagnosis is suggested by respiratory symptoms which are refractory to usual treatment.[44] Lobectomy may be required if medical management does not alleviate it.[44]

In an attempt to prevent development of atelectasis, children old enough to cooperate should be trained how to cough prior to surgery. Similarly, principles of postural drainage should also be taught in the preoperative period so as to be more effective postoperatively.

Liberal use of antacids should be encouraged in a child on corticosteroids, since the increased stress of surgery may lead to peptic ulceration or bleeding. Topical anesthetics and antihistamines tend to be contact or Type IV sensitizers, especially in asthmatics with coexisting eczema. Topical antibiotic lotions or ointments containing penicillin or other antibiotics which can potentially be used systemically also should be avoided for the same reason. Neomycin, which is not used systemically, is a particularly potent sensitizer.

Allergic or pseudoallergic reactions to a local anesthetic can present as localized swelling, erythema, hive formation, and pruritis and may interfere with optimal healing of that area of skin or be confused with a local infection. Skin tests are of limited value, and it is better to carefully record the offending anesthetic; and for subsequent procedures, substitute an agent from the group that contains paraaminobenzoic acid esters (procaine, tetracaine, chloroprocaine) for one of the non–cross-reacting group composed mainly of amides (lidocaine, mepivacaine, prilocaine) or vice versa. If a child has had reactions to both groups of local anesthetics, diphenhydramine (Benadryl) is a less effective, but useful, substitute.

Catgut (in fact, derived from sheep intestine!) allergy has been well documented in the ophthalmologic literature characterized by pruritis, chemosis, and hyperemia of the conjunctiva from 72 hours to seven days after an operation.[45,46] Although in the cases cited the ultimate outcome of the operation was not affected, a local tissue hypersensitivity explained some of the unusual and alarming postoperative eye reactions observed. The role that suture material might play in local inflammatory reactions at other surgical sites is only conjecture, but is a consideration that merits further investigation. We know of no descriptions of allergic reactions to silk suture material in silk-sensitive individuals but, theoretically, this may also occur.

It is clear from the previous discussions in this chapter that the most important principle to prevent a complication in the allergic child, especially the asthmatic, is the use of vigorous and appropriate pre- and postoperative medical care. Ideally, the asthmatic should be symptom-free prior to a surgical procedure. The concept of round-the-clock management should be pursued not only before but after the operation.

REFERENCES

1. Minden, P., and Farr, R.S.: The allergic child. In Gellis, S.S. and Kagan, B.M., eds. Current Pediatric Therapy. Philadelphia: W.B. Saunders, 1970, vol 4.
2. Coombs, R.R.A. and Gell, P.G.H.: Classification of allergic reactions responsible for clinical hypersensitivity and disease. In, Clinical Aspects of Immunology, ed 2. Philadelphia: F.A. Davis, 1968, pp 575–596.
3. Minden, P. and Farr, R.S.: The management of allergic disorders in children. Pediat Clin N Amer 16:305–320, 1969.
4. Sheldon, J.M., Lovell, R.G., and Mathews, K.P.: A Manual of Clinical Allergy, ed 2. Philadelphia: W.B. Saunders, 1967.
5. Sherman, W.B.: Hypersensitivity—Mechanisms and Management. Philadelphia: W.B. Saunders, 1968.
6. Samter, M., ed.: Immunological Diseases, ed 2. Boston: Little, Brown, 1971, vol 2.
7. Ayres, S.M.: Patient advice during acute air pollution episode. Arch Environ Health 22:591–592, 1971.
8. Ayres, S.M.: Clean air facilities—a proposal by an authority. Industr Med and Surg 37:591–592, 1968.
9. Levine, B.B. and Zolov, D.M.: Prediction of penicillin allergy by immunological tests. J Allerg 43:231–244, 1969.
10. Abraham, G.N., Petz, L.D., and Fudenberg, H.H.: Immunohaematological cross-allergenicity between penicillin and cephalothin in humans. Clin Exp Immun 3: 343–357, 1968.
11. Grieco, M.H.: Cross-allergenicity of the penicillins and the cephalosporins. Arch Intern Med 119:141–146, 1967.
12. Reisman, R.E., Rose, N.R., Witebsky, E., and Arbesman, C.E.: Penicillin allergy and desensitization. J Allerg 33:178–187, 1962.
13. Mushin, W.W., Rosen, M., and Jones, E.: Halothane hepatic complications. Brit Med J 3:18–22, 1971.
14. Paronetto, F. and Popper, H.: Lymphocyte stimulation induced by halothane in patients with hepatitis following exposure to halothane. New Eng J Med 283:277–280, 1970.
15. Aach, R. and Kissane, J.: Massive hepatic necrosis following multiple exposures to halothane. Amer J Med 45:589–600, 1968.
16. Samter, M. and Beers, R.F., Jr.: Intolerance to aspirin. Clinical studies and consideration of its pathogenesis. Ann Int Med 68:975–983, 1968.
17. Farr, R.S.: Presidential message. The need to reevaluate acetylsalicylic acid (aspirin). J Allerg 45:321–328, 1970.
18. Ramirez, M.: Horse asthma following blood transfusion. JAMA 73:984–985, 1919.
19. Smith, D.T.: The diagnostic and prognostic value of the second strength dose of PPD (5.0 micrograms). Am Rev Resp Dis 101:317–319, 1970.
20. Smith, R.E. and Wolnisty, C.: Allergic reactions to tetanus, diphtheria, influenza and poliomyelitis immunization. Ann Allerg 20:809–813, 1962.

21. Ansell, G.: Adverse reactions to contrast agents. *Invest Radiol* 5:374–384, 1970.
22. Peters, G.A., Hodgson, J.R., and Donovan, R.J.: The effect of premedication with chlorpheniramine on reactions to methyl-glucamine iodipamide. *J Allerg* 38:74–83, 1966.
23. Van Dellen, R.G. and Thompson, J.H., Jr.: Absence of intestinal parasites in asthma. *New Eng J Med* 285:146–148, 1971.
24. Rey, M. and Rey, H.A.: *Curious George Goes to the Hospital.* Boston: Houghton Mifflin, 1966.
25. Chase, F.: *A Visit to the Hospital.* New York: Wonder Books, 1958.
26. Donaldson, V.H. and Rosen, F.S.: Hereditary angioneurotic edema: A clinical survey. *Pediatrics,* 37:1017–1027, 1966.
27. Ellis, E.F. and Henney, C.S.: Adverse reactions following administration of human gamma globulin. *J Allerg* 43:45–54, 1969.
28. Talamo, R.C., Levison, H., Lynch, M.J., Hercz, A., and Hyslop, N.E.: Symptomatic pulmonary emphysema in childhood associated with hereditary alpha-1-antitrypsin and elastase inhibitor deficiency. *J Pediat* 79:20–26, 1971.
29. Bates, D.V., Macklem, P.T., and Christie, R.V.: *Respiratory Function in Disease,* ed 2. Philadelphia: W.B. Saunders, 1971, pp 22–23.
30. Bau, S.K., Aspin, N., Wood, D.E., and Levison, H.: The measurement of fluid deposition in humans following mist tent therapy. *Pediatrics* 48:605–612, 1971.
31. Falliers, C.J., McCann, W.P., Chai, H., Ellis, E., and Yazdi, N.: Controlled study of iodotherapy for childhood asthma. *J Allerg* 38:183–192, 1966.
32. Hirsch, S.R., Vierner, P.F., Zastrow, J.E., and Kory, R.C.: The expectorant effect of glyceryl guaiacolate: A controlled in vitro and in vivo study. *J Allerg* (abstr.) 45:115–116, 1970.
33. Bierman, C.W.: Pneumomediastinum and pneumothorax complicating asthma in children. *Amer J Dis Child* 114:42–50, 1967.
34. Wintrobe, M.M., ed: *Harrison's Principles of Internal Medicine,* ed 6. New York: McGraw-Hill, 1970.
35. Reisman, R.E.: Asthma induced by adrenergic aerosols. *J Allerg* 46:162–177, 1970.
36. Paterson, J.W., Conolly, M.E., Davies, D.S., and Dollery, C.T.: Isoprenaline resistance and the use of pressurised aerosols in asthma. *Lancet* 2:426–429, 1968.
37. Keighley, J.F.: Iatrogenic asthma associated with adrenergic aerosols. *Ann Int Med* 65:985–995, 1966.
38. Spector, S.L. and Farr, R.S.: Comparison of varying doses of albuterol and placebo aerosols for the relief of bronchospasm. *J Allerg and Clin Immun* (abstr) 49:128, 1972.
39. Tamer, M.A., Modell, J.H., and Rieffel, C.N.: Hyponatremia secondary to ultrasonic aerosol therapy in the newborn infant. *J Pediat* 77:1051–1054, 1970.
40. Blumenthal, J.S., Blumenthal, M.N., Brown, E.B., Campbell, G.S., and Prasad, A.: Effect of changes in arterial pH on the action of adrenalin in acute adrenalin-fast asthmatics. *Dis Chest* 39:516–522, 1961.
41. Striker, T.W., Stool, S., and Downes, J.J.: Prolonged nasotracheal intubation in infants and children. *Arch Otolaryng* 85:210–213, 1967.
42. Morgan, A.P.: The pulmonary toxicity of oxygen. *Anesthesiology,* 29:570–579. 1968.
43. More hazards of oxygen, editorial. *New Eng J Med* 279:379–380, 1968.
44. Dees, S.C. and Spock, A.: Right middle lobe syndrome in children. *JAMA* 197:78–84, 1966.
45. Apt, L., Costenbader, F.D., Parks, M.M., and Albert, D.G.: Catgut allergy in eye muscle surgery. I. Correlation of eye reaction and skin test using plain catgut. *Arch Opthalmol* 63:30–35, 54–59, 1960.
46. Apt, L., Costenbader, F.D., Parks, M.M., and Albert, D.G.: Catgut allergy in eye muscle surgery. II. Correlation and comparison of eye reaction and skin test after the use of plain and chromicized catgut. *Arch. Opthalmol* 65:474–480, 1961.

Index